Textbook
of
Colour Doppler Imaging

Textbook
of
Colour Doppler Imaging

Satish K Bhargava
MD(Radiodiagnosis) MD(Radiotherapy)
DMRD FICRI FIAMS FCCP FUSI FAMS
Head, Department of Radiology and Imaging
University College of Medical Sciences
(University of Delhi) and GTB Hospital
Dilshad Garden, Delhi

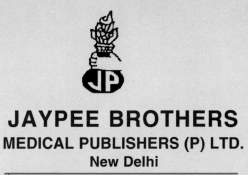

JAYPEE BROTHERS
MEDICAL PUBLISHERS (P) LTD.
New Delhi

Published by

Jitendar P Vij

Jaypee Brothers Medical Publishers (P) Ltd

EMCA House, 23/23B Ansari Road, Daryaganj

New Delhi 110 002, India

Phones: 23272143, 23272703, 23282021, 23245672, 23245683

Fax: 91+011-23276490   e-mail: jpmedpub@del2.vsnl.net.in

Visit our website: http://www.jpbros.20m.com

Branches

- 202 Batavia Chambers, 8 Kumara Krupa Road, Kumara Park East,
  Bangalore 560 001, Phones: 2285971, 2382956 Tele Fax: 2281761
  e-mail: jaypeebc@bgl.vsnl.net.in

- 282 IIIrd Floor, Khaleel Shirazi Estate, Fountain Plaza
  Pantheon Road, **Chennai** 600 008, Phone: 28262665 Fax: 28262331
  e-mail: jpmedpub@md3.vsnl.net.in

- 4-2-1067/1-3, Ist Floor, Balaji Building, Ramkote
  Cross Road, **Hyderabad** 500095, Phones: 55610020, 24758498
  Fax: 24758499   e-mail: hyd2_jpmedpub@sancharnet.in

- 1A Indian Mirror Street, Wellington Square
  Kolkata 700 013, Phone: 22451926 Fax: 22456075
  e-mail: jpbcal@cal.vsnl.net.in

- 106 Amit Industrial Estate, 61 Dr SS Rao Road, Near MGM Hospital
  Parel, **Mumbai** 400 012 , Phones: 24124863, 24104532 Fax: 24160828
  e-mail: jpmedpub@bom7.vsnl.net.in

Textbook of Colour Doppler Imaging

© 2004, Satish K Bhargava

This book has been published in good faith that the material provided by the contributors is original. Every effort is made to ensure accuracy of material, but the publisher, printer and editor will not be held responsible for any inadvertent error(s). In case of any dispute, all legal matters to be settled under Delhi jurisdiction only.

First Edition: 2004

ISBN   81-8061-032-2

Typeset at   JPBMP typesetting unit
Printed at   Greatway Prints, Delhi

Dedicated to
My loving late wife
Kalpana
and my son
Sumeet
Whose inspiration and sacrifice
have made possible to bring out this book

Contributors

Satish K Bhargava MD(Radiodiagnosis)
MD(Radiotherapy) DMRD FICRI FIAMS
FCCP FUSI FAMS
Head Deptt of Radiology and Imaging
Univeristy College of Medical Sciences
(University of Delhi) and GTB Hospital
Dilshad Garden, Delhi

Suchi Bhatt MD(Radiodiagnosis)
Lecturer, Deptt of Radiology and Imaging
University College of Medical Sciences
(University of Delhi) and GTB Hospital
Dilshad Garden, Delhi

Leena Gupta MBBS
Resident, Deptt of Radiology and Imaging
University College of Medical Sciences
(University of Delhi) and GTB Hospital
Dilshad Garden, Delhi

Rohini Gupta MBBS
Resident, Deptt of Radiology and Imaging
University College of Medical Sciences
(University of Delhi) and GTB Hospital
Dilshad Garden, Delhi

Shefali Gupta MD(Radiodiagnosis) DNB
Sr Resident, Deptt of Radiology and Imaging
University College of Medical Sciences
(University of Delhi) and GTB Hospital
Dilshad Garden, Delhi

Vipul Gupta MD(Radiodiagnosis)
Asstt Prof, Deptt of Neuro-Radiology
All India Institute of Medical Sciences
Ansari Nagar, Delhi

Gurpreet Gulati MD(Radiodiagnosis)
Asstt Prof, Deptt of Cardiac-Radiology
All India Institute of Medical Sciences
Ansari Nagar, Delhi

Shashank Jain MBBS
Resident, Deptt of Radiology and Imaging
University College of Medical Sciences
(University of Delhi) and GTB Hospital
Dilshad Garden, Delhi

Jaideep Malhotra
MD FICOG FIAJAGO FICMCH FICMU
Malhotra Nursing and Maternity Home (P) Ltd
Agra

Narendra Malhotra
MD FICOG FIAJAGO FICMCH FICMU
Malhotra Nursing and Maternity Home (P) Ltd
Agra

Vanaj Mathur DMRD(Consultant Sonologist)
Malhotra Nursing and Maternity Home (P) Ltd
Agra

Gopesh Mehrotra MD(Radiodiagnosis)
Reader, Deptt of Radiology and Imaging
University College of Medical Sciences
(University of Delhi) and GTB Hospital
Dilshad Garden, Delhi

Sakshi Mittal MD(Radiodiagnosis)
Senior Resident, Deptt of Cardiac Radiology
All India Institute of Medical Sciences
Ansari Nagar, Delhi

Poonam Narang MD(Radiodiagnosis)
Assoc Prof, Deptt of Radiology
Maulana Azad Medical College and
Associated GB Pant Hospital
New Delhi

Bharat Parekh MD(Radiodiagnosis) FICRI
Secretary, IMA College of Radiology and
Imaging and Consultant Radiologist
ECLAT Poly Clinic
Mumbai

OP Sharma
MD(Radiodiagnosis) PhD(Radiology) FICRI
Prof, Deptt of Radiodiagnosis and Imaging
Institute of Medical Sciences
Banaras Hindu University
Varanasi

Sanjiv Sharma MD(Radiodiagnosis)
Head, Department of Cardiac-Radiology
All India Institute of Medical Sciences
Ansari Nagar, Delhi

Deep N Srivastava MD(Radiodiagnosis)
Additional Prof, Deptt of Radiodiagnosis
All India Institute of Medical Sciences
Ansari Nagar, Delhi

AK Srivastava MSc
Physicist
Department of Radiology and Imaging
University College of Medical Sciences
(University of Delhi) and GTB Hospital
Dilshad Garden, Delhi

Sanjay Thulkar MD(Radiodiagnosis)
Assistant Prof, Deptt of Radiodiagnosis
All India Institute of Medical Sciences
Ansari Nagar, Delhi

Lalendra Upreti MD(Radiodiagnosis) DNB
Associate Prof, Deptt of Radiodiagnosis
University College of Medical Sciences
(University of Delhi) and GTB Hospital
Dilshad Garden, Delhi

GP Vashisht MD(Radiodiagnosis) FICRI
Director, Deptt Radiology and Imaging
Batra Hospital and Medical Research Centre
Delhi

Shalini Verma MBBS DMRD
Sr Resident, Deptt of Radiology and Imaging
University College of Medical Sciences
(University of Delhi) and GTB Hospital
Dilshad Garden, Delhi

Anju Yadav MD(Radiodiagnosis)
Sr Resident, Deptt of Radiology and Imaging
University College of Medical Sciences
(University of Delhi) and GTB Hospital
Dilshad Garden, Delhi

Preface

Colour Doppler sonography has been in use for more than three decades now and has constantly evolved to its present status of being the minatory of the vascular laboratory. It has unparalled application in assessing cerebral, abdominal and peripheral vasculature. Colour Doppler is now widely applicable in intravascular, and interventional procedures. This added a new dimension of its role in therapeutic radiology. Its role in differentiating benign versus malignant lesions is increasing day by day. The extent and severity of the disease process and haemodynamic alteration caused by it can be confidently estimated. In fact all sonographers, must now be familiar with Doppler imaging, as blood flow assessment is used virtually every time an ultrasound examination is carried out.

Colour Doppler sonography is a combination of Doppler ultrasound and gray scale ultrasound to provide simultaneous realtime visualization of soft tissues structures and blood flow over the entire scan field. Interpretation of this information required a sound knowledge of the basic technical principles of colour Doppler imaging and the pathophysiology involved in the disease process. This book is a sincere effort to provide a clear scenario of the fascinating world of colour Doppler sonography. It deals with the basic fundamentals of colour Doppler sonography and its application in the specific body regions. The extensive text covered in this book itself portrays the burden borne by this aspect of imaging. An attempt has been made to provide an update knowledge of the subject. Use of contrast medium in vascular ultrasonography has been highlighted in this book. A satisfactory number of illustrations have been included in each chapter to provide an interesting insight into the subject.

This is the first Indian book on colour duplex sonography. I feel that this sincere effort will be critically analysed, appreciated and appraised.

Satish K Bhargava

Acknowledgements

I am grateful to my colleagues and friends who gave timely support and stood solidly behind me in our joint endeavour of bringing out this book which was required keeping in view of wide acceptability of ultrasound in developing countries like ours. My special heartfelt thanks are due to the sincere and hardworking staff of M/s Jaypee Brothers particularly Mr Jitendar P Vij, Chairman and Managing Director, Mr RK Yadav, Publishing Director, Mr PS Ghuman, Production Manager, Mr RK Majumdar, artist, Ms Mubeen Bano. It is indeed the result of the hard work of the staff of M/s Jaypee Brothers and the contributors who have always been keen desire to work with `smiling faces and with polite voices as a result of which this book has seen the light of the day.

Contents

1

The Story of Doppler

Satish K Bhargava
AK Srivastava

Doppler colour flow mapping a new and exciting advances in cardiac ultrasound is a method whereby blood flow is imaged and displayed on 2D image.

The first discription of the physical principle used in colour flow devices is attributed to Johann Christian Doppler, an Austrian Mathematician and Scientist who lived in the first half of the nineteenth century. Doppler's first descriptions concerned changes in wavelength of light as applied to astronomical events. In 1842, he presented a paper entitled "on the coloured light of double stars and some other Heavenly Bodies" in which he postulated that certain properties of light emitted from stars depend upon the relative motion of the observer and the wave source. He suggested that the coloured appearance of certain stars was caused by their motion relative to the earth, the blue ones moving toward earth and the red ones moving away. He drew an analogy of a ship moving to meet or retreat from incoming ocean waves. The ship moving out to sea would meet the waves with more frequently than a ship moving towards the shoreline. Interestingly Doppler never extrapolated his postulates to sound waves.

There was immediate criticism of Doppler. Just like today, critics abounded. Among them was Buys Ballot who in 1844 stated he simply did not believe Doppler. There is rather amusing account of the difficulties Buys Ballot encountered in attempting to disclaim the Doppler effect. In 1845, he borrowed a steam locomotive from Dutch Government and arranged for a trumpet player to ride a fiat car as it approached and then left a station. Two other trumpet players were positioned on the ground one to either side, where an observer with the ability to appreciate perfect pitch listed to all the trumpets playing the same note. Following a hail-storm and other delays, the experiment finally took place. The note was higher in pitch as it departed when compared with trumpets on the ground. Aside from verifying Doppler's observations, this experiment proved that "getting started in Doppler" was difficult to understand even then.

Even with this scientific verification, Buys Ballot and others continued to level strong criticism. Those struggling to understand the Doppler principle will be interested to know that while Doppler's postulate concerning frequency shift from moving objects was ultimately shown to be correct his extrapolation about colour shift of light from stars was later proven to be wrong. He incorrectly assumed that all the stars emitted white light. In reality the colours and lines of the various stars are a function of thin surface temperature rather than their direction or velocity of movement.

We are familiar with the Doppler effect in everyday life. For example an observer stationed on a highways overpass easily notices that the pitch of the sound made from the engine of a passing automobile changes from high to low as the car high frequency sound termed as ultrasound that is reflected off the moving red blood cells and then returned at a different frequency dependent upon the speed and direction of the moving blood. The result information is displayed as various wave for on the velocity spectral analysis. The clinical uses of blood flow imaging systems have expanded immensely since the first measurement of flow in the heart that was performed by Satomura in 1956.

Despite its wide spread use, Doppler methods and principle are difficult to understand and implement without considerable training and experience.

approaches and then passes into the distance. The engine is emitting the same sound as it passes beneath, but the observer notices a change in pitch dependent upon the speed of automobile and its direction.

Doppler effect is now employed in modern astronomy. It has practical application in radar detection of storm and is used in modern weather forcasting. It can help to form the "radar trap" used by police on modern highways to detect speeding automobiles in developed countries.

The medical applications of Doppler are dependent upon the use of ultrasound and have been in practice for sometime. Doppler systems emit a burst of very

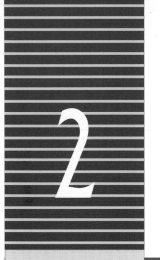

Basic Haemodynamics

AK Srivastava
Satish K Bhargava

INTRODUCTION

Doppler ultrasound uses to display change in sound frequency caused by moving blood. Consequently before discussing Doppler ultrasound and its application to imaging. It is necessary to describe the nature of blood flow.

Just as hydrodynamics describes the motion of fluids especially of water and interaction of fluid with its boundaries, haemodynamics is the term used to describe a collection of mechanism that influences the active and changing or dynamic circulation of blood. Circulation is of course a vital function. Blood is a mixture of plasma and cellular constituents mostly erythrocytes.

Hydrodynamic principles are applicable to blood vessels that are normally accessible to Duplex sonography (larger than 1 mm in diameter). But blood flow is influenced by many factors, include cardiac function, elasticity of vessels walls, vessel curvature and branching. Some of the factors can, however, be measured in reasonable simple term, but many other cannot be measured because they are difficult to quantify and generally are not well-understood.

With these limitation in mind, this chapter presents the basic principles of the dynamics of blood circulation and many factors that influence blood flow and the haemodynamics of occlusive disease. These considerations are helpful in understanding the normal physiology of blood circulation and the abnormalities that can occur in the presence of vascular obstruction.

Physical Aspects

Flow between two points which is the movement of a fluid in certain direction, can arise only when there is differences in energy level between these two points.

Usually, the difference in energy level is reflected by a difference in pressure, and circulatory system generally consists of a high pressure, high energy, arterial reservoir and a venous pool of low pressure and energy. These reservoirs are connected by a system of distributing vessels (smaller arteries) and by the resistance vessels of the microcirculation, which consists of arterioles, capillaries and venules.

During flow, energy is continuously lost from the blood because of the friction (viscosity) between its layers and particles. The viscosity of blood determines mainly by its haematocrit.

Due to this internal friction both pressure and energy levels therefore decrease from arterial to the venous ends. The energy necessary for the flow is continuously restored by the pumping action of the heart which forces blood to move from the venous system into the arterial pressure and the energy difference needed for flow to occur. The high arterial energy level is result of the large volume of blood in the arterial reservoir. The function of the heart and blood vessel is normally required to maintain the volume and pressure in arteries within limit required for smooth function. This is achieved by maintaining a balance between the amount of blood that enters and leaves the arterial reservoir.

The amount that enters the arteries is the cardiac output. The amount that leaves depend on the arterial pressure and on the total peripheral resistance which is controlled in turn by the amount of vasoconstriction in the microcirculation.

Under normal condition, flow to all the body tissues is adjusted according to tissues particular need at a given time.

This adjustment is accomplished by alteration in level of vasoconstriction of arterioles within the organ supplied. Maintenance of normal volume and pressure in arteries thus allows both for adjustment of blood flow to all parts of the body and for regulation of cardiac output.

Laminar Flow

In most vessels, blood moves in concentric layers or laminar hence, the flow is said to be laminar. Each infinitesimal layer flows with a different velocity (Figs 2.1a and b).

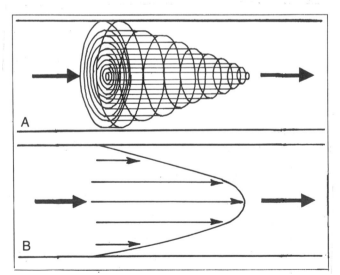

Figures 2.1a and b
Principle of laminar flow in a vessel with a circular cross-section (a) the flow velocity within individual fluid layers (concentric cylinders) increases with distance from the vessel wall, and (b) laminar flow velocity profile in longitudinal section. The tips of the individual velocity vectors describe a parabola. Flow velocities are highest at the centre of the vessel

KEY POINTS

– Flow between two points in certain direction occur only when there is difference in energy level (Pressure) between these two points.
– In blood flow energy levels continuously decrease due to viscosity and this loss of energy inflow is continuously restarted by pumping action of heart.

In theory, a thin layer of blood is held stationary next to vessel wall at zero velocity because of an adhesive force between blood and the inner surface of vessel. The next layer flows with a certain velocity but its movement is delayed by the stationary layer because of friction between the layers generated by the viscus properties of the fluid. The second layer in turn delays the next layer which flows at a greater velocity. The layer in the middle of the vessel flow with highest velocity (Fig. 2.2) and the mean velocity across the vessel is half of the maximal velocity. Because rate of change of velocity is greatest near the wall and decreases towards the center of vessel, a velocity profile in the shape of a parabola exist along the vessel diameter.

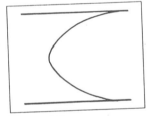

Figure 2.2
Parabolic profile of laminar flow

Loss of energy during blood flow occurs because of friction, and the amount of friction and energy loss is determined in large part by the dimension of the vessels. In small vessel especially in the microcirculation even the layer in the middle of the lumen are relatively close to the wall and are thus delayed considerably, resulting in a significant opposition or resistance to flow.

In large vessels, by contrast a large central core of blood is far from the wall and the frictional energy loss are minimal but frictional and energy loss increases if laminar flow is disturbed.

The relation between flow volume per unit time q, viscosity η, length of vascular segment l, vessel radius r and pressure difference (P_2-P_1) at proximal and distal end of tube is described by Hagen and Poiseuille's law as expressed in equation (1):

$$P_2 - P_1 = \frac{8\ln q}{\pi r^4} \qquad \textbf{(1)}$$

By analogy with Ohm's law

$$V = RI$$

$$R = \frac{8\ln}{\pi r^4}$$ Where R is resistance to flow

This means even a small changes in radius can result in large changes in flow.

For example a decrease in radius by one half would lead to increase in flow resistance by a factor of 16 or would lead to 95 per cent decrease in flow.

Because the length of the vessels and the viscosity of blood do not change much in the cardiovascular system, alteration in blood flow occur mainly as a result of changes in the radius of the vessels and in the difference in the pressure energy level available for flow.

Poiseuille's equation can be written as:

$$R = \frac{P_2 - P_1}{q}$$

Hence by measuring pressure difference and blood flow (q) the resistance can thus be calculated.

The major part of the total resistance of vascular system originates from the arterioles—the part of arterial vascular tree with the largest capacity for vaso motor regulation.

Resistance can be thought of as the pressure difference needed to produce one unit of flow and can thus be considered as an index of the difficulties in forcing blood flow through vessel.

As discussed in earlier section regarding laminar flow. In colour Doppler sonographic imaging a laminar flow velocity profile is present when the lightest shades of a colour are located along the centre of a vessel, indicating central high velocity flow. At the same time, flow close to the vessel wall is coded in darker shades of same colour representing lower flow velocity.

Poiseuille's law applicable with precision only to constant laminar flow of a simple fluid (such as water) in a rigid tube of uniform bore. In blood circulation these conditions are not met.

Instead, the resistance is influenced by the presence of numerous interconnected vessels with a combined effect similar to that observed in electrical resistance.

In the case of vessels in series, the overall resistance is equal to the sum of the resistances of the individual vessels, whereas in the case of parallel vessels, the reciprocal of the total resistance equals the sum of the reciprocal of the individual vessel resistances.

Thus the contribution of any single vessel to the total resistance of vascular bed or the effect of change in dimension of vessel, depend on the pressure and relative size of other vessel link in series or in parallel.

The mean flow velocity of a fluid originating from a reservoir or a vessel with a large diameter in comparison to the mean flow velocity in more distal segment with a reduced diameter will be lower than in distal segment due to the reduction in cross sectional area. This effect is based on the principle of continuity, i.e. there is no loss or gain of fluid volume (volumetric flow is independed of the vessel cross sectional area). The flow velocity profile in the initial portion of the segment is very flat (entrance effect, plug flow) except for a large velocity gradient in the boundary layer along the vessel walls, further along the distal segment the flow gradually reaches its steady-state parabolic velocity profile.

The opposite effect occurrs when there is a sudden increase in the cross-section in vessel area (exist effect).

The flow velocity profile elongates as velocity gradient between the central and peripheral laminae increases. Eventually the parabolic flow velocity profile will be restored. The more drastic increase in lumen diameter, the greater the likelihood of flow separation near the vessel walls. This is characterised by localized zones of flow reversal.

This must be differentiated from turbulence. Thus type of physiological flow separation occurs for example in carotid bulb where the CCA bifurcates into the internal and external carotid arteries.

Flow separation is also commonly observed distal to a vascular stenosis especially when there is a sudden increase in the vessel diameter.

Disturbed Flow and Turbulence

Various degree of deviation from orderly laminar flow occur in the circulation under both normal and abnormal conditions. Factors responsible for these deviations include the following:

1. The flow velocity, which changes throughout the cardiac cycle as a result of acceleration during systole and deceleration in diastole.

2. Alteration in the lines of flow, which occurs whenever a vessel changes dimension including variations in diameter associated with each pulse, and

3. The types of flow, which are distorted at curves, bifurcations and in the branches that take off at various angles.

Depending on the viscosity and density of fluid as well as the cross sectional area of vessel lumen, the volume flow rate increases proportionally as predicted by the Poiseuille's law, when the pressure difference along the vascular segment increases. If the cross- sectional area of lumen remain constant, for example, the flow rate must increase. If the flow velocity is increased beyond a certain value, the initial laminar flow is destabilized. At first the fluid laminae are no longer continually directed parallel to vessel walls. Wave like irregularities develop in the laminae creating a pattern known as disturbed flow." As the flow velocity continue to increase, vortices may form near the vessel walls. Since the Doppler angles related to individual fluid, particles are no longer identical, an unhomogenous distribution of different shades of colour appear in CDS image across the vessel lumen. Same pixel may under go a complete flips, even in disturbed flow, depending on the angle between the total vectors (vector sum of all the flow vectors) and the direction of the ultrasound beam. This will only occur if the angle between the total flow vector and ultrasound beam is closer to 90°.

When the flow velocity exceed a critical value, the entire lumen is filled with fluid components where individual velocity vectors are randomly aimed in all the directions. This chaotic, flow pattern is the result of turbulence. Total velocity vector, however still points in the main flow direction. The flow velocity profile in a region with turbulent flow is very flat, resulting a large velocity gradient near the vessel walls. Turbulent flow can be recognised in CDS by a mixture of different colour pixels next to one another represents flow in different directions.

The existence of turbulent flow depend on the vessel diameter d = 2r (r—radius) the average flow velocity v, across the lumen, the density of the fluid and viscosity of the fluid. The factor than affect the development of turbulence are expressed by the dimensionless Reynolds number (Re)

$$Re = \frac{qv2r}{\eta}$$

The Reynolds number is dimensionless. Because density and viscosity (η) of blood are relatively constant, the development of turbulence depends mainly on the size of the vessels and on the velocity of flow. In a tube model, laminar flow tends to be disturbed if Reynolds number exceed 2000. However, in the circulatory system, disturbances and various degrees of turbulences are likely to occur at lower values because of body movements, pulsatile nature of blood flow, changes in vessel dimensions, roughness of the endothelial surface and other factors.

Turbulence develops more readily in large vessels under conditions of high flow and can be detected clinically by the findings of brutes or thrills. Bruits may same times may be heard over the ascending aorta during systolic acceleration in normal individuals at rest and are frequently heard in state of high cardiac output and blood flow, even in more distal, such as femoral artery. Distortion of laminar flow velocity profile can be assessed using ultrasound flow detectors, and such assessments can be applied for diagnostic purpose. For example, in arteries with severe stenosis, pronounced turbulence is a diagnostic feature observed in post-stenotic zone. Turbulence occurs because a jet of blood with high velocity and high kinetic energy suddenly encounters a normal diameter lumen or lumen of increased diameter (because of poststenotic dilatation) where both the velocity and energy level are lower than in stenotic zone.

During turbulent flow, the loss of pressure energy between two parts in a vessel is greater than that which would be expected from the factors in Poiseuille's equation and parabolic flow velocity profile is flattened.

KEY POINTS

Normal flow can be characterized as parabolic flow, however, due to presence of stenosis or drastic increase in diameter of lumen of vessel, flow profile may be disturbed or may be called as turbulant flow.
- Localized zones of flow reversal may also occur in normal flow near the bifurcation of arteries. Such flow separation occur, for example, in carotid bulb where CCA bifurcate into internal and external carotid arteries. This normal flow must be differentiated from turbulence.

Pulsatile Flow

Compared with continuous flow, the analysis of discontinuous pulsatile flow is considerably more complex.

With each heart beat, travel stroke volume of blood is injected into the arterial system, resulting in a pressure wave that travels throughout the arterial tree. The speed of propogation amplitude and slope of pressure wave changes as it traverses the arterial system. These boundary condition gives rise to two basic Doppler system (i) Low resistance, and (ii) High resistance.

Pressure change from cardiac activity The pumping action of heart maintains a high volume of blood in the arterial end of the circulation as large pressure amplitude developed in the left ventricle during each cardiac cycle, the aorta and large vessel reduce the pressure amplitude that are transmitted to the arterial tree.

Because of the intermittent pumping action of the heart, the pressure and flow vary in a pulsatile manner.

During the rapid phase of ventricular ejection the volume of blood at the arterial end increases, raising the pressure to systolic peak. During the latter part of systole, when cardiac ejection decreases, the outflow through the peripheral resistance vessel exceeds the volume being ejected by the heart and pressure begin to decline. This decline continues to flow from the arterioles into the microcirculation. Part of the work of heart leads directly to forward flow, but a large portion of energy of each cardiac contraction results in distention of the arteries that serve as reservoir for storing the blood volume and energy supplied to the system. The storage of energy and blood volume provides for continuous flow to the tissue during diastole.

Arterial Pressure Wave

The pulsatile variation in blood volume and energy occurring with each cardiac cycle are manifested as a pressure wave that can be detected throughout the arterial system. The amplitude and shape of arterial pressure wave depend on a complex interplay of factors, which include the stroke volume and time course of ventricular ejection, the peripheral resistance, and the stiffness of the arterial walls. In general, an increase in any of these factors results in an increase in the pulse amplitude (i.e. pulse pressure, difference between systolic and diastolic pressures) and

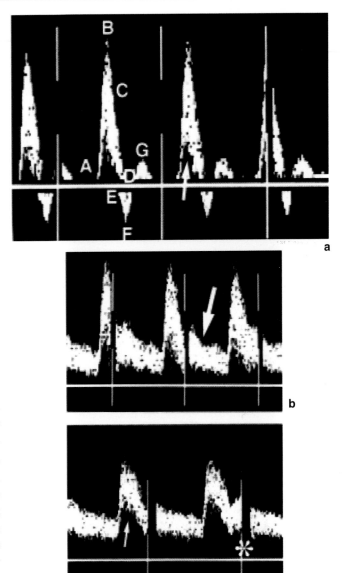

Figures 2.3a to c
Influence of the peripheral flow resistance on Doppler spectra recorded from the brachial artery (a,b) and internal carotid artery (C) in a healthy subject. (a) Triphasic spectrum at rest. High peripheral vascular flow resistance (peripheral-artery pattern) with a sharp systolic velocity increase (A-B), a rapid drop in velocity in late systole (C-D), diastolic flow reversal (E-F), and late diastolic forward flow (G). Note the spectral window below the systolic peak (white arrow), (b) after exercise , a pronounced forward-flow component appears in diastole (white arrow) due to the decrease in peripheral flow resistance. The spectral pattern is intermediate between a and c, and (c) low peripheral vascular flow resistance. The spectrum displays a high diastolic forward flow and less pulsatility than in a and b (parenchymal artery pattern). The empty systolic window (arrow) indicates undisturbed flow. Periodic refreshing of the colour Duplex image creates a brief, intermittent void in the spectral waveform(*)

frequently in a concomitant increase in systolic pressure. For example—increased stiffness of the arteries with age tends to increase both the systolic and pulse pressures.

The arterial pressure wave is propagated along the arterial tree distally from the heart. The speed of propogation, or pulse wave velocity, increases with stiffness of arterial walls and with the ratio of the wall thickness and diameter.

In mammalian circulation, arteries become progressively stiffer from the aorta towards the periphery. Therefore, the special propagation of the wave increases as it moves peripherally. Also the gradual increase in stiffness tend to decrease wave reflection and has a beneficial effect is that the pulse and systolic pressure in the aorta and proximal arteries are relativily lower than in peripheral vessels. The pressure against which the heart eject the stroke volume associated cardiac walls are accordingly reduced.

Pulsatile Flow Pattern

Pulsatile changes in pressure are associated with corresponding acceleration of blood flow with systole and deceleration in diastole. Although energy stored in the arterial walls maintains a positive arteriovenous pressure gradient and overall forward flow in the microcirculation during systole, temporary cessation of forward flow or even diastolic reversal occurs frequently in position of human arterial system.

So, in principle pulsatile flow is laminar. However, the flow velocity profile of pulsatile blood flow is subjected to extensive changes during the cardiac study as discussed earlier.

The reason for this is that blood flow is opposing a resistance based on inertial forces which dump quick pulsatile change of motion. The flow velocity profile is flat during acceleration phase and approximates a parabolic shape only as long as same forward flow persists after the acceleration phase ends. If transient flow reversal occur it begin near the vessel wall where the lowest flow velocity prevail during antegrade flow and propagate towards the centre of the vessel.

The flow is particularly unstable during this phase, and turbulence can develop even at very low Reynolds number.

Effect of Arterial Obstruction

As in continuous flow, the changes from laminar to turbulent flow is marked by transitional phenomena referred to as "disturbed flow". Unlike continuous flow, the Raynolds number in pulsatile flow varies over the cardiac cycle due to changes in flow velocity and vessel diameter.

Even in each physiologic conditions, this can give rise to periodic turbulence during certain parts of the cardiac cycle. The development of turbulence in pulsatile flow is also influenced by the shape of the flow velocity profile and the heart rate.

Haemodynamics at Stenosis

Arterial obstruction can result in reduced pressure and flow distal to the site of blockage, but the effect on pressure and flow are greatly influenced by a number of factors proximal and especially distal to the lesion.

Encroachment on lumen of an artery by arteriosclerotic plaque can result in diminished pressure and flow distal to the lesion but this encroachment on the lumen has to be relatively little resistance to flow compared with the resistance vessels with which they are in series.

A basic understanding of flow dynamic is essential for the correct interpretation of most phenomena encountered in Doppler studies of arterial system—prestenotic, interstenotic and poststenotic changes in absolute and relative flow velocities and flow pattern are the variables that lead to a correct diagnosis and permit a quantitative assessment of pathologic finding regardless of Doppler technology used.

Principle of Continuity in Assessing the Severity of Stenoses

Volume flow (flow rate/time) in a particular vessel remains constant in any given segment of the vessel except at sites where part of the flow volume is directed from the original channel at an arterial branching of the vessel.

Volume flow q is expressed by:

$$q = A \times v$$

Where q = Volume flow/time
A = Cross-sectional area of vessel
v = Average flow velocity in a given cross-section of the vessel.

If the vessel has a circular cross-section the above equation changes to

$$q = \pi r^2 v$$

Where r = vessel radius

The principle of continuity is expressed (Fig. 2.4) by:

$$q_1 = q_2$$
$$q = A_1v_1 = A_2v_2$$

or

$$\frac{A_1}{A_2} = \frac{v_2}{v_1}$$

Where $q_{1,2}$ = Volume flow/time at position 1 and 2

$A_{1,2}$ = Cross-sectional area of vessel with a position 1 and 2

$v_{1,2}$ = Average flow velocity in a given cross-section of the vessel at position 1 and 2

A reduction in the lumen diameter necessarily leads to an increase in the flow velocity.

For example 50 per cent reduction in diameter corresponding to 75 per cent reduction in area leads

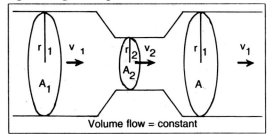

Volume flow = constant

Figure2.4

The principle of continuity. The flow velocity v_{1-2} changes according to the variations in the cross-sectional area A_{1-2} of the vessel. The flow volume in the vessel remains constant at all positions. Thus, the increase in flow velocity can be used in determining the reduction in luminal cross-section area and calculating the degree of stenosis (see text)

to an increase in flow velocity by a factor of 4. Based on the relative increase in flow velocity the degree of stenosis can be calculated as far as the continuity equation is valid.

$$X = 100\left(1 - \frac{100}{Y}\right)$$

Where X = Degree of stenosis in %
Y = Relative velocity increase in %

or

$$X = 100\left(1 - \frac{v_1}{v_2}\right)$$

Where v_1 is prestenotic velocity
v_2 Intrastenotic velocity

Thus detection and determination of the severity of vascular stenosis with Doppler ultrasound is based on recording the relative velocity increase or Doppler frequency shift that is produced by the stenosis. Very severe flow rate—limit lesion can also reduce intrastenotic flow velocity to such a degree that the absolute interstenotic flow velocity is less than that associated with a moderate, non-flow reducing stenosis.

As the degree of stenosis increases, the velocity measured by Doppler frequency analysis are lower than theoretically predicted as a consequence of intrastonic energy losses due to friction that was neglected in the above equation.

During haemodynamic evaluation of severity of stenoses by Duplex sonography it is presumed that vascular segment of interest can be visualised in longitudinal section. The scan-plane must pass precisely through the centre of prestenotic and intrastenotic areas to ensure that maximum flow velocities are obtained for use in the calculation. Prominent vascular calcification, entering gas or bone and obesity are physical obstacle that can prevent direct visualisation of the stenotic area. In these cases Duplex ultrasound permits only an approximate indirect assessment of the severity of the vascular obstruction.

In vessels that do not show significant branching in the area near the stenosis, flow velocities should be measured at the interstenotic and immediate prestenotic levels for quantifying a stenosis.

Although continuity equation is still valid, the relative distribution of volume flow is unpredictable if the stenosis is located at a bifurcation or an arterial branching. The degree of stenosis can be determined from velocity measurements only by measuring both intrastenotic flow velocity and the flow velocity at a more distal site in a segment having normal lumen size, well away from stenotic jet or turbulence. Alternatively, the degree of proximal stenoses of internal carotid artery can be estimated from empirically derived ratios of the maximum systolic velocities at the prestenotic and intrastenotic levels.

There are two basic method in Duplex sonography for determining the severity of a stenoses on the basis of flow velocity. See Figures 2.5a to c.
1. By Doppler spectrum analysis
2. By evaluation of the colour encoded flow velocities in CDS.

As a basic rule, the maximum flow velocity in a given vascular segment should be measured at the time of maximum systolic forward flow. The maximum flow velocity can be derived from Doppler spectrum or determined by using a special colour in the colour

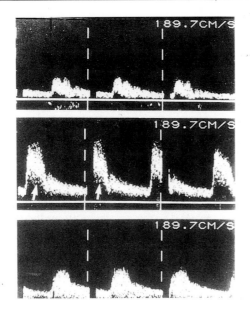

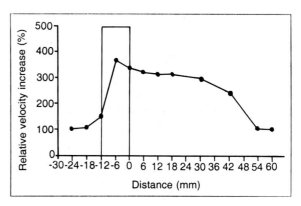

Figures 2.5a to c
(a) Prestenotic spectrum from common carotid artery
(b) Intrastenotic spectrum shows a mark elevation of flow velocity
(c) Poststenotic spectrum shows filling in the systolic window

Figure 2.6
Measurement of the flow velocities across a stenosis causing a 75% concentric area reduction (= 50% diameter reduction) in a vascular phantom. Luminal diameter is 6 mm proximal and distal to the stenosis. Length of the stenosis is 12 mm proximal and distal to the stenosis. Length of the stenosis is 12 mm. The shaded box indicates the vicinity of the stenosis (−12 to 0 mm). The Doppler sample volume was positioned mid-stream, and the velocities were calculated from the Doppler spectrum (maximum systolic velocity). The graph shows a typical progression of velocity changes across the stenosis (relative to the prestenotic value). The relative velocity increase does not quite reach the theoretically predicted value of 400% due to frictional losses. The poststenotic jet extends several centimetres distally past the stenosed segment

duplex image to tag the highest flow velocities. The use of maximum systolic velocities permits the most accurate assessment of the degree of stenoses. If the time averaged velocities are used, the severity of the lesion will be underestimated due to entrance effects and changes in the flow velocity profile during pulse cycle.

It must be pointed out that it is absolutely mandatory to perform a Doppler angle correction when flow velocities are calculated from Doppler frequency shift. It is only possible to use the Doppler frequency shift in calculating the degree of stenosis if crossover angle between the longitudinal vessel axis and the individual ultrasound beam are the same in both position.

Interstenotic and Poststenotic Flow Changes

Due to increased flow velocity, the interstenotic Reynolds number can rise tremendously only in the case of severe lesion. This may lead to disturbed flow or even turbulent flow within stenosis (Fig. 2.6). Distal to stenosis, the maximum flow velocity continues to be elevated (Poststenotic jet) atleast in certain zone of the vascular cross-section with exit effects playing a significant roles. Zone of retrograde inherently

laminar flow can develop near the vessel wall distal to a stenosis (flow separation and flow reversal (Figs 2.7a to e). These stationary eddy current close to the vessel walls may propogate distally depending on the flow velocity and degree of stenosis.

The poststenotic Reynolds number may far exceed the intrastenotic Reynolds number as the flow enters the poststenotic lumen at elevated velocities. This may cause marked turbulence to develop in the poststenotic segments in addition to zones of flow reversal along the vessel walls. This may extend distally for a distance several times the normal vessel diameter. Besides the

---

KEY POINTS

Turbulence and flow reversal can be easily recognised in color duplex imaging using Doppler frequency analysis.

Turbulent flow produces spectral broadening and spectral window is completely filled with simultaneous occurrence of positive and negative Doppler frequency shift.

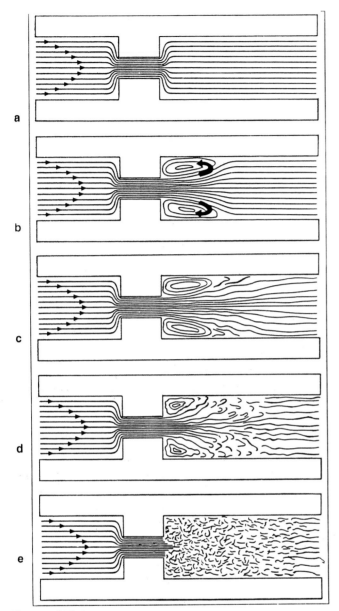

Figures 2.7a to e
Schematic representation of poststenotic flow changes as a function of physical boundary conditions. The prestenotic flow velocity increases from a to e while the degree of stenosis remains constant. In principle, the progression of changes from a to e is characteristic of all factors that would produce an increase in the Reynolds number, (a) low prestenotic flow velocity. There are no poststenotic flow disturbances, (b) with a slight increase in prestenotic flow velocity, zones of flow reversal (curved arrows) develop near the vessel walls, but the flow remains generally laminar, and there is no turbulence, (c) when the prestenotic flow velocity is increased further, wave-like irregularities develop in the laminae (disturbed flow) in addition to flow reversal, (d) at a high prestenotic flow velocity, turbulence develops distal to the stenosis from the zones of flow reversal. Flow is still disturbed at some distance from the stenosis, and (e) a very high prestenotic flow velocity is associated with severe poststenotic turbulence

pressure drop across the stenosis, turbulence is partially responsible for the energy loss resulting in a volume flow reduction associated with severe stenoses.

Turbulence and flow reversal are easily recognised in colour duplex imaging using Doppler frequency analysis. Turbulent flow produces broadening of the Doppler spectrum that may completely fill in the systolic window beneath the spectrum envelope and simultaneous occurrence of positive and negative Doppler frequency shifts.

The location and extent of local flow reversal and turbulence depend in a complex way on the geometry of the stenosis, the degree of stenoses, the surface structure of vessel walls, the prestenotic flow velocity, the viscosity of the blood and pulsatility of the flow. There are no general rule for determining the severity of stenosis from the length and extent of flow reversal and turbulence.

The main value of a colour coded presentation of these phenomena is that it permit the identification of a vascular stenosis when the lesion itself is obscured by vessel wall calcification or calcified plaque.

VENOUS HAEMODYNAMICS

The pressure remains in the vein, after the blood has reversed the arterioles and capillaries, is low when the subject is in the supine because their large diameters, medium and large veins, offer little resistance to flow and blood more readily flow from the small veins to right atrium where the pressure is close to atmospheric pressure.

Flow and pressure changes during the cardiac cycle. Figure 2.8 shows changes in the pressure and

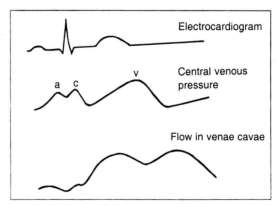

Figure 2.8
Schematic representation of normal changes in pressure and flow in the central veins associated with the cardiac cycle. a = a wave; c = c wave; v = v wave

flow in large veins such as the venae cava that occur during the phases of cardiac cycle. Such oscileation in pressure and flow at times be transmitted to more peripheral vessels.

There are three positive pressure waves (Fig. 2.8). These can be distinguished in central nervous venous pressure and reflect corresponding changes in pressure in atria.

One wave 'a' is caused by atrial contraction and relaxation. The upstroke of 'c' wave is related to the increase in pressure when the atrioventricular values are closed and bulge during isovolumetric ventricular contraction. The subsequent down stroke results from the fall in pressure caused by pulling the atrio-ventricular valve rings towards the apex of heart during ventricular contraction. The upstroke of 'v' wave results from a passive rise in atrial pressure during ventricular systole when the atrioventricular valve are closed and atria fill with blood from the peripheral veins. The 'v' wave downstroke is caused by fall in pressure that occurs where the blood leaves the atria rapidly and fills the ventricles soon after the opening of atrio-ventricular valve early in ventricular diastole.

In abnormal condition such as congestive heart failure or tricuspid insufficiency venous pressure is increased. This elevation of venous pressure may lead to the transmission and cardiac phasic charges in pressure and flow to the peripheral vein of the upper and lower limb. Such phasic changes may occasionally be found in healthy well-hydrated individuals probably because a large blood volume distends the venous system.

Venous Effect of Respiration

Respiration has profound effect as venous pressure and flow during inspiration, the volume in the veins of thorax increases and the pressure decreases in response to reduced intrathoracic pressure. Expiration leads to the opposite effect, with decreased venous volume and increased pressure. The venous response to respiration is reversed in the abdomen where the pressure increases during inspiration because of the descend of diaphragm and decreases during expiration as the diaphragm ascends. Increased abdominal pressure during inspiration decreases pressure gradient between peripheral veins in the lower extremities and the abdomen thus reducing flow in the peripheral vessels.

During expiration, when extra-abdominal pressure is reduced, the pressure gradient from lower limb to abdomen is increased and flow in the peripheral veins rises correspondingly.

In the veins of the upper limbs, the changes in flow with respiration are opposite to those in the lower extremities because of reduced intrathoracic pressure inspiration. The pressure gradient from the veins of upper limb to right atrium increases when flow increases. During expiration flow decreases because of the resulting increase in intrathoracic pressure and the corresponds rise of the right atrial pressure. The respiratory changes in flow in upper limb may be influenced by changes in pressure with the upper part of the body elevated venous flow tends to step at the height of inspiration and resumes with expiration, probably because of the compression of subclavian vein at the level of the first ribs during contraction of accessory muscles of respiration.

Venous Obstruction

Venous obstruction can be acute or chronic. In the case of severe chronic obstruction, oedema may occur.

Acute obstruction, usually associated with thrombosis may lead to potentially fatal pulmonary embolism.

Doppler flow detection and Duplex scanner may be used for this purpose.

The presence or absence of obstruction is also gauged by increasing flow towards the examination in site by squeezing the limb distally or by activating the distal muscle group and thus increasing venous flow towards the flow detecting probe.

Absence of increased flow sound attenuation and increased flow is associated with obstruction between the probe location and the site from which the enhancement of venous flow is attempted.

When volumes are competent, flow in peripheral veins, is towards the heart.

When there are incompetent veins proximally, there may be retrograde filling in the peripheral veins such as these in ankle region from the more proximal veins in addition to normal filling from capillary beds.

The presence or absence of the retrograde flow may be detected by listening with a Doppler flow detecter and squeezes the limb proximally.

Doppler Principle and Instrumentation

Satish K Bhargava
AK Srivastava

INTRODUCTION

Ultrasound imaging is especially useful in cardiovascular system because of its ability to produce images of cardiac anatomy and flowing blood through many points of vascular system. Approaches to the identification of the moving structure including relative pulse echo imaging, motion mode (M mode) display of reflected ultrasound pulse, and the Doppler's shift method.

The Doppler method has a number of application in clinical medicine, including detection of foetal heart beat, detection of air embolism, blood pressure monitoring, detection and characterization of blood flow and localization of blood vessel occlusion.

Over 30 years ultrasound scanner have exploited the Doppler effect to detection in above mentioned areas. The first measurement of flow in heart was performed by Satumora in 1956, currently available technique include continuous wave Doppler, pulse wave Doppler, colour flow imaging and newest colour amplitude imaging (power Doppler).

Doppler Effect

When there is relative motion between a source and a detector of ultrasound, the frequency of the detected ultrasound differs from that emitted by the source.

If the source and detector are moving away from each other, the frequency measured by the observer will be lower than the frequency detected by stationary observer. If they are moving towards each other, the frequency will be higher.

In daily life everyone has probably noticed the Doppler shift effects (Fig. 3.1). The sound coming from the siren of a police car moving towards an observer is at higher pitch than the sound measured by another observer when the police car is moving away from him. When the

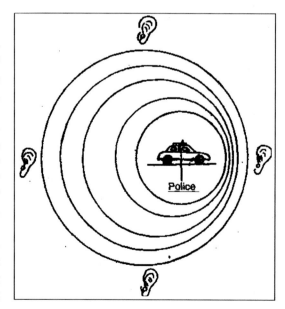

Figure 3.1
Due to the movement of the source and the observer relative to one another the frequency of the observed and transmitted signals differ

car is passing an observer, a sudden jump in the sound frequency can be clearly heard. Exactly same thing would be noticed in the opposite case, when an observer is moving towards a stationary sound source, passes it and then moves away from source. If the emitter and observer are moving towards one another, the perceived wavelength is shortened, resulting in the perception of a higher frequencies. If the emitter and observer moving away from one another, the perceived wavelength is longer than in stationary case resulting in perception of a lower frequency.

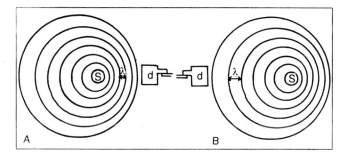

Figures 3.2a and b
(a) Source moving towards a stationary detector
(b) source moving away from a stationary detector

The shift in frequency is illustrated in Figure 3.2. In Figure 3.2A an ultrasound is moving with velocity v_s, towards the detector. After sometime following production of one particular wave front, the distance between the wave front and the source is $(C - v_s)/t$ where C is velocity of sound in the medium. The wavelength (λ) of the ultrasound in the direction of motion is shorten to:

$$\lambda = \frac{C - v_s}{fo}$$

Where fo is frequency of ultrasound from the source.

$$f_B = \frac{C}{\lambda} = \left(\frac{C}{(C - v_s/fo)} \right)$$

f_B – frequency observed

$$f_B = fo \left(\frac{C}{C - v_s} \right)$$

The shift in frequency f_D is then

$$f_D = f_B - fo = fo \left(\frac{v_s}{C - v_s} \right)$$

If the emitter and observer are moving away from each other the results in perception of lower frequency. In general,

$$f_B = fo \, \frac{C + V_{observer}}{C - V_{source}}$$

f_B	=	Observed frequency
fo	=	True frequency
C	=	Speed of sound
Vobes	=	Velocity of observer
vs	=	Velocity of source

If the source and detector are at the same location and ultrasound is reflected from an object moving towards the location with a velocity V_{source}, the object acts first as a moving receiver as it receives the ultrasound signal and then act as a moving source as it reflects the signal. As a result, the ultrasound signal received by receiver exhibit a frequency shift.

$$F_D = 2fo \, \frac{v}{c}$$

This is because $f_B = fo \left(\frac{c + v}{c - v} \right)$

$$f_B = fo \left(1 + \frac{2v}{c} \right)$$ when $v < c$ using Taylor series ignoring the higher form

hence $f_B - fo = f_D = 2fo \, \dfrac{v}{c}$

If an object is moving towards the source, Shift in frequency is positive

i.e. $\quad f_D = 2fo \, \dfrac{v}{c}$

If object is moving away from source and detector,

the $\quad f_D = -2fo \, \dfrac{v}{c}$

or Doppler shift is negative.

Negative sign indicates that frequency of detected ultrasound is lower than that emitted by the source.

The above discussion has assumes that ultrasound beam is parallel to the motion of an object. If the source and observer are not moving directly away from or towards each other but an angle θ the equation becomes,

$$f_D = 2fo \, \frac{v \, Cos \, \theta}{C}$$

This technique is used to study motion, primarily that of circulatory system. Since RBCs are not continuous and act as rough surface and therefore act as a scatter of US beam. This scattering is known as Rayleigh Tyndall scattering and caused by RBCs in blood.

RBCs are particulate components of blood that interact with the ultrasound (Platelets are small in size and WBCs are too few in number)

A typical arrangement is illustrated in Figures 3.3a and b. An ultrasound transducer is placed in contact with the skin surface. It transmits a beam where frequency is f_o. The receiver frequency f_r will differ from fo when echos are picked up from moving scatter such as RBCs. The Doppler frequency f_D is defined as the difference between received and transmitted frequency and is given by:

$$f_D = f_r - f_o = \frac{2f_o \, n \, \text{Cos} \, \theta}{C}$$

Where θ is called Doppler angle. This angle strangely influences Doppler shift for a given reflector velocity.

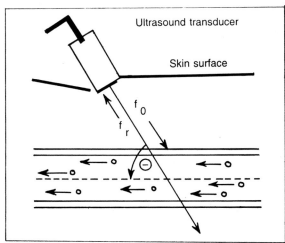

$$F_D = f_r - f_o = \frac{2\,f_o\,v}{c}\cos\theta$$

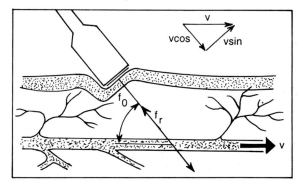

Figures 3.3a and b
Arrangement for detecting Doppler signals from blood. The angle θ is the Doppler angle, which is the angle between the direction of motion and the beam axis, looking toward the transducer

The reference frequency used is for clarity, always transducer central frequency, although this is by no means necessary. In most diagnostic ultrasound system, a reference frequency about 25% lower than the central frequency is used in order to improve the penetration and the velocity range.

A factor of 2″ occurs in the equation in the numerator because the sound must make two trips. One trip goes from transducer to receiver in motion (erythrocytes acts as receiver) and ultrasound wave from transducer will be perceived as Doppler shifted. Second trip from moving reflector (erythrocytes will act as a transmitter in motion relative to stationary receiver transducer). Solving the equation for v results in,

$$v = \frac{f_D \, C}{2f_o \, \text{Cos} \, \theta}$$

The actual determination of Doppler angle may be very difficult. However, when interpreting the measured shift it must never be forgotten that the effect is angle and reference frequency dependent. Only by measuring the Doppler angle, the reference frequency and Doppler shift, can the blood flow velocity be calculated.

Theoretically, no Doppler shift occur when probe is exactly perpendicular to the direction of motion this is because $\theta = 90°$ and cos 90° = 0. In practice small Doppler shift may be detected when probe appear to be perpendicular to the direction of flow in vessel because some portion of beam is not perpendicular to the motion as a result of divergence of ultrasound beam.

When flow is directed toward the transducer $\theta = 0$ and hence Cos $\theta = 1$. Hence Doppler frequency detected for the orientation would be maximum.

As mentioned earlier absolute measurement of reflector velocity require that Doppler angle is accurately determined.

Uncertainty in the measurement of Doppler angle particularly at large angles, introduce error in velocity computation. A 5 degree error for 70 degree Doppler angle causes the velocity estimation to deviate by 25 per cent. A decrease in the Doppler angle to 40 degree reduces this deviation to 8 per cent for same uncertainty of 5 degree in the angle measurement.

As a general guideline, Doppler signals from superficial blood vessels (e.g. carotids) should be acquired at angle between 30 and 60 degrees whenever possible.

The lower angular limit is recommended because total internal reflection occurs at the vessel wall blood boundary for small angles and sound beam does not reach the moving blood. The accurate measurement of Doppler angle is difficult for tortuous vessels that radically change direction. Some Doppler instrument allow the operation to specify the direction of flow on an image and then instrument automatically calculate the Doppler angle.

Determining the volumetric flow of blood in the units of cubic centimetre per second requires an estimation of the area of vessel as well as Doppler angle. Volumetric flow Q is the product of average velocity v and cross section area of A of vessel

$$Q = vA$$

In clinical measurement of volumetric flow, several source of error reduces the accuracy below which what would be expected is based upon intrinsic precision of Doppler shift measurements. The measurement of vessel area is typically based upon the measurement of vessel diameter in the image.

However, the angle at which the image plane cut through the vessel may cause either under estimation or over estimation of diameter. Also the Doppler unit may not sample the average velocity in a vessel. Flow in a vessel is not same throughout. It is usually greatest at the centre and decreases to zero at the vessel wall. Complex flow profile are possible, particularly if a stenosis, bifurcation or plaque formation is present. An accurate estimation of average velocity require sampling of velocity at different radii within the vessel point across the stream. It is possible to make some

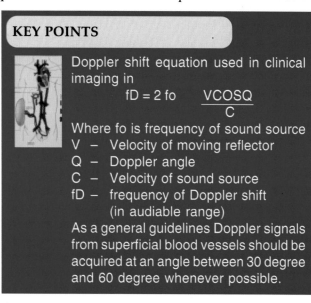

KEY POINTS

Doppler shift equation used in clinical imaging in

$$fD = 2\,fo\ \frac{VCOSQ}{C}$$

Where fo is frequency of sound source
V – Velocity of moving reflector
Q – Doppler angle
C – Velocity of sound source
fD – frequency of Doppler shift
      (in audiable range)
As a general guidelines Doppler signals from superficial blood vessels should be acquired at an angle between 30 degree and 60 degree whenever possible.

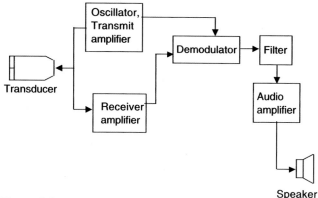

Figure 3.4
Block diagram of CW Doppler instrument

simplifying assumption. For example—in laminar flow the average velocity is half the maximum value.

Instrumentation

The most basic Doppler system through which first Doppler blood velocity measurements were performed is continuous wave Doppler system. CW Doppler operation is used in a variety of instruments, ranging from simple, inexpensive hand-held Doppler unit to "high end" Duplex scanner in CW Doppler may be one of the several operating modes.

A simplified block diagram of the necessary component of CW Doppler system is presented in Figure 3.4.

Such a system requires a separate transmitter and receiver. For example one can use two piezoelectric transducers mounted in same enclosure depicted in Figure 3.4. The transmitted sound wave and receiving pattern of receiver are very directional. To obtain maximum sensitivity for detecting returning echo signals the beam regions of the transmitter and receiver are caused to overlap. This overlap is achieved by inclining the transducer elements. The region of beam overlap defines the most sensitive region of the transducer. The transmitter continuously excites the ultrasonic transducer with a sinusoidal electric signal of frequency f_o producing incident ultrasound beam echo returning to the transducer have frequency f_r. These signals are amplified in the receiver and then sent to a demodulator to extract the Doppler signal. Here the signal are multiplied by reference signal from the transmitting, producing a mixture of signals, part having a frequency (fr+fo) and part having a frequency (fr-fo). The sum frequency (fr+fo) is very high, twice the ultrasound frequency and easily removed by electronic filtering. This leaves signals with frequency (fr-fo) at the output, which is the Doppler signal. It is possible to eliminate signal of certain frequency ranges that might be due to respiratory motion of the liver or another organ or due to pulsating, vessel wall. This is done in the instruments that have additional electronic filters in their circuitry. For example—by applying high pass filter.

The lower cut-off frequency of such wall filter is usually operater selectable.

Doppler frequency for blood flow lies within the audible range which is generally the case for most Doppler signals results from blood flow by using Doppler shift equation. This is because speed of interface for biological system are relatively small (0.5 to 200 cm/sec) compared with velocity of sound in tissue.

Basic CW Doppler units usually have only a few controls, but operators should be familiar with these on their own equipment.

Transmit power to vary the amplitude of signal from the transmitter to transducer thus changing the sensitivity to weak echos, some simple units omit this control, keeping the transmit level constant.

Directional Doppler

A basic CW Doppler instrument allows detection of magnitude of Doppler frequency, but it provide no information of whether flow is towards or away from the transducer that is whether Doppler shift is positive or negative.

A common technique for determining flow direction is to use Phase V quadrature detection technique in the Doppler device which allows forward and reverse flow to be separated.

After the received echo signal are amplified, they are split into two identical channels for demodulation. The channels differ only in that the reference signals from the transmitter sent to the demodutalors are 90 degree out of phase. Two separate Doppler signal are produced. They are identical except for a small phase difference occur between them, and thus phase difference can be used to determine whether the Doppler shift is positive or negative.

Since the frequencies used in medical ultrasound and velocity encountered in the human body, combine to produce Doppler frequency shift in audible range. It is customary to send the Doppler signal directly to loudspeakers. An experienced sonographer can gain significant diagnostic information from the audio output.

Another way of processing the Doppler signal is to digitize it in an analogue to digital converter (ADC) and then use, for example—Fast Fourier Transform (FFT) to extract the spectral information (See in next chapter).

Continuous wave instruments are good for superficial vessel such as carotid. They are also very sensitive to weak signal such as might be found in digital artery of a finger. CW system has no limit on the maximum velocity measures and can therefore measure any velocity correctly (lack of aliasing). Other advantage includes the high accuracy of Doppler shift estimate with the narrow frequency band width that is used.

However system suffer from one major constraint. Since information received from entire ultrasound beam, it is impossible to determine the depth of specific blood vessel. Hence an error-some velocity measurement may result if several vessels are insonated simultaneously in the same area since any motion within the sample path of transmit and receive transducer will result in a Doppler shift. This sample volume starts near the transducer face and usually extends into the tissues as the beam will penetrate. In addition to this, technique prone to object motion within the beam path.

Pulsed Wave Doppler

Pulsed wave Doppler unit use the echo ranging principle to provide quantitative depth information of the Doppler signals from different depth, allowing for detection of moving interface and scatter only from within a well-defined sample volume (Fig 3.5). This sample volume can be positioned any where along the axis of the ultrasound beam.

The principal components of pulsed wave Doppler instrument are shown in Figure 3.5. One transducer is used in pulse echo format similar to imaging technique with the exception that spatial pulse length is usually longer to minimum of 5 cycle/pulse to 25 cycle/pulse is used to achieve better narrow band frequency characteristic for a more accurate determination of frequency shift. In conventional B-mode images no. of cycle/pulse is 2-3 cycle/pulse with this system same transducer element both sends and receivers sound, similar to non-Doppler systems.

Depth selection is achieved with use of electronic gating. Here transducer is excited with a short

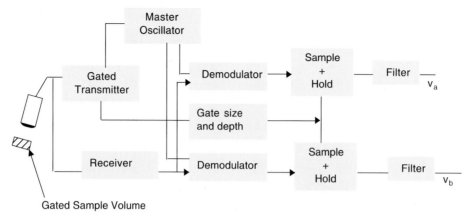

Gated Sample Volume

Figure 3.5

Principal components of a pulsed Doppler instrument. The transducer is excited by a brief pulse; echo signals are amplified in the receiver and sent to the quadrature demodulators. A portion of the demodulated waveform is held in the sample and hold unit, which forms the Doppler signal by using several pulse-echo sequences. V_a and V_b are signals representing flow towards and away from the transducer

duration burst and then no sound sent for brief period of time that is transducer is silent for a period of time to listen for echoes before another burst of ultrasound is generated. This differs from continuous wave Doppler where one transducer continuously excited.

Here in PW, scattered and refleted echo signal are detected by same transducer as mentioned earlier. Detected signal is amplified by receiver and applied to demodulator. The output of demodulator is then applied to a sample and hold circuit, which integrates a portion of the signal selected by range gate. Which means received signal is electronically gated for processing so that only those echoes detected in a narrow time interval after pulse, corresponds to a specific depth that contribute to the Doppler signal all other echos are rejected by the electronics.

The delay time before the gate is turned on determine the axial location of the sample volume or depth, the amount of time the gate is activated establishes the axial length of sample volume. The depth of tissue being examined for flow is determined by varying the length of time after sound is transmitted before gate is turned on. Gate parameter such as position and duration are controlled by operator and can be adjusted. The sample length is between 1-15 mm. The lateral dimension of sampling volume are dictated by beam width which is influenced by transducer frequency and focussing characteristics. The received echo must be evaluated to determine if the reflector is moving. This is accompanied by comparing the phase of the echo with a reference signal for which phase is synchronized with the transmitter pulse. Two waves are described as being in phase if their maximum, minimum and zero point occur concurrently.

The echo from stationary reflector has the same phase as the reference signal where as the echos from moving structure undergoes a phase shift via the Doppler effect.

The system is repeatly pulsed. The pulse repetition frequency (PRF) is the frequency at which sound pulses are transmitted.

Hence in Pulsed Wave mode, range discrimination is obtained, since the time of flight of a received echo can be converted into a specific depth. This assures propagational velocity of ultrasound in tissue to be known and received signal sampled accordingly.

One sample per period is acquired until enough data for an accurate estimation of Doppler shift have been collected, (typically 64-128 sample). The technique is known as range gating.

KEY POINTS

Basic Doppler systems used in Doppler sonography is

– Continuous wave Doppler
– Single gated Pulsed Wave Doppler
– Multi gated pulsed Wave Doppler
– Duplex Doppler
– Colour Flow imaging
– Power Doppler Imaging

A comparison of CW and PW methods is given in Table 3.1.

CW versus PW Doppler ultrasound	
Table 3.1 *CW Doppler*	*PW Doppler*
+ sensitive	+ range resolution
+ inexpensive	+ variable sample volume size
+ high signal/noise ratio	+ stepping stone to more advanced modalities
+ low accoustic output	– lower signal/noise ratio
– no range resolution	– high output power
– prone to object motion within beam path	– range velocity ambiguity

Limitation of Doppler systems: The use of CW and PW Doppler ultrasound raises a number of problems and ambiguities all of which influence the performance of Colour Flow Images (CFI) system as well.

Even when only one vessel is studied and only one frequency is emitted a range of Doppler frequencies will be received. This phenomena is known as spectral broadening. It is due to either to flow profile variation within the vessel (i.e. many different velocities are detected) or to transit time effect. The latter is a fundamental uncertainty inherent in Doppler measurement.

It is due to the finite period of time that each erythrocyte contributes to the back scattered signal, when it passes through the beam. Thus, even a single scatterer moving at constant velocity will give to a spread of frequencies.

An echo must have returned to the receiver before the next pulse is transmitted, if the depth of origin is to be unambiguously determined. The maximum depth accessible is therefore limited by the propagation or velocity and the inter-pulse duration of the system (i.e. 1/PRF).

Further more there is a limit to the maximum velocity measurable. This is due to digitization applied. If the Doppler signal changes too rapidly then it is impossible to reconstruct the correct Doppler shift frequency.

This is known as aliasing.

A common way that aliasing is manifested on a Doppler spectral display is displayed in Figure 3.6.

The Doppler spectrum wraps around the display with high velocities being converted to reversed flow immediately at the point of aliasing and still high

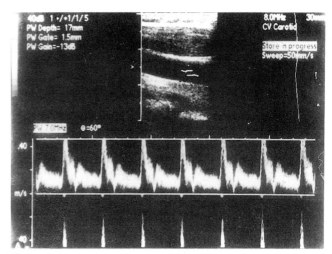

Figure 3.6
Manifestation of aliasing on a spectral display

velocities in the flow signal appearing as progressively lower velocities.

To avoid aliasing the Nyquist sampling rate theorem must be fulfilled. This theorem states that

$$f_D \leq \frac{f_s}{2} = \frac{PRF}{2}$$

Where f_s is system's sampling frequency (equal to PRF). Hence at a minimum the PRF must be at least 2 times the frequency of Doppler signal to construct the signal sucessfully.

When PRF equals $2 \times f_D$ this is known as Nyquist limit. Hence $PRF \geq 2 \,|\, f_D |$

If the frequency of Doppler shift is above Nyquist limit then aliasing occur. An amalogy would be a person who is trying to count a train of moving boxcars. This person keeps his eyes closed and opens them periodically for a brief look at the boxcars. He must open his eyes with a high enough frequency so that he sees each boxcars otherwise he may arrive at a count that is too low. The PRF must be high enough to sample the vessel adequately so that Doppler information is accurate.

To measure reflector moving with high velocity and producing large Doppler shift a high PRF is necessary.

But a high PRF limits the depth that can be sampled because a certain time is required to collect the echoes arising from that depth before the next pulse is sent out.

So while the maximum velocity measurable, v max increases with increasing PRF, the maximum depth measurable, dmax decreases.

The ambiguities in maximum depth and velocity measurable are often combined into one expression.

$$v_{max} < \frac{C^2}{8\ fo\ d_{max}}$$

If the flow to be studied is known to be unidirectional, then relationship be $C^2/4dfo$.

The maximum depth and velocity are inversely related and this equation is therefore independent of PRF. As sample volume depth increases the maximum detectable Doppler signal frequencies increases and hence the maximum reflector velocity that can be detected decreases. At any depth lower ultrasound frequencies permit detection of greater velocities than high frequencies.

The trade off between maximum velocity and depth measurement constitute an important compromise inherent in PW Doppler system.

In practice aliasing can be avoided or at least limited by changing a number of parameters as shown in Table 3.2.

Techinque for avoiding aliasing
Increase PRF
Increase the beam/vessel angle
Reduce the depth
Reduce the transducer frequency
Change the base-line
Use CW instead

Table 3.2

One such example is shown in Figure 3.8 wherein base line has been increased to correct aliasing which is shown in Figure 3.5.

An additional problem affects all Doppler scanner is the angular dependence when converting the Doppler shift from a frequency (in Hz) to a velocity in (m/s). The correct angle of incidence may not be known. Suppose as an example the true angle is 50° but it is estimated to be 45°. The error in velocity is 10 per cent. At 70° the same uncertainly results in a 25 per cent error, while at angle less than 20 degree. These errors are insignificant.

MULTIGATED PW DOPPLER SYSTEMS

A single gated PW Doppler system limit the information to one particular location or depth along the scan line. In order to obtain data from several depth simultaneously a so called multigated (MG) PW Doppler system must be employed. Multigate PW

systems typically contain 64-128 gates with a minimum axial length of 1mm for each sample volume.

Basically after demodulation the received signal is directed to a number of parallel processing channel. Each has a slightly different range gate setting. This allows number of adjacent sample volumes to be positioned across a vessel in Figure 3.7. The problem of locating a vessel is greatly reduced.

Since the assessment of the blood flow velocity is performed simultanesouly in each sample volume, the velocity distribution along the vessel cross section can be determined as a function of time. The velocity profile will be influenced by the presence of for example plaques or stenosis and can be therefore a useful diagnostic tool.

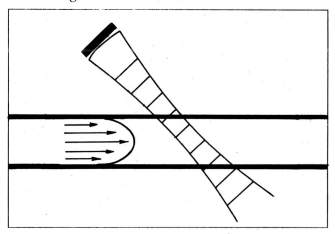

Figure 3.7
Velocity profile measurement using a multigated (MG) Doppler system

Duplex Doppler Systems

In spite of the advantage afforded by MG Doppler system, orientation and locating the desired vessel remain a problem. One way to overcome this is to combine 2D B-mode scan with flow information from Pulsed wave Doppler data.

The first such combined system were referred to as Duplex Doppler scanner.

This is because without some visual guidance to the vessel of interest, PW Doppler would be of little use.

In Duplex system a PW Doppler beam is visualized across the B-mode image with a sample volume position indicated by a cursor. This permits vessels to be easily selected for further evaluation. For example as shown in Figure 3.8 with the duplex image at the

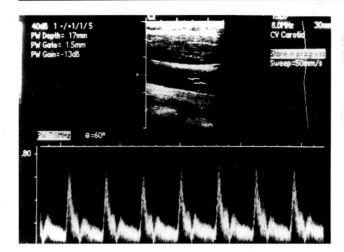

Figure 3.8
Correction of aliasing by increasing the velocity scale on the machine

top and spectral data in the form of sonogram at the bottom. Notice how the location of the sample volume alters the measured spectra (low velocity at the vessel wall and higher flow in the centre).

An advantage of a Duplex system is that the angle of incidence can be estimated from the B-mode. Thus Doppler frequency shift can be transferred to flow velocity estimates. The assessment of the angle of incident rest on the number of assumption such as flow parallel to the vessel wall and no curvature of the vessel in the scan plan. These assumptions are however rarely fulfilled. Due to error, one should always have a beam flow angle between 30 to 60 degree. Other errors include vessel being off axis or curving compared to the scan plan. This problem also occur in CFI system. The error in velocity measurement due to z plane misalignment or slice thickness have been found to be less than 5 per cent at optimal setting but upto 20 per cent error has been measured in non-optimal circumstances.

In spite of the name "Duplex" the B-mode and Doppler scanning do not occur simultaneously. It takes significantly longer to acquire Doppler data than B-mode data, and early Duplex scanner often "froze" the B-mode completely when obtaining flow information.

The loss of realtime imaging was a major drawback. More recently Duplex system employed mechanical that might lower the frame rate but will not freeze the image. It is however relatively straight forward to employ different frequencies for imaging and Doppler.

Currently realtime Duplex imaging is achieved with an electronically controlled transducer which can switch between imaging and Doppler fast enough to maintain an acceptable frame rate. Even though it is more complicated to obtain different transmit frequencies for Doppler and B-mode (it require employing very broad band transducer). Such systems have many advantages when compared to their mechanical counterpart.

4

Doppler Spectral Analysis

AK Srivastava
Satish K Bhargava

For many structures of interest, Doppler signal is in the audible rangle. For same applications, adequate clinical analysis may be made simply by listening to the signals. The listener then characterizes the flow according to the qualities of audible signal. However great deal of information may be obtained by analysing the signal quantitively. Which is done by using digital technique called FFT (Fast Fourier Transformation technique).

If blood flow were continuous rather than pulsatile. If blood vessel followed straight lines and were uniform in caliber, if the blood following at the same velocity at the periphery and in the centre of the lumen, and if the vessels were disease-free, then each blood vessel would produce a single Doppler ultrasound frequency shift, and frequency spectrum is not needed.

But in case of blood flow, Doppler signal is fairly complex because flow is pulsatile and vessels are not always straight moreover flow is slower at the periphery than in the centre of the vessels and vessel lumen may be distorted by other sclerosis and other pathology. This is why, blood flow produces a mixture of Doppler frequency shift that changes from moment to moment and from place to place within lumen. Spectrum shows the mixture of Doppler frequency present from vessel at that moment of time.

Separate a complicated signal into its individual frequency components so that relative contribution of each frequency components to the original signal can be determined (Fig. 4.1a).

The Doppler frequency spectrum is same what called power spectrum because the power or strength of each frequency is shown (Fig. 4.1b) by brightness of pixels. The power of given frequency shift in turns, proportional to number of RBCs produced at that particular frequency shift. If RBCs are large at a particular velocity then corresponding Doppler frequency shift is displayed as brighter on display on the otherhand if small number of RBCs moving at a particular velocity then frequency shift corresponding to that velocity will be darker.

The Doppler frequency/velocity spectrum information can be presented in both frequency (kHz) and velocity. Velocity information is computed by assessing Doppler angle as shown (Fig. 4.1a) and then instrument automatically calculate velocity via Doppler equation (as discussed in Chapter 3).

As discussed in earlier section, Doppler angle between 60-30 degree is required because above 60 degree, any error in estimating Doppler angle may lead to large error in estimation velocity whereas less than 30 degree may cause total internal reflection.

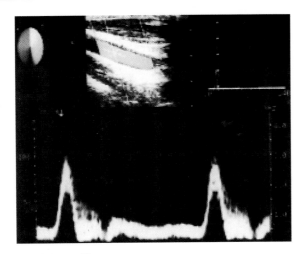 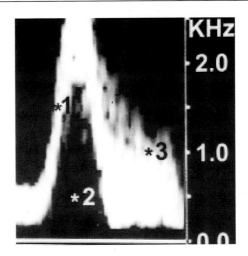

Figures 4.1a and b
The Doppler spectrum display. The following information is presented on the display screen [(a) entire display; (b) magnified Doppler spectrum]. B-mode image The image of the vessel, the sample volume, and the Doppler line of sight are shown at the top of the display screen. Time: The time is represented on the horizontal (x) axis of the Doppler spectrum in divisions of a second. Frequency shift and velocity: The Doppler frequency shift (jHz) and the velocity (cm/sec) are shown on the vertical (y-axis) scales of the spectrum. Flow direction: The direction of flow is shown in relation to the spectrum baseline. For peripheral vascular work, flow away from the transducer is shown above the baseline, and flow towards the transducer is shown below the baseline. This relationship may be reversed by the operator. The distribution of velocities within the sample volume is illustrated by the brightness of the spectral display (z-axis). To better understand the z-axis concept, examine the magnified spectrum shown in B and imagine that the spectral display is made up of tiny squares called pixels (for picture elements). You cannot see the pixels in this image, because they are purposely blurred together to smooth the picture. The pixels are there, however, and each corresponds to a specific moment in time and a specific frequency shift and velocity. The brightness of a pixel (z-axis) is proportionate to the number of blood cells causing that frequency shift at that specific point in time. In this example, the pixels at asterisk 1 are bright white, meaning that at that movement, a large number of blood cells have a velocity corresponding to a frequency shift of +1.5 kHz. The pixels at asterisk 2 are black, meaning that at that movement, no (or very few) blood cells have a velocity corresponding to a frequency shift of +0.5 kHz. The pixels at asterisk 3 are gray, meaning that at that a moderate number of blood cells have a velocity coresponding to a +0.5 kHz frequency shift at that moment

When operating Duplex instrument always uses velocity mode rather than frequency mode for two reasons. First velocity measurment compensates for variation in vessel alignment relative to skin surface as shown in Figure 4.1a.

Secondly Doppler frequency shift is inherently linked to output frequency of transducer but velocity is independent of transducer frequency.

Secondly the actual shape or size of sample volume may be somewhat different from the linear representation shown on Duplex information.

Third, the Doppler spectrum displays flow information only within the sample volume and does not provide information about flow in other portion of the blood vessel that are visible on the ultrasound image.

Sample Volume

The frequency spectrum shows blood flow information from a specific location called the Doppler sample volume. Three characteristics of sample volume must be know first since it is value which is 3-Dimentional but displaced on two-dimension, thickness of sample volume cannot be shown which can lead to error of localization. Doppler signals may be obtained from vessel that are orginally within the sample volume but are not shown on 2D display.

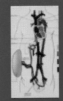

KEY POINTS

Doppler spectrum is a quantitative representation of Doppler Shift information obtaining using Fast Fourier Transformation Technique (FFT). A great deal of information is obtained by analysing the spectra such as nature of spectra to sham normal flow and disturbed flow, spectral broadening or spectral window.

Direction of Flow

Direction is displayed relative to the direction of transducer. Flow in one direction is displayed above the baseline and flow in other direction is displayed below the baseline. The apparent direction may be reversed either by moving the transducer around and by pressing the button on the instruments. The arbilrary choice of this may lead to significant diagnostic error. If accurate flow direction is necessary comparison must be made in direction of known vessel in which direction of flow is already known by the operator.

Wave Form

In arteries each cycle of cardiac activity produces a distinct "wave" on the Doppler frequency spectrum.

The shape of Doppler frequency spectrum defines the flow property. These wave forms are illustrated in Figures 4.2a to c.

In case of low pulsatility Figure 4.2a, wave form shows broad systolic peaks and forward flow

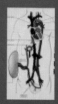

throughout diastole. The carotid, vertebral, renal and coeliac arteries all have low pulsatile waveform in normal individuals because these vessel feed circulatory systems with low resistance to flow. Here flow is always forward and therefore waveform is

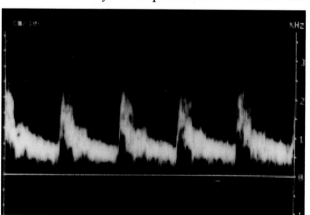

a

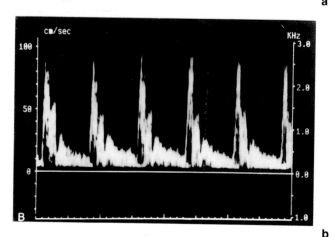

b

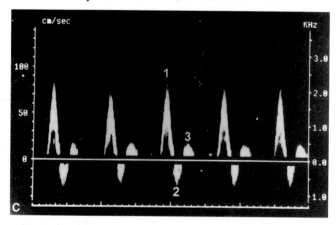

c

Figures 4.2a to c
Pulsatility (a) low pulsatility is indicated by a broad systolic peak and persistant forward flow throughout diastole (e.g. internal carotid artery), (b) moderate pulsatility is indicated by a tall, sharp and narrow systolic peak, and flow reversal earlier diastole and absence of flow late in diastole, (c) in this classic triphasic example: The first phase (1) is systole, and the second phase (2) is brief diastolic flow reversal and the third phase (3) is diastolic forward flow and relatively little diastolic flow, high pulsatility is characterized by a narrow systolic peak flow reversal

always displaced in one direction either positive or negative.

Moderate pulsatility as shown in Fig. 4.2b, wave form shows tall and sharp sytolic peak but forward flow throughout diastole. Examples of moderate pulsatility are few in carotid and superior, mesenteric artery (during fasting).

High Pulsatility flow the waveform as shown in Fig. 4.2c have tall, narrow and sharp systolic peaks and reverse or absent diastolic flow. The example of high pulsatility is the triphasic flow pattern seen in an extremity arteries of a resting individuals. Since only a low flow rate is required at rest in these vessels is the arterioles are most vasocontricted.

A sharp systolic peak (first phase) is followed by brief flow reversal (second phase) and then by brief forward flow (third phase). These show that circulatory system with high resistance to blood flow, when body is at rest.

In most clinical situation qualitative assessment of pulsatility is sufficient but in some situation we may need it. For example, CDS greatly simplifies the identification of blood vessels and vascular pathology. Stenosing plaques are easily identified by the narrowing of the perfused vessel human and typical stenotic flow abnormalities. The total occlusion of a vessel is manifested by the complete absence of colour flow signal. The quantification of vascular stenosis can be accomplished with the help of colour coded images alone by noting the relative interstenotic velocity increase. But when the conditions are less than ideal, their qualitative information is must.

Envelope Traces of the Doppler Spectrum

So called envelopes are commonly used in a simplified description of spectral wave forms and in the measurement of flow velocities.

The traces or curve may be drawn by machine itself or traced manually. An envelope is obtained by drawing a trace along the time axis connection to selected desplayed Doppler frequency shift. The most common used envelopes trace to the maximum and mean frequency over time.

Various envelopes in Doppler spectrum analysis are showed in Figures 4.3a to c.

1. *Maximum frequency shift (A):* This is the highest Doppler frequency shift at each moment in time in the Doppler spectrum. In order to eliminate noise generally, the frequency below which a certain

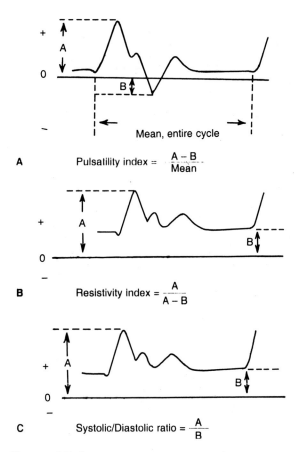

Figures 4.3a to c

Pulsatility measurements. (a) the pulsatility index (b) the resistivity index (Pourcelot), and (c) the systolic/diastolic ratio

percentage (e.g. 95%) of all measure frequency shift tall is selected.

2. *Minimum frequency (B):* The lowest Doppler frequency shift at each moment in time in Doppler spectrum.
3. *Mean frequency shift:* Arithmetic mean of all Doppler frequency shift at each moment in time.

Normal value for pulsatility measurement vary from one location in the body to other. In additions to this pathological and physiological process may alter arterial pulsatilies patterns seen in extremity arteries during rest converted to a low-resistance, monophasic pattern after vigorous excercise, this pattern is distinctly abnormal in a resting patient and in that circumstances indicate arterial insufficiency in addition to this slowed ventricular emptying valvular reflex, valvular stenosis and other factor may significantly afffect arterial pulsatility.

Acceleration is other important flow feature evident in Doppler arterial wave forms. In most normal situation flow velocity is an artery accelerate very rapidly during systole and flow peak reached within few microsecond after ventricular contraction begin.

Rapid flow acceleration produces an almost vertical deflection of the Doppler wave form at the start of systole. If however, severe arterial obstruction is present, proximal to the point of Doppler examination, systolic flow acceleration may be slowed substantially as shown Figures 4.4a and b.

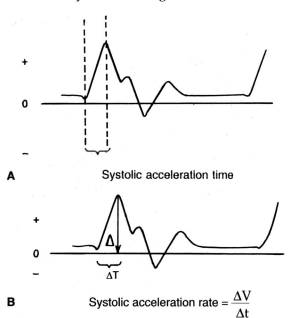

A   Systolic acceleration time

B   Systolic acceleration rate = $\dfrac{\Delta V}{\Delta t}$

Figures 4.4a and b
Acceleration measurements: (a) acceleration time and (b) acceleration index

Quantitative measurement of acceleration is achieved by measuring the acceleration time and acceleration index as shown in Figures 4.4a and b.
1. Systolic acceleration time
2. Systolic acceleration rate = $\dfrac{\Delta V}{\Delta t}$

Vessel Identity

Doppler wave form are particularly helpful in identifying the internal and external carotid arteries which have low and moderate pulsatility respectively. Pulsatility is also of value for differentiating among portal veins, hepatic veins and hepatic arteries within the liver.

Systolic Window

When in Doppler spectral analysis no frequency shift detected within a certain range of frequencies this region remains black in conventional gray scale display when flow is laminar for example the great majority of blood cells are moving at a uniform speed and spectrum displays a thin line that outline a clear space which is known as spectral window. See Figures 4.5a and b.

Thus systolic window is said to be empty or clear. The systolic window represents the frequency below the minimum detected Doppler frequency shift within each time increment. When a small volume is used the size of systolic window indicates the degree of laminar flow present.

The larger the band width of measured Doppler frequency shifts, the smaller the systolic window.

An increased band width of measured Doppler shift represents the increased degree of flow disturbance based on non-uniform orientation of velocity vector of individual flow element in sample volume.

Especially in poststenotic spectra, the window may be completely filled in Figures 4.6a to d.

In disturbed flow, blood cell is less uniform as discussed which is manifested by spectral broadening or widening.

The degree of spectral widening is proportional to severity of flow disturbances as shown in Figures 4.6a and d.

Although disturbed blood flow often indicates vascular disease but flow disturbances also occur in normal vessel.

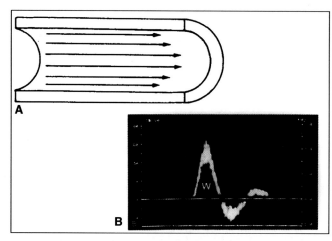

Figures 4.5a and b
Laminar flow. (a) Illustration of parallel lines of blood cell movement, (b) Doppler spectrum during laminar flow. At all times, the blood cells are moving at similar velocities. As a result, the spectrum is a thin line that encloses a well-defined black "window" (W)

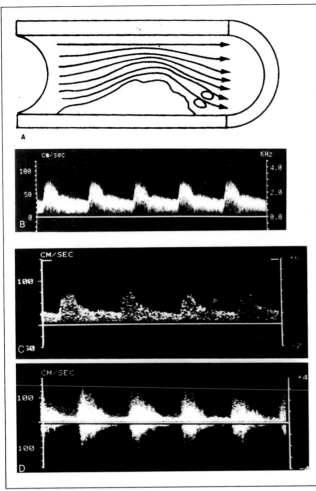

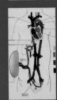

Figures 4.6a to d

Disturbed flow. (a) disturbed flow illustration, (b) minor flow disturbance is indicated by spectral broadening at peak systole and through diastole, (c) moderate flow disturbance causes fill-in of the spectral window, and (d) severe flow disturbance is characterized by spectral fill-in, poor definition of spectral borders, and simultaneous forward and reversed flow. The audible Doppler signal has a loud, gruff character when flow is severely disturbed

Kinks, curves and arterial branching may produce normal flow disturbance as shown in carotid flow where prominent area of reversed flow is normal occurance (Figs 4.7a and b).

Diagnosis of Arterial Obstruction

Five main catagories of information are used in this process:

a. Increased stenotic zone velocity

b. Disturbed flow in poststenotic zone

c. Proximal pulsatility changes

d. Distal pulsatility changes

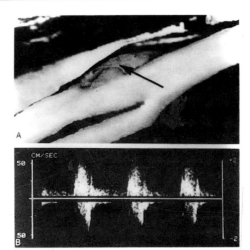

Figures 4.7a and b

Normal bifurcation flow disturbance. (a) flow reversal in the bulbous portion of the common and internal carotid arteries causes localized flow reversal (arrow), and (b) simultaneous forward and reverse flow is evident in the bulbous region on the Doppler spectrum

KEY POINTS

To analyse Doppler traces, Doppler indices are used which reflect the main characteristic of Doppler wave form. These are usually incorporated into the softwave of the ultrasound machine.

$$\text{Pulsatility index} = \frac{A - B}{\text{Mean}}$$

$$= \frac{\text{Peak systolic} - \text{End diastolic}}{\text{Mean velocity}}$$

$$\text{Resistivity index} = \frac{A}{A - B}$$

Systolic/diastolic ratio = A/B

A/B ratio is simple to use and calculate but it can account for reverse flow it is commonly used in obstetrics for fetal and umbilical vessel evaluation.

RI High diastolic flow leads to low value of RI. This does not handle reverse diastolic flow. commonly used to evaluate renal transplant.

PI-Can reflect both reverse diastolic flow and a wide range of velocities. Commonly used to evaluate the extremities and carotids.

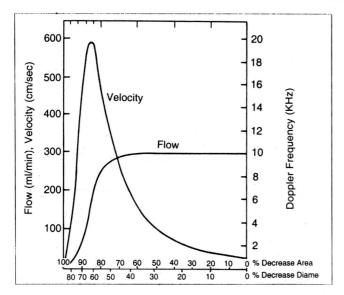

Figure 4.8

Relationship among velocity, flow, and lumen size. This graph refers specifically to internal carotid artery stenosis, but the principles illustrated apply to stenoses in other arteries throughout the body. Note that peak systolic velocity in the stenotic internal carotid lumen (labelled velocity) increases exponentially as the lumen diameter decreases (from right to left). The highest velocities correspond to approximately 70% diameter reduction. With greater stenosis severity, peak systolic velocity falls off rapidly to zero (because of rapidly increasing flow resistance). In contrast to velocity, volume flow (labelled flow) remains stable until the lumen diameter is reduced by about 50%. With further reduction in lumen size, volume flow falls off very rapidly to zero. Finally, note the relationship of per cent diameter and area reduction, as shown at the base of the figure. Fifty per cent diameter reduction equals about 70% area reduction, and 70% diameter reduction equals about 90% area reduction!

e. Indirect effects of the obstruction such as colla-
   teralization.

The term stenotic zone refers to narrow portion of the arterial lumen. For determining the severity of arterial stenosis, the single most valuable Doppler finding is increased velocity in the stenotic zone (Fig. 4.8). This is because blood must move more quickly if the same volume is to flow through the narrow lumen as through the larger, normal lumen.

Amount of increased velocity is directly proportional to the severity of luminal narrowing.

Three stenotic zone velocity measures are commonly used to determine the severity of arterial stenosis.

1. Peak systolic velocity which is the highest systolic velocity within stenosis A

2. End diastolic velocity which is the highest end diastolic velocity B

3. Systolic velocity ratio which compares peak systole in stenosis with peak systole proximal to the stenosis (normal portion vessel).

Peak systole in the stenotic zone is the first Doppler parameter to become abnormal as an arterial lumen becomes narrowed.

Shown in Figure 4.8 peak systole rises steadily with progressive narrowing but ultimately, the flow resistance becomes so high that peak systole falls to normal or even subnormal levels. This drop in velocity can cause under estimation of degree of stenosis.

Low flow velocity may also lead to false diagnosis of arterial occlusion, if the flow velocity is so low that Doppler signal cannot be detected with ultrasound.

The region of maximum velocity within stenotic zones may be quite small and that reason, the sonographer must search the stenotic lumen with the sample to locate the highest flow velocity. If highest flow velocity is overlooked then degree of stenosis may be underestimated.

End diastolic velocity also increase in proportion. So the degree of stenosis narrow is less then 50 per cent. Then this velocity may remain largely normal.

With moderate stenosis (50-70%) diameter reduction end diastolic velocity is above normal.

End diastolic velocity is particularly good marker for severe stenosis because the parameter is not elevated.

The systolic velocity ratio, as defined is an additional important parameter for the diagnosis of arterial stenosis. This ratio is used clinically for measurement of internal carotid renal and extremity artery stenosis as discussed earlier.

Poststenotic Flow Disturbance

The poststenotic zone is the region immediately beyond arterial stenosis where flow disturbances are commonly present.

As the flow stream from the stenotic lumen spreadout in the poststenotic zone, the laminar flow pattern is lost and flow become disorganised which generate disturbed Doppler spectral pattern (Figs 4.9a to d) with forward and reversal flow.

The maximum flow disturbance occurs with one cm beyond the stenosis and in very severe stenosis, soft tissue adjacent to this position of artery may vibrate causing a visible bruit on CDI.

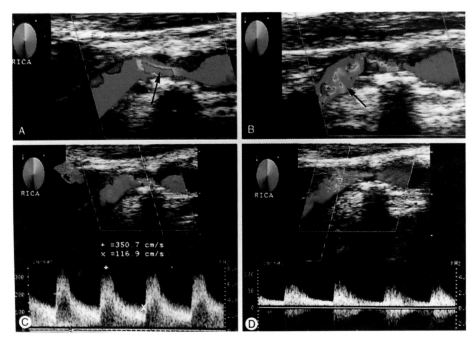

Figures 4.9a to d
Local effects of arterial stenosis. (a) high velocities present in the narrowed portion of the arterial lumen generate an area of aliasing (arrow) within the stenotic lumen, (b) disturbed flow in the poststenotic area generates a mixture of colours (arrow), (c) Doppler spectral analysis shows markedly elevated velocity at peak systole (350.7 cm/sec) and end diastole (116.9 cm/sec), and (d) severe flow disturbance is evident in the poststenotic region, as indicated by simultaneous forward and reverse flow, spectrum fill-in, and poor definition of the spectrum margins

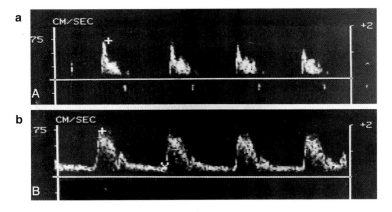

Figure 4.10
Increased common carotid artery pulsatility due to internal carotid artery occlusion

About two cm beyond the stenosis the flow disturbance becomes less visible and spectral broading diminises. Normally laminar flow pattern usually is reestablished with three cm beyond the stenosis. Severe flow disturbance however with simultaneous forward and reverse flow does not occur in normal vessel and therefore an important sign of high grade stenosis.

In some cases, stenosis may be obscured by plaque calcification and in such instances poststenotic disturbed flow may be the only sign of severe arterial stenosis.

Proximal Pulsatility Changes

Arterial obstruction causes increased pulsatility in portion of the artery proximal to the stenosis. For example with severe internal carotid artery obstruction the Doppler spectrum in the common carotid artery has high pulsatility feature rather than normal low pulsatility pattern.

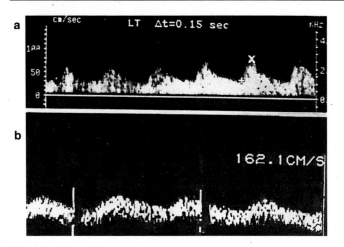

Distal Pulsatility Changes

Doppler waveform abnormalities seen distal to stenosis also have considerable value in the diagnosis of arterial stenosis.

Doppler waveform distal to severe arterial obstruction has the damped appearance (Figs 4.11a and b).

Figures 4.11a and b
(a) The acceleration time is prolonged (0.15 sec) in the left kidney due to severe proximal renal artery stenosis, and (b) severely damped dorsalis pedis artery waveform distal to femoral/popliteal artery occlusion. Normally, this waveform distal to femoral/popliteal artery occlusion

Which means the systolic acceleration is slowed, the systolic peak is rounded, the maximum systolic velocity is lower than normal and the diastolic flow is increased.

5

Colour Flow Imaging (CFI)

AK Srivastava
Satish K Bhargava

After devising multigated Doppler systems (*See* Chapter 3) that acquire flow data along an entire scan line, and Duplex system which overlap a Doppler beam on a B-mode image, the next step seems logical overlay a B-scan with flow information from all depths, i.e. along the entire A line and expand the number of A lines to cover a region of interest. This is the principle of all CFI systems. This imaging is one of most important development in ultrasound imaging. This imaging method superimposes a blood flow image on a standard gray scale, ultrasound image, permitting instantaneous visual assessment of blood flow. The estimated velocity of each sample volume is mapped in a colour representing the direction of flow as well as its magnitude (via the colour and hue).

Typically shades of red and blue are used for flow towards and away respectively, from the transducer. There are however, numerous other colour maps available from different manufacture. The variance of velocity estimate, i.e. spectral broadening of the Doppler signal can be included as a third colour often green (Figs 5.1a and b).

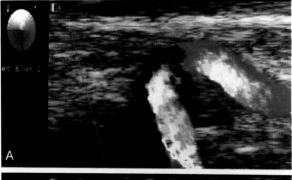

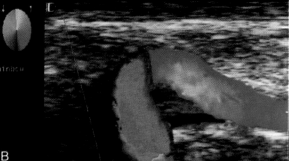

Figures 5.1a and b
Colour flow schemes. A variety of colour schemes are used in colour-Doppler instruments. (a) with this scheme, progressive increase in the frequency shift changes the image colour from red to pink to white, or from dark blue to light blue to white, depending on the flow direction, and (b) with this scheme, the colour changes from red to yellow or from blue to green, as the frequency shift increases

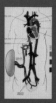

KEY POINTS

CFI (Colour Flow Imaging Technique) superimposes blood flow Doppler data on a standard gray scale US image. It is customary to show flow in one direction as red and flow in other direction as blue. Magnitude of velocities is displayed indifferent shades of colour. In case of increased velocity, shades of colour are shown from darker shades of red or blue toward lighter shades of red or blue.

Principles of Colour Flow Imaging

Gray scale ultrasound instrument use only two pieces of information from each echo that returns from the patient's body: the distance from echo to the transducer and strength of echo.

The echo signal typically contains other information such as a Doppler frequency shift, but this information is disregarded. Colour Doppler instruments are different from gray scale instrument because they use the Doppler shift information in addition to time of flight and amplitude information. For each echo show on colour Doppler image, the instrument makes fine determination.

1. How long has it taken for the sound beam to travel to and from the site of the echo? This indicate the distance of echo reflector from the transducer.
2. How strong is the echo? The strength or amplitude of ultrasound signal determines how brightly the echo is displayed as the image (for both gray scale and colour Doppler components).
3. Is a Doppler frequency shift present? If so, the echo is represented in shades of colour.
4. What is magnitude of the Doppler frequency shift? The magnitude of the Doppler shift is proportionate to the blood flow velocity and the Doppler angle. Different frequency levels are shown as the image as different colour shades or hues.
5. What is the direction of the Doppler shift?

The instrument determines whether flow is towards or away from the transducer by noting whether the echo has a higher or lower frequency than the ultrasound beam sent from the transducer. A higher Doppler frequency means flow is towards the transducer and low Doppler frequency means flow is away from transducer. It is customary to show flow in one direction in blue and flow in the other direction in red. However, the operator can select other colour schemes if desired.

The way to show colour has two different ways:

1. *Shifting line method* Different colours are used to represent different frequency levels (e.g. blue, green, yellow, white with increasing frequency).

2. *Changing shades method* Here same colour is used but the colour gets lighter as frequency increases (e.g. dark red, light red pink and white).

These colour images are shown in Figure 5.1b.

Even though CFI systems may appear to constitute a logical extension of PW Doppler and Duplex Doppler, they do infact represent a fundamentally different hardwave structure. The reason for this is the time! In a PW system 64-128 samples are acquired per Doppler waveform over approximately 10 msec.

Even if each A line was processed enough in parallel channel to cover all depth along the scan line, there would not be sufficient time to record 128 Doppler A line and B-mode image in realtime.

Consequently CFI systems are limited to 6-32 samples per range gate, i.e. 6-32 burst transmitted in each direction. This time limit puts severe constraint on all filters and estimators involved in the processing scheme. Hence digital filters and early digitisation are essential in CFI system to get sufficient fast and short responses.

In Figure 5.2, a block diagram of a basic CFI system is presented. The left most column represent a PW system while middle column is the colour Doppler processor. Notice how the digitisation takes place as early as possible.

Since strong stationary and quasi stationary echo are not filtered out before digitisation a very powerful ADC is required. The right most column depict B-mode circuity.

In Doppler instrument only one parameter such as mean Doppler shift is extracted and shown. Hence this method is less time consuming for estimating the mean velocity along the entire A line, without resorting to parallel processing must be devised. This is the last of CFI estimater.

Frequency estimation technique used in most CFI system is known as auto correlation method. Here the phase of autocorrelation function is calculated as a function of the interpulse duration time (i.e. 1/PRF).

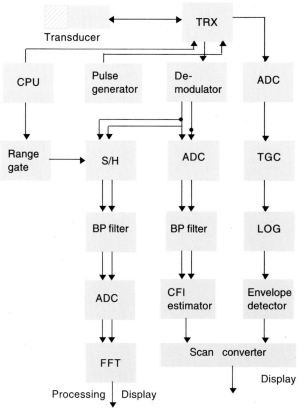

Figure 5.2
Block diagram of integrated CFI scanner. The second column from the left represents the PW Doppler system, the third the colour flow system, and the right-band coloumn the B-mode system. Abbreviations are explained in the text

This is equivalent to comparing echo segment from consecutive A lines to one another and allows the phase change caused by Doppler shift of the RBCs to be estimated.

The mean Doppler shift and thus mean velocity can be calculated from the phase shift.

The autocorrelation can estimate the Doppler shift along an A line with as few as 3-4 samples. This requires all stationary echoes which are much stronger than blood flow signals to be removed efficiently. The calculations are performed in approximately one msec at PRF of 4 kHz.

An alternative estimation based on line domain correlation has been developed. In this method the velocity estimate is based on maximising the cross-correlation between small segments of two consecutive A lines.

Time domain flow imaging (under the name colour velocity imaging) is not widely used by ultrasound equipment manufacturer. One major advantage of this technique is that it is much less susceptible to aliasing.

To get a realtime B-mode image as well as to visualize rapid flow changes, it is necessary to switch rapidly between imaging and Doppler acquisition.

Linear or phased arraw transducer with their electronic switching and beam steering capabilities are therefore the most common choice for CFI systems. Mechanical transducers have been employed in the past, but these are becoming increasingly rare on today's scanner.

Another problem is how to combine the pulse echo and Doppler data acquisition. In synchronous systems the received signal is split into two separate processing schemes, one for imaging and other one for Doppler. But requirement for optimal Doppler and optimal pulse echo are not similar. Therefore, even though very high frame rates are feasible, this is achieved at the expense of resolution and general image quality.

Alternatively, pulse echo and Doppler data can be acquired independently (an asynchronous system). This scheme allows the B-mode imaging and the Doppler pulses to be optimised separately. However, other compromises are required.

In every other pulse is used for imaging and alternatively Doppler, the available PRF is halved. This mean a reduction in the maximum velocity measurable.

On the other hand, if many Doppler burst are employed interrupted by a single imaging pulse, the possible B-scan frame rate is reduced. Instead, a complete time sharing scheme is used. A whole image scan is performed and Doppler information is then collected over a time period which retains a resonable frame rate (15 frame/sec).

Asynchronous data acquisition will mean missing the Doppler signal in periods during which B-mode image is being performed. Hence it is necessary to generate a substitute signal. This is done by either repeating the last bit of Doppler acquisition or by synthesising a Doppler filter signal. In CFI systems, the period of flow data acquisition can be minimised by reducing the overall number of Doppler scan times, the axial resolution and region of interest.

Problems in CFI

As describes CFI system are based on the principles of PW Doppler scanner. Hence aliasing is recurring problem specially since much lower PRF is used. Another problem arises because one simple characteristic, Doppler frequency representing the blood velocities in the sample volume over a one msec period is displayed, separated by long dead times.

A frame rate of 10 is not uncommon in CFI scanners which means a rate of 10 interrogation and displays per sample volume per second.

Solid tissue motion is another CFI artifacts. This is called flash artifacts is usually of very short duration, which makes it easy to recognise, although the artifact may obscure low flow particularly in the abdomen.

Since all colour coding is performed relative to transducer, multiple flow beam angles may constitute a problem. Very tortuous vessel will be colour coded in a wide range of lines, often with flow both towards and away from the transducer. This phenomena is less noticeable in linear arrays where the angle of incidence is constant. In transducer with a sector shaped field of view even a straight vessel perpendicular to the transducer surface will be coded in multitude of hues. Due to very limited number of samples available for CFI estimater, these are more qualitative than their spectral counter parts (FFT) based processor as in CW, PW and MG Doppler system consider a PW Doppler system. The sonogram provides a display of all Doppler frequency detected in a sample volume in each 10 msec period with 64-128 samples per Doppler waveform and display at a rate of 100 display per second. conversely in CFI system one Doppler shift is found for each 100 msec. More quantitative blood velocity information is then obtained from PW system.

CLINICAL ADVANTAGES OF COLOUR FLOW IMAGING AND ITS LIMITATION

Technical Efficiency

Perhaps the greatest advantages of colour flow imaging is technical efficiency. When moving blood is encountered, the vessel lights up even if the vessel is too small to be resolved on the gray scale image. Because vessels stand out in vivid colour, they may be located and follow much more easily than with gray scale instruments. Further more basic judgement about blood flow can be made easy with colour flow imaging. One can quickly determine the presence or absence of flow, the direction of flow and the presence of local flow disturbances and therefore sonographer can quickly examine long vascular segments such as vascular bypass graft, with relative ease.

Furthermore, colour flow imaging facilitates the examination of vessels such as calf veins and renal arteries.

Assistance in sorting out abdominal anatomy. Another advantage of colour flow imaging simplifies differentiation between vascular and non-vascular structure, which is particularly useful in the abdomen. One of the most obvious application is sorting out porta hepatis anatomy. The bile ducts, which do not exhibits flow, may be differentiated visually from the hepatic artery and portal vein, in which flow is seen.

Flow assessment in entire lumen, a major advantage of colour flow imaging is the depiction of blood flow throughout a large segment of a vessel, rather than solely at the Doppler sample volume. Because flow features are visible over a large area, localized flow abnormalities are readily apparent and are less likely to be overlooked than with gray scale Duplex methods.

The sonographer is immediately made aware of the location of any flow abnormalities which speeds up the examination and permit rapid assessment of long segment of vessels for obstruction and other pathology.

Visual measurement of stenoses As compared with gray scale ultrasound, colour flow imaging makes it easier to define the residual lumen in stenotic vessels permitting more precise visual measurement of arterial stenoses. Direct, visual stenosis measurement remain problem prone however, due to vessel tortuosity and acoustic shadows from calcified plaque.

KEY POINTS

Advantage of CFI

1. Its greatest advantage is that when US encounters with moving blood even very small vessel are displayed by providing colour.
2. Presence or absence of flow can be easily recognised.
3. CFI simplifies differentiation between vascular and non-vascular structure.
4. Flow assessment in entire lumen.

Disadvantage of CFI

1. Reduced flow rate.
2. Display mean velocity
3. Aliasing occur such as the PW Doppler system.

Differentiation of severe stenosis and occlusion The ability of colour flow imaging to detect low velocity flow in a tiny residual lumen may facilitate the differentiation between occlusion of an artery and near occlusion with a tricle of residual flow.

Limitation of Colour Flow Imaging

Flow information is qualitative because:
1. Flow image is based on the average Doppler shift within the vessel, rather than the Peak Doppler shift. Average Doppler shift is not helpful for actually putting a number on a stenosis. Furthermore average Doppler shift is lowered by flow disturbances.
2. It is not corrected for Doppler angle.
3. Only a few frequency levels are shown.

Because colour flow images are qualitative, Doppler spectrum analysis must be used to derive quantitative flow data.

Low PRF and Frame Rate

A very large number of data must be processed by the colour flow instrument to give each pixel and each television frame. Because of long processing time it may lead to serious effect on the gray scale and colour. Doppler images are therefore acquired with reduced PRF and reduced frame rate.

Reduced PRF may have the following effect:
1. The B-mode image may be degraded because fewer data are available to build up the image.
2. Doppler alasing may occur due to Nyquist limits.
3. Low PRF and low FR may limit the visualisation of rapidly moving cardiac or vascular event. For example, cardiac valve motion may be less clearly seen with colour flow scanning than with the gray scale scanning.
4. Low frame rates may produce image flicker. If the frame rate is reduced below 15 frame/sec in the lumen, eye no larger blurs the ultrasound images into a moving pictures.
5. *Flow detection is angle dependent* Blood flow is not detected with colour flow device in vessel that are perpendicular to the ultrasound beam. A false positive diagnosis of vascular occlusion may occur if a vessel is approximately perpendicular to the ultrasound beam. This is particularly severe problem when curved array scanner are used for colour Doppler imaging.

6. *Flow direction is arbitrary* Colour of vessel on the CFI is not an absolute indication of flow direction. The colour is assigned relative to the transducer. The operator may reverse the colour scheme (arteries blue, vein red) simply by reversing the orientation of transducer or by pushing a button on the instrument. To determine the true direction of flow, the operator must closely observe the orientation of the vessel relative to the transducer or refer to a vessel in which the flow direction is known such as aorta.
7. *Colour flash* With CFI, anything within the FOV that moves to the transducer is shown in colour.

   In the abdomen peristaltic motion, cardiac motion or transmitted pulsation from great vessels may generate blotches of colour on the ultrasound image called colour flash which can obscure structure of interest.

   The colour flash problem is particularly apparent in the upper abdomen because the heart motion.
8. *Visible bruit* It is a peculiar, but useful flow phenomenon that can be seen with colour flow imaging. A martage of colour is seen within the soft tissue adjacent to the blood vessel; this colour effect is caused by vibration of the vessel. This vibration in-turn is caused by a severe flow disturbance within the vessel; A visible bruit suggests severe arterial stenosis but caution is advised in interpreting, this finding because several flow disturbances may sometime occur in the absence of a significant stenosis.

Optimizing Colour Flow Image Quality

CFI is derived from weak scattered US waveform RBCs. Hence flow detection is particularly susceptible to ultrasound instrument settings. The following set of rule may help sonograph to obtain adequate flow information when it is difficult.

Doppler angle Since this angle affect the CFI so when flow is absent in vessel one can move the colour flow box or transducer to improve the Doppler angle.

Velocity range If the instrument is set to detect arterial velocities, it is not sensitive to venous velocities or vice versa. Hence use proper PRF to take care of velocity range to level appropriate for the vessel of interest.

FOV If depth of field is shown on image, always use optimal depth.

Colour box size It is best to use a small colour box especially when examining vessels deep within the body.

Power and gain If gray scale image is priortised the colour flow image suffer and vice versa. If any trouble in detecting flow, shift the image processing priority towards colour.

Thump control It refers to electronic filtering that removes colour artifacts generated by the heart or vascular pulsations. Thump control is not needed in smaller peripheral vessels and should be set as low as is practical.

Wall filtering If wall filter is set too high, low frequency signals generated by low velocity flow are eliminated. The wall filter is designed to eliminate low frequency noise but if it is set too high, it also eliminates flow information. It may a major problem for detection of venous flow or evaluating small intrarenal arteries.

Very slow flow Power Doppler may be more sensitive to the presence of slow flow than standard colour Doppler imaging and it may be useful to switch to these modality when vessel appears occluded.

Power Doppler Flow Imaging

As it name implies, this is a Doppler method, but differs from standard Doppler methods. In that

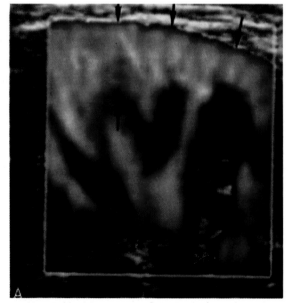

Figure 5.3
Colour amplitude image of a kidney. (a) conventional colour flow image shows the presence of a range of frequency shifts in the cortical region of the kidney and noise in the tissue

power or intensity of Doppler signal is measured and mapped and thus ignores the velocity of Doppler signal detected from each location.

In power Doppler system the density of red blood cells is depicted as opposed to their velocity (Fig. 5.3).

The amplitude and this intensity or a power of back scattered signal depends on the number of RBCs present within the sample volume, the size of vessel and the attenuation of intervening tissue. Since the Doppler frequency shift information is not utilised, power Doppler images is non-directional and does not suffer from aliasing.

The advantages of this modality over colour flow imaging are therefore:

1. Power Doppler imaging is said to be more sensitive in detecting blood flow. 10-15 dB of improved sensitivity have been reported. Hence smaller vessels and vessels with flow slow can be imaged. The reason, why smaller vessels are visualised in power Doppler is that the display dynamic range has been increased by sacrificing part of the available information (velocity and direction) and by increasing the persistence of the display flow signals. This allows the colour priorities to be increased then producing the apparent increase in sensitivity.

   Since more dynamic range can be used because of noise that would overwhelm the standard colour flow imaging can be arising a uniform background colour, e.g. light blue. Hence anything that represents noise is blue (Fig. 5.4) and anything that represents flow is another colour (usually gold).

2. As described earlier power Doppler imaging is not affected by aliasing. Even the aliased portion of signal has the power and can be displayed as flow (Fig. 5.5).

3. Power Doppler is significantly less angle dependent (unless the angle becomes so close to perpendicular that the Doppler signal are below the flow detectability thershold of colour processor) so, angle affects are usually ignored.

4. Power Doppler display improves in functional lumen definition. The difference between Doppler frequency shift from a sample volume close to the vessel wall and from one partially overlapping the wall will be very small. However, the number of red blood cells isonated within the two sample volumes will be quite different and therefore, so will the amplitude of the back scattered signals.

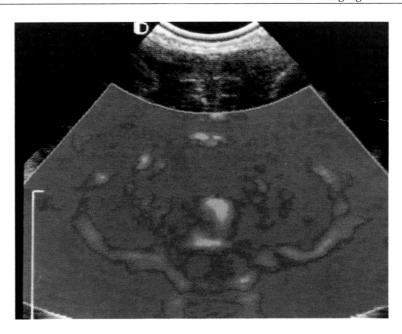

Figure 5.4

This power Doppler image of the cramial vasculature uses a blue back ground which enhances flow detection because noise is converted to a uniform blue colour

5. Power Doppler imaging has one final advantage that has been appreciated since the advent of ultrasound constrast agents. Power Doppler imaging is less subject to blooming than the standard colour Doppler imaging. Blooming is the spread of colour outside of the blood vessel that occurs when amplification of Doppler signal is too great.

Blooming is particular problem when contrast agent is used to improve the detection of blood flow.

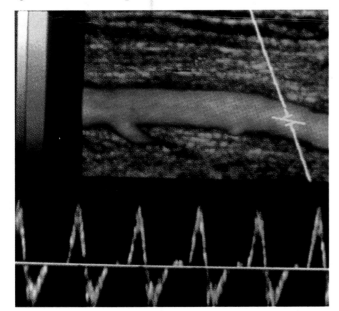

Figure 5.5

Quantitative spectral information can be obtained in power Doppler mode

Intravenous injection of the echo-enhancing agent greatly increases the Doppler signal intensity, causing over amplification and severe blooming. With power Doppler blooming does not occur.

In spite of its potential advantages over colour Doppler, power Doppler imaging has two major limitations.

1. Frame rate is slow, which render this imaging method useless for rapidly moving vessels, rapidly moving patients (especially children) and areas subject to respiratory or cardiac motion.

    To compensate motion induced artifacts power Doppler significantly increase weighted temporal averaging (high frame to frame averaging). This technique reduces motion artifacts but increases the display response time (i.e. colour map seems to lag behind the gray scale image).

2. Power Doppler imaging does not provide flow direction information and therefore cannot assess effects such as pulsatility and flow reversal.

The power Doppler depicts the density of red blood cells in vessel and should be used as an adjunct to conventioned mean frequency velocity based colour flow imaging.

Harmonic Imaging

Harmonic imaging relies on inherent property of microbubbles to resonate at specific frequency once they have encountered the ultrasound beam. Each compound has a specific resonant frequency and various subharmonic frequencies. The resonant frequency is largely dependent upon the particle size. Extensive studies on animal suggest that this may be a method to further enhances the effect of contrast agents.

Harmonic Imaging requires an ultrasound machine which can transmit the sound beam at a specific frequency and receive at the resonant frequency. The resonant frequency is twice that of the transmitting frequency. The signal to noise ratio is improved because in theory only the echoes arriving back to the transducer from the object are displayed. That means that images are displayed from contrast fill objects other are removed from the display.

This is important particular useful when conventional US imaging is limited by motion artifacts examples include imaging of heart and vessels seen in renal artery, located deep in the abdomen adjacent to the pulsating aorta.

6

Contrast Agents in Ultrasound

Satish K Bhargava
Suchi Bhatt
Shefali Gupta
Rohini Gupta

INTRODUCTION

The major motivation and need for the current rapid rate of development of contrast agents for ultrasound lies in the nature of the current performance limits of ultrasound and colour Doppler. At present most Duplex and colour Doppler imaging systems are capable of detecting flow from vessels whose lumina lie below the resolution of the image. The detection of such unresolved flow using Doppler systems can be demonstrated simply by using a Duplex scanner to create a power Doppler image of the kidney in which vessels not visible on gray scale image become visible using Doppler mode. These vessels are the arcuate and the interlobar branches of the renal arteries. Their diameter is known to be less than 100 μm and therefore below the resolution limits of the image. However, as we progress distally, the blood flows more slowly as the rate of bifurcation increases giving lower Doppler shift frequencies and the quantity of blood in a given volume of tissue also decreases, weakening the back scattered echo. Eventually a point is reached at which the vessel cannot be visualised and the Doppler signals cannot be detected.

Two factors determine where that point will lie. Doppler shift frequency and echo strength.

First the velocity of blood must be sufficient to produce a Doppler shift frequency that is distinguishable from that produced by the normal motion of tissue and second the received intensity of the backscattered ultrasound must provide adequate signal strength for detection by the transducer above the acoustic and electric noise of the system. Using a higher frequency ultrasound helps in both aspects. The Doppler shift frequency corresponding to a given flow velocity increased in proportion to the transmitted sounds frequency and the backscattered intensity increases with the fourth power of transmitted frequency as predicted by the Rayleigh relationship.[1] In practice the penetration of sound through tissue places an upper limit on the ultrasound frequency that can be used.

For deeper vessels of the abdomen ultrasound frequencies above 5 MHz produce blood echoes whose amplitude at the skin surface is too small for detection by most current systems. In this and many other applications involving small vessels, it is the strength of the backscattered echo rather than Doppler shift frequency that defers the smallest vessel from which Doppler signals can be detected. It also defines the scale of vasculature. It is possible to detect in a neovascularised mass or a collateral vessel to a vascular occlusion. For larger vessels the effect of increasing the echo from blood is to enhance the signal to noise ratio which again determines detectability in such vessels as the renal artery or the middle cerebral artery when approached transcranially. There is then clear clinical potential for contrast agents capable of enhancing the echo of moving blood especially in systemic arterial system.

The principal requirements for an ultrasound contrast agent are that it to be easily introduciable into the vascular system, be stable for the duration of the diagnostic examination, have low toxicity and modify one or more acoustic properties of tissues that determine the ultrasound imaging process.

The essential mechanisms whereby microbubbles act as echoenhancers are same as pertain to scattered echoes elsewhere the echo intensity is proportional to change in acoustic impedance as the sound beam crosses from blood to the gas in bubbles. The impedance mismatch at such an interface is very high and essentially all the incident sound is reflected though all will not travel back to the transducer. However, though the reflection is near complete by itself. This would not produce a very effective enhancing agent because microbubbles are very small and present in only small numbers. The reflectively is proportional to the sixth power of the particles diameter and directly to their concentration.

Rather the intense echogenicity of microbubbles results from the fact that they resonate when insolated and this makes them behave as though much larger and thus more echogenic than a rigid bubble of the same diameter (10^{14} × or larger). Maximising this resonance is a critical aspect of this design. Obviously the microbubbles must be made small enough to cross the capillaries (< 7 μ) and like any other mechanical resonance system, the critical frequency depends on their diameter. It is a most fortunate coincidence that microbubbles in this size range happen to have their resonance frequencies in the 2-15 MHz. This most fortunate coincidence makes microbubbles such extremely effective reflectors that even in the low concentration after they have been dispersed throughout the systemic circulation, they produce some 20 dB of enhancement in echo strength-an increase of some 100 folds. Range of ultrasound frequencies that are used for clinical diagnosis microbubbles at (1-7 μ diameter) do not diffuse across the endothelium. So there is no interstitial phase of enhancement. Thus, they are essentially markers for the blood pool (or for any other body space into which they have been placed) and their distribution is similar to those of tagged red cells. Typically the effective duration of vascular enhancement is a few minutes after which the microbubbles dissipate although, this model is complicated by evidence that some microbubbles are taken up by the phagocytic cell systems and these have liver/spleen specific effects.

The techniques for making microbubbles have been devised both to control their size and to make them sufficiently stable to provide a clinically useful enhancement time of at least a few minutes.

Levovist

It consists of galactose ground into tiny crystals whose irregular surfaces act as nidation sites on which air pockets form when it is suspended in water. A trace of palmitic acid is added as a surfactant to stabilise the resultant microbubbles which therefore are in effect tiny soap bubbles.

Optison

It represents another class of microbubbles with a shell formed by sonicating a solution of human serum albumin. The resulting capsules are filled with a per-fluorocarbon gas (perfluoropropane) whose high molecular weight shows dissolution and thereby prolongs the enhancement for several minutes.

Sonovue

It is a family of microbubbles whose membrane consists of phospholipids. In this case, the gas is sulphur hexafluorides[5, 6] which diffuses slowly like perfluoro compounds.

KEY POINTS

- Arcuate and interlobar branches of renal arteries and arteries less than 100 μ) has low resolution to make image.
- Hence shift frequency and echo strength determines the visualization of small vessels.
- Contrast agents increases both above and hence act as echo enhancer.
- Echo enhancers are microbubles— levovist, optisan, sonovue.
- Non-vascular use—tubal patency in infertility, ureteric reflux in children with urinary tract infections.
- Vascular use—cardiac, transcranial, carotid and renal.

Extensive preclinical and clinical trials have demonstrated an excellent safety profile for intravenous injection of microbubbles. The total amount used is minute (less than 200/ml in the case of a dose of Levovist and their small size makes embolisation most unlikely.

The main unwanted effect is a mild and transient local discomfort at the injection site which results from the high osmolality of this agent.

THE IMPACT OF CONTRAST ENHANCEMENT

The arrival of the contrast agent some seconds after peripheral venous injection in the portion of the systemic vasculature is marked by a dramatic increase in signal strength. In spectral Doppler, this is seen as intensifying of the gray scale of the spectrum for spectral Doppler examinations that fail because of lack of signal strength, the effect of the contrast agent is to rescue the examination.

In colour Doppler, the parameter mapped to colour is the estimated Doppler shift frequency, which corresponds to the relative blood flow velocity. Colour should therefore remain unaltered by contrast enhancement, what does change is the range of locations from which colour signals are detected. The effect of contrast agent is to raise the signals from small vessels above that threshold to that point at which they are effectively detectable on a colour image. Thus more vessels appear in a contrast enhanced ultrasound image.

Studies have demonstrated the capacity of contrast agents to increase the technical success rate of Doppler ultrasound, for example—in clinical transcranial Doppler studies of middle cerebral artery administration of 10 ml of levovist in concentration of 200, 300, 400 mg/ml resulted in dose dependent increases in both surgical intensity and duration of enhancement. At a concentration of 400 mg/ml Levovist increased the Doppler signal by approximately 25 dB. The time to peak enhancement was between 30 and 60 seconds and duration of enhancement was reported to be sufficiently long to be clinically useful.[2]

If the target vessel is large than the flow detectable, the impact of the agent may be to shorten the examination time. In one study Levovist halved the examination time for the Duplex investigation of renal artery stenosis.[3] Yet another study[4] suggested improved accuracy in measuring peripheral vascular velocity when contrast is used.

In a satisfactory colour Doppler study of the abdomen one use of the agent might simply be to enable a higher ultrasound frequency to be used, exploiting the agent to counter the higher tissue attenuation. In such a case, contrast enhancement translates into higher spatial solution.

Alternatively the colour system may be set to use fewer pulses per scan line (that is a lower ensemble length) while still achieving the same sensitivity to blood flow by means of contrast enhancement. The agent will then provide the user with a higher frame rate.

An important general concept in the practical use of microbubble enhancing agents is their fragility, so that, they are readily destroyed by the insolating beam. In some situation strategies to preserve them improve their visualisation significantly. The most important example is in echocardiography where the entire microbubble population generally passes through the ultrasound beam. A major increase in both the amount and duration of enhancement can be achieved by scanning intermittently (triggered by ECG) rather than continuously such approaches allow gray scale visualisation of myocardial perfusion.

If the bubbles in a tissue slice are deliberately destroyed, then their reappearance is related to the rate of inflow of fresh bubbles which depends on the tissue flow rate. This destruction-reperfusion approach has been used for the myocardium and can be expected to be useful also in kidney and other abdominal organs.

As microbubbles resonate in the ultrasound beam they behave like a musical instrument and emit harmonic signals at double their resonance frequency. If a scanner is modified to detect these harmonic signals and use them to form the image or Doppler trace, the confusing clutter signal from tissue stationary or moving are suppressed and a cleaner image or trace is produced.

In harmonic mode, echoes from the contrast agent are received preferentially by means of a bandpass filter whose centre frequency is at the second harmonic. Echoes from the solid tissues as well as from red blood cells themselves are suppressed.

The particular potential application of this entirely new diagnostic method is the detection of blood flow in small vessels surrounded by tissue that is moving - in the branches of coronary arteries or in the myocardium[5] itself as well in the parenchyma of abdominal organs.[6]

Another way to improve the signal/clutter ratio[8] is to use a pair of pulses to form each B-mode line, the second of each pair being inverted in phase. The final image line is formed by summing the two resultant echo trains. Since the echoes from linear reflectors such as tissue, are inverted they cancel out but the non linear response of the microbubbles means that their echoes are not exactly symmetricel in the compression and expansion phase and so they do not cancel out. This phase inversion. scan mode has similar effect in reducing clutter as the harmonic mode but with the important advantage of retaining the full spatial resolution of B mode which is compromised in the latter because a narrow band pulse must be used.

CLINICAL APPLICATIONS

Non-vascular Use

Contrast agents have been used to evaluate tubal patency in infertility and ureteric reflux in children with renal tract infections.

Echovist is installed into the uterine cavity via a small foleys catheter and using transvaginal sonography tracking of the echogenic contrast along the tubes and into the adnexal peritoneum is observed to estabalish tubal patency (Figs 6.1 to 6.3). Some false negative results may be obtained due to tubal spasm and it does not offer the same anatomical detail as HSG when tubal surgery is an option. However, it a simple OPD procedure and is radiation-free.

For vesicoureteric reflux, Levovist is instilled into the bladder as for conventional MCU. The lower ureters and renal pelvis are examined transabdominally as the bladder is filled to stimulate micturation. Sensitivity seems to be higher than for X-ray MCU, perhaps because there are no time constraints on imaging and the level of reflux can be assessed using the same criteria. Avoidance of radiation is an obvious advantage though the posterior urethra is not well seen. So, it may not be possible to replace the initial investigation in boys. For girls and for all follow-up studies, the US MCU has become standard in many paediatric departments.

VASCULAR USES

Cardiac

The use of contrast media is to opacify the cardiac chamber. This improves delineation of the left ventricular endocardial border and allows better

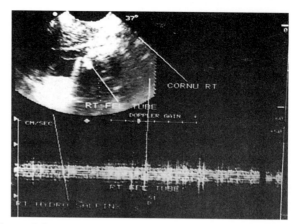

Figure 6.1
Hydrosalpinx-contrast agent (Agitated Haemecele) with Duplex mode

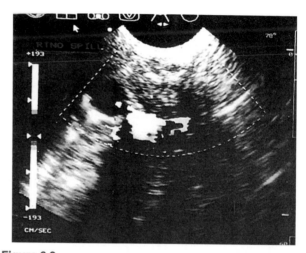

Figure 6.2
Colour mode—Patent tube

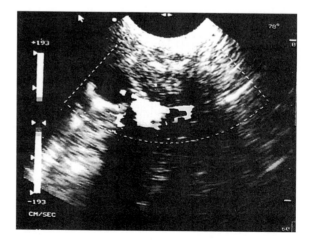

Figure 6.3
Distal turbulence demonstrated by contrast agent (Agitated Haemecele)

KEY POINTS

- Transcranial, carotid, renal, portal vein, peripheral, arterial, IVC, venous.
- Functional uses of contrast Doppler
- Mature scar—no vascularity while tumour recurrence shows marked vascularity.
- Hepatocellular carcinoma—fill in arterial phase while regenerating nodule and adenocarcinoma fill slowly.

estimates of left venticular function and measurement of ejection fraction. In many cardiology unit micro-bubble enhanced echocardiography has replaced isotope studies (particularly the MUGA scan) for left ventricular function. It is cheaper, quicker and avoids ionising radiation.

The development of means to detect microbubbles in the myocardial capillaries is making myocardial perfusion estimates possible and ultrasound contrast stress echo studies are becoming more widely used. The possibilily of studying the coronary arteries directly is also becoming an option.

TRANSCRANIAL DOPPLER

Transcranial Doppler (TCD) is a typical field where Doppler signals are routinely difficult to obtain because of the attenuation by the skull. Microbubbles improve signal intensity overcoming these technical difficulty. It allows a more complete depiction of the cerebral arterial system and basal veins. It is especially useful in depicting lesion with low blood flow velocities and low flow volume.

Cavernomas appear as echogenic areas with slow flow on Doppler. Flow within cavernomas themselves is undetectable but after Levovist enhancement, mean peak systolic flow velocities of 10 to 15 cm/sec are seen. Contrast enhanced TCD may therefore be especially useful in the intensive care unit as well as intra operatively and during postoperative follow-up.

As long as, there is good ultrasonic window through the temporal bone arteriovenous malformations can be detected without the need for enhancement because of their high velocity flows which is often bi-or multidirectional. Microbubbles may enhance delineation of the entire malformation and reveal even occult AVM.

Aneurysms, characteristically identified as sharp systolic bidirectional Doppler signal with a machine like noise may be detected on unenhanced TCD but can be diagnosed with higher accuracy and at a smaller size with contrast enhanced TCD. Enhanced Doppler can be expected to assist in the management of subarachnoid haemorrhage in detecting possible sources of haemorrhage and in monitoring arterial spasm.

The diagnosis of cerebral vascular stenosis is based on demonstrating aliasing on colour Doppler supported by characteristic changes in the Doppler frequency spectrum especially high velocities. In patients with poor signal transmission through the temporal bone, microbubble enhancement reduces the failure rate and may be especially helpful in distinguishing high grade stenosis from occlusion. Low volume flow at high grade stenosis may be missed on transcranial ultraosound because the signals are weak, exactly as with the extracranial carotid arteries.

The increased signal intensity after microbubble enhancement allows a complete three-dimensional reconstruction of the circle of Willis and improves the delineation of tumour feeding vessels and the identification and localisation of highly vascularised areas within the tumour. Additionally 3D display may rescue the examiner dependence of vascular ultrasound by allowing off line analysis. It may also help overcome some of the limitation of access to cerebral vessel by allowing display of reformatted sections in planes that cannot be obtained directly.

To date harmonic imaging has been disappointing in transcranial Doppler because the stimulation of microbubbles to resonate in a non-linear mode depends upon achieving a higher acoustic intensity than for simple resonance and this is difficult to achieve through the attenuating skull bone. The recently described technique of wideband harmonic imaging seems to be less dependent on sound pressure suggesting a potential for transcranial imaging.

CAROTID DOPPLER

Echo enhancement by contrast allows carotid Doppler to be performed by less skilled operators and with inexpensive scanners so the technique could become more widely used. Enhancement may also lead to better delineation of plaque ulcers. The ability to improve demonstration of trickle flow in very light stenosis is of undoubted clinical value because these patients benefit from endarterectomy whereas surgery is of no benefit once the internal carotid artery has occluded.

RENAL DOPPLER

Preliminary studies have shown that Levovist improves the diagnosis of significant renal artery stenosis by substantially reducing the failure rate for both the main renal arteries and for changes in intrarenal waveforms. This resulted in fewer false negative and false positive results when compared to digital subtraction angiography. This could increase the value of ultrasound screening for renovascular hypertension to the extent that microbubble enhancement becomes a routine part of investigation. Ultrasonic diagnosis of renal vein thrombosis is difficult because access to the renal veins may be limited and also because the process commonly starts in small veins at lobar level and then propogates to the main renal vein. By this stage collaterals open up both at the capsule and in the renal hilum thus the demonstration of venous signal at renal hilum does not completely exclude renal vein thrombosis. Better delineation of the venous anatomy following enhancement may prove to be an important application of microbubbles though there are no reports on this use.

Microbubble enhancement provides valuable added confidence in the diagnosis of acute transplant occlusion affecting the surgical anastomosis.

PORTAL VEIN DOPPLER

Echo enhanced Doppler provides useful information in a failed Doppler study. Enhancement allows a decision between a technical failure and true absence of flow. This situation is common is cirrhosis because of the highly attenuating liver and because the portal vein flow velocity may be very low. A confident diagnosis of portal vein patency can be achieved more often so that DSA can be avoided in some cases.

PERIPHERAL ARTERIAL DOPPLER

Signal strength is improved by microbubble enhancement and this is likely to prove helpful in improving signals from segments where shadowing from calcific plaques attenuates the signals and from very light stenoses where the flow velocity drops (trickle flow). In addition contrast speeds up to procedure. Levovist has been shown to improve the signals from leg arteries in a clinical trial but the diagnostic advantage has not been evaluated systematically.

IVC

IVC thrombosis is occasionally difficult to diagnosis especially in the infrarenal portion which is often obscured by intestinal gas. A microbubble enhancing agent might be very useful here and for the same reason, in the iliac veins in the pelvis. Echovist injected into a vein in the foot improves visualisation of the cava and of the flow disturbances around caval filters. Whether a microbubble injected into a distant (artecubital) vein would also be useful has not been studied systematically.

PERIPHERAL VENOUS DOPPLER

Unenhanced Doppler may fail in the diagnosis of deep vein thrombosis especially where the leg is swollen or obese and in diagnosis of below knee deep vein thrombosis. As with other vascular beds these problems amount to between a few and 10 per cent.

A problem with microbubbles is the dilution of contrast agent because of the large volume of these capacitance vessels as reflected in the partial success reported for Echovist injections directly into veins of foot when compared to limited value of Levovist injected into an antecubital vein. Since this is such an important clinical problem, action research continues and it may be that infusion techniques will improve the clinical usefulness of microbubble agents for DVT.

FUNCTIONAL USES OF CONTRAST DOPPLER

The clinical applications can be divided into those that interrogate the entire haemodynamics of an organ and those that study only one region, for example, a tumor. There have been two main whole organ studies looking at the liver and the transplanted kidney.

For the liver either the inflow or the outflow can be chosen and in both the principle is to separate the venous from the arterial signals because the normal balance whereby some 25 per cent of hepatic flow is arterial is shifted towards much higher proportions in diseases where there is arteriovenous shunting especially cirrhosis and malignancy.[7]

The inflow measurements were originally made by estimating the flow in the hepatic artery and portal vein using conventional spectral Doppler to obtain the mean flow velocity and multiplying this by the vessels area to obtain the Doppler perfusion index: unfortunately the excellent results initially reported have proved to be difficult to reproduce but a microbubble enhanced DPI promises to be more easily reproduced. In this method a bolus of contrast is tracked using a power Doppler gate that covers both artery and vein and the relative slopes of the two arrival curves is used to derive the two values. In the outflow method a spectral Doppler gate is placed over a hepatic vein and the relative slopes of the two arrival curves is used to derive the two values. In the outflow method a spectral Doppler gate is placed over a hepatic vein and the arrival time of an iv bolus is measured. In both cirrhosis and metastatic disease the arrival time is much earlier than in patients with chronic hepatitis or controls and this may allow early detection and avoid the need for biopsies. For the transplant kidney a spectral Doppler gate that covers the artery and the vein and is used to track the arrival time of the bolus and from these the true arteriovenous transit can be calculated.[8] It seems to be longer in rejection than in acute tubular necrosis and so unnecessary biopsies might be avoided.

The regional approach has been used for malignancies seeking to improve differential diagnosis by revealing features of neovascular isation for example in the liver.[9]

Many studies in the breast show that the arrival time in cancers is earlier than in benign masses though some cases of benign breast change have been confusing especially those that have an inflammatory component.[10]

The lack of vascularities in mature scars in comparison to the marked vascularity of tumour recurrence has emerged as a proven clinical tool for this problem. In liver a variety of temporal patterns have been described that are generally similar to those seen in triple phase CT. Malignancies especially hepatocellular carcinomas fill during the arterial phase a few seconds after injection while regenerating nodules and haemangiomas fill slowly, the latter typically from the periphery and usually in complete (Figs 6.4a to d). Focal nouldar hyperplasia shows similar temporal features to malignancies though their liver specific phase discriminates them well (Figs 6.5a to c).

An interesting way to make use of the fragility of microbubbles is to set up an infusion for steady blood level, apply a destructive pulse to a region of interest and then with non-destructive interrogating pulse watch for reperfusion as the slice fill with micro-

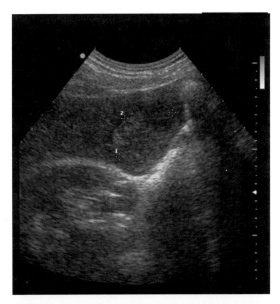

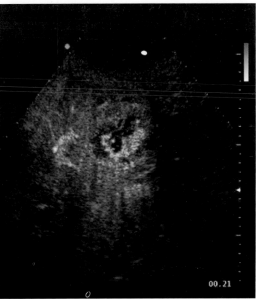

Figures 6.4a and b
Hepatocellular carcinoma (a) grey scale image shows a well-defined mixed echogenicity mass lesion in the liver, (b) early arterial phase image of the lesion after contrast administration shows peripheral enhancement

bubbles. This reperfusion kinetic method has been applied to the myocardium where it shows great promise as a way to detect regional perfusion defects caused by anastomotic failures or by rejection.

The liver specific phase of microbubbles seen after the agent has cleared from larger vessel is an example of tissue targeting. It occurs with agents that are phagocytosed by the RES such as (sonovist and sonazied) but also with Levovist. Clinically this phase

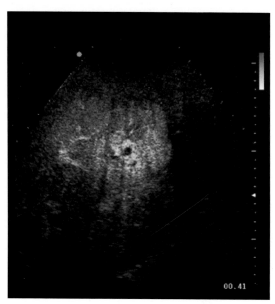
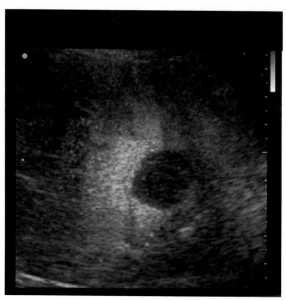

Figures 6.4c and d
Hepatocellular carcinoma (c) progressive centripetal enhancement in the lesion is evident in late arterial phase, (d) in the late phase, surrounding liver enhances more than the lesion from which contrast has been washed out, leading to increased lesional conspicuity

is significant because many lesions particularly malignancies do not take up the agents and so are highlighted as microbubble poor spaces.[11]

In this phase the microbubbles are not moving so convertional Doppler does not detect them and they are not obvious on gray scale. Non-linear modes such as colour Doppler stimulated acoustic emission (SAE) or the phase inversion mode (PIM) imaging are needed for their depiction. The effect is transient especially with a fragile agent such as Levovist because it depends on bubble destruction and so special scanning approaches have to be used taking care to minimise inadvertent exposure to ultrasound. Allowing the vascular phase to clear (3 min with Levovist) then scanning with slow sweeps through the region of interest and then reviewing the images in the cine loop is one practical approach. The scanner needs to be set for maximum output power using a low frequency and with the transmit few at the region of interest maximising the SAE effect but it may also be possible to employ phase inversion techniques in a non-destruction mode. The effects can be produced in all subjects but are weaker when sound attenuation is high and with Levovist fade over 30 min: the best effect is achieved 5-15 min after injection.

SAE reveals most types of focal lesion as colour defects and the increase in conspicuity is striking (Figs 6.6a and b). In a specific study where 2 blinded observers scored the SAE signal intensity. Both scored all 15 metastases as low SAE with significantly more signal in 4 haemangiomas and in other benign lesions. One observer was able to distinguish haemangiomas from metastases completely, while the other scored an overlap in only one case (a metastasis with moderately high SAE). Scores similar to the surrounding liver were seen in 2 cirrhotic nodule, 2 focal fatty change and 4 focal nodular hyperplasia. High SAE activity seemed to corrleate with a benign aetiology and scanning in SAE mode improved specificity. Initial evaluation of suspected cases of FNH in SAE mode might replace sulphur colloid radionuclide scanning.

PIM provides better spatial resolution so that new lesions smaller than 1 cm in diameter can be seen.[12] It exploits the non-linearity of microbubble behaviour based on the fact that bubbles are easily expanded by a negative pressure but progressively resist compression by increased pressure. Thus they respond differently to the compression and rarefaction phases of the ultrasound wave and this information can be extracted by summing the echoes from each scan line from two pulses of inverted phase. Tissue returns opposite signals which cancel out but microbubbles give different signals and do not cancel completely. The system has a reduced frame rate but selects for the location of the microbubbles and retains the spatial

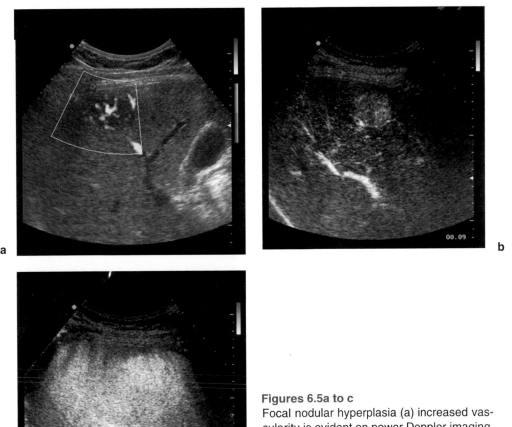

a

b

c

Figures 6.5a to c
Focal nodular hyperplasia (a) increased vascularity is evident on power Doppler imaging, (b) increased vascularity is also seen in early arterial phase, after contrast administration. A branch of right hepatic artery is also well visualized, (c) late arterial phase image shows progressive contrast enhancement

resolution of gray scale imaging. In a preliminary study of 12 patients being screened for liver metastases strong gray scale signals filling the liver parenchyma were elicited while metastasis appeared as defects even if they were isoechoic on conventional ultrasound.

A multicenter study including 128 patients suspected of having liver metastases confirmed these results with greatly improved sensitivity especially for small (subcentimeter) lesions, fewer false positives and detection of some lesions that were too small to be detected on CT but were seen on Gadolinium enhanced MRI.

Although focal diseases in the liver is the most important application, these agents also collect in normal spleen and this has proved to be useful in distinguishing splenunculus from lymphadenopathy and in detecting small intrasplenic masses such as in lymphoma.

Limitations of both these methods include their transient effect fall off in the far field and artefacts such as shadowing. A difficulty with liver specific phase imaging using Levovist is obtaining proof of the nature of the defects seen because the transient effect makes biopsy almost impossible.

This may be resolved with the more persistent agents undergoing clinical trials.

SAE has relatively poor spatial resolution but has the advantage of intrinsic segmentation since it uses the colour Doppler circuitry the colour signals can easily be separated from the gray scale component so that the exact correspondence between the bubble signature and the lesion or tissue seen on gray scale is apparent. PIM has the same spatial resolution as gray scale but the bubble and tissue components are inextricably enlarged and so the two signals cannot be separated.

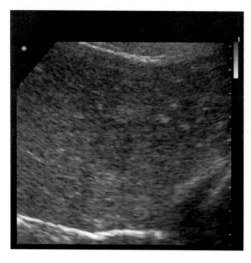 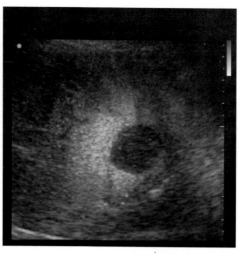

Figures 6.6a and b
(a) A baseline sonogram shows an ill-defined hypoechoic lesion is the liver, (b) after contrast administration lesion appears as a colour defect and becomes more conspicuous

A recently introduced mode, Agent Detection Imaging (ADI) offers a combination of both features. A development of SAE but using power Doppler it depicts the bubble destruction signature as a colour overlay with the same spatial resolution as the underlying gray scale scan. It offers the combination of excellent spatial resolution and the ability to view the background and the bubble signals together or separately so that the precise location of the microbubbles can be determined.

The therapeutic potential of microbubbles is a topic of active research.[13,14] They may be used in two ways, to enhance the effects of High Intensity Focussed Ultrasound (HIFU) by increasing the amount of energy deposited or by acting as vehicles for therapeutic agents. In this mode, the loaded microbubbles are ruptured at the desired site by applying sufficiently intense sound to achieve a local high concentration of agent, thrombolytic agent or an anticancer drugs.

REFERENCES

1. Burns PN: Interpreting and analyzing the Doppler examination. In Taylor KJW, Burns PN, Wells PNT (Eds)New York : Raven Press: 55-99, 1995.
2. Bauer A, Becker G, Krone A, Frohlich T: Transcranial duplex sonography using ultrasound contrast enhancers. *Clin Radiol* **51**: 19-23, 1996.
3. Missouris CG, Allen CM, Balen FG: Non invasive screening for renal artery stenosis with ultrasound contrast enhancement. *J Hyperten* **14**: 519-24, 1996.
4. Tschammler A, Viesr G, Schindler R: Ultrasound contrast media *in vitro* studies. *J Ultrasound Med* **12**: S33 1993.
5. Porter TR, Xie F, Kriesfeld D: Improved myocardial contrast with second harmonic transient ultrasound response imaging in humans using intravenous perfluorocarbon exposed sonicated dextrose albumin. *J Am Cell Cardiol* **27**: 1479-1501 1996.
6. Kono Y, Moriyasu F, Yawada K: Conventional and harmonic gray scale enhancement of the liver with sonication activation of a US contrast agent. *Radiology* 201, 1996.
7. Albrecht T, Blomley MJ, Casgron DO: Non invasion diagnosis of hepatic cirrhosis by transit time analysis of ultrasound contrast agent. *Lancet* **353**: 1579-83, 1999.
8. Blomley M, Albrecht T, Eckersley R: Renal arterio venous transit time measured noninvasively using bolus injections of microbubble contrast. *Radiology* **209**: 461, 1998.
9. Wilson SR, Burns PN, Muradati D: Harmonic hepatic US with microbubble contrast agent: initial experience showing improved characterisation of haemangioma, hepatocellular carcinoma and metastasis. *Radiology* **215**: 153-61, 2000.
10. Albrecht T, Patel N, Cosgrove DO: Enhancement of bower Doppler signals from breast lesions with the ultrasound contrast agent Echogen emulsion: subjective and quantitative assessment. *Academic Radiology* **5 (Suppl)**: S195-98; discussion S199, 1998.
11. Albrecht T, Blomley M, Wilsons: Improved detection of metastatic liver lesions using pulse inversion harmonic imaging with Levovist a multicenter study. *Radiology* 1685, 2000.
12. Harvey C, Blomely M, Eckersley R: Improved detection of hepatic malignancies using pulse inversion mode in the late phase of enhancement with the ultrasound contrast agent Levovist (SHU 508A): early experiences *Radiology* (Submitted) 1999.
13. Ho SY, Barbarese E, D'Arrigo JS: Evaluation of lipid coated microbubbles as a delivery vehicle for Taxol in brain tumor therapy. *Neurosurgery* **40**: 1260-66: discussion 1566-68, 1997.
14. Porter TR, Leveen RF, Fox R: Thrombolytic enhancement with perflurocarbon exposed sonicated dextrose albumen microbubbles. *American Heart Journal* **132**: 964-68, 1996.

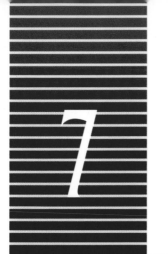

Cerebrovascular Doppler Sonography

Gopesh Mehrotra
Leena Gupta
Satish K Bhargava

Doppler ultrasound is the principal investigation for patients with possible carotid disease. Indications for Doppler ultrasound of neck arteries are:

1. Transient ischaemia (TIA's) < 24 hrs
2. Reversible ischaemic neurological deficit (rind)
3. Pre-operative-in high risk groups
4. Mild stroke in younger patients, in resolution
5. Non-focal symptoms possibly vascular (atypical cases)
6. Pulsatile masses
7. Following endarterectomy
8. Suspected trauma or dissection, including the trauma to vertebral vessels
9. As screening measure
10. Subclavian steal syndrome
11. Posterior fossa ischaemia

A completed stroke does not warrant a carotid Doppler examination as endarterectomy is not likely to be offered, whereas definite benefit is shown for patients with severe stenosis with symptomatic ischaemia who undergo endarterectomy in terms of risk for subsequent stroke trials. For asymptomatic bruits value of surgery is less clear.

To know the degree of significant stenosis in relation to need for carotid surgery were conducted in North America and Europe. These two trials differed somewhat in methodology and also in the results. Whereas North American trial demonstrated some improvement by surgery for the patients with stenosis greater than 50 per cent and definite improvement for stenosis greater than 70 percent the European trial put the percentage at 60 per cent, above which the surgery reduced the risk of stroke. Also because of different methods of measuring stenosis the 70 per cent stenosis in the European trial corresponded to 50 per cent reduction in North American trial. Whereas North American trial compared diameter of stenosed vessel with the normal vessel more distally whereas in European trial, stenosed vessel diameter was compared with the expected normal vessel diameter at the same level. Both trials compared the results with angiography of stenosis which remains the gold standard despite being interobserver assessment, invasive and with interobserver variability.

Patients who are to undergo surgery for peripheral or coronary artery disease, aneurysms or other vascular disease are also at risk and hence candidates for carotid Doppler sonography.

Following endarterectomy, reocclusion may develop over next 24-40 hrs, neointimal hyperplasia between 1-2 years or restenosis over seven years. Therefore follow-up with carotid ultrasound is mandatory.

Technique For carotid arteries the patient lies supine with pillow under shoulders and neck turned to opposite side to open the anterior triangle of the neck. Generally 7-10 MHz frequency transducer is used and transverse scanning from sternoclavicular region up in the neck is first done, followed by longitudinal scanning to outline both carotid arteries. (Fig. 7.1) particular scan plane can be recommended and variety of planes might be used to define the anatomy optimally. In the region of carotid bulb reverse flow may be seen, helping the identification and minimising the time required. Spectral Doppler is required to assess and quantify the abnormal flow. In the colour mode the position of maximum Doppler shift is sought and cursor is placed accordingly. The angle of insolation and gate range is optimised. The velocity setting and wall filters are adjusted and maximum shift is located by obtaining waveforms.

It is important to identify external carotid artery separate from the internal carotid artery, more importantly in the presence of disease, where the distinction may be even more difficult as the significant disease alters the waveform characteristics, blurring the distinction between external carotid and internal carotid flow. In such situations, tapping the superficial temporal artery over zygoma induces the fluctuations in blood flow only in the external carotid artery. Scanning the orbit for the reversal of flow in the ophthalmic artery confirms the significant carotid artery occlusion.

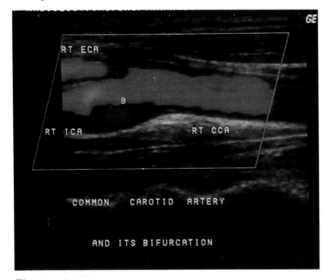

Figure 7.1
Normal longitudinal colour Doppler flow image of the common carotid artery and its bifurcation with flow reversal bone (blue area) appearing at early systole or peak systole

Common carotid and internal carotid artery show laminar flow on colour image (Fig. 7.2).

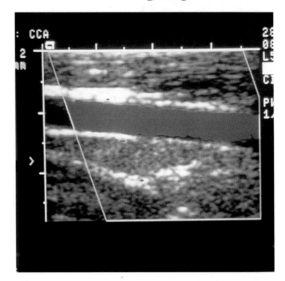

Figure 7.2
Colour Doppler image of common carotid artery showing uniform filling of lumen, suggesting presence of laminar flow

The external carotid artery may normally be identified by appearance of cervical branches low in the neck, location and particular waveform characteristics such as more pulsative flow with little flow in diastole (Fig. 7.3) (high resistance pattern) and the prominent dicrotic notch. As against this internal carotid artery shows less pulsatile flow with relatively high diastolic flow and localised widening of bulb at the origin (Fig. 7.4). Waveform of CCA resembles that of ICA (Fig. 7.5).

The intimal thickness is best measured when the carotid artery is in longitudinal section with the

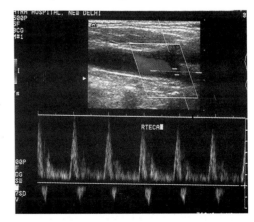

Figure 7.3
Waveform of normal external carotid artery showing triphasic waveform characteristic of arteries supplying muscular bed

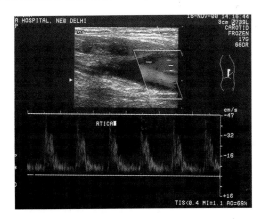

Figure 7.4
Normal waveform of right internal carotid artery persistent flow is seen during diastole. Spectral window can also be appreciated

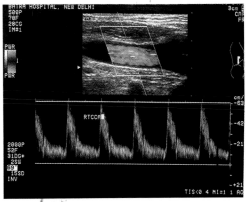

Figure 7.5
Pulse Doppler of normal carotid artery shows sharp systolic peak with antegrade flow during diastole

ultrasound beam orthogonal to it, and is taken on the far wall, in the magnified image. The cursors are placed between luminal margin of the inner line and the inner margin of the outer line. The normal values are taken to be less than 0.8 mm.

For the vertebral arteries during the longitudinal scanning in carotid plane the scan plane is rotated laterally till it comes to overlie the lateral masses of cervical vertebrae, the vertebral artery being visible in between the gaps. The artery can also be sought for, low in the neck between the vertebral column and subclavian artery or high in posterior neck when it passes around the lateral mass of atlas.

The direction of flow in the verterbal arteries should be noted to identify the phenomenon of the subclavian steal. This phenomenon can be unmasked in the latent cases by asking patient to do some muscular work by arm or inducing the reactive hyperemia in the arm

muscles or by occluding brachial artery with a pressure cuff for 2-3 minutes and then releasing the cuff.

Abnormal findings The normal and abnormal flows can be quickly distinguished. The colour Doppler is helpful. Though colour variations may be seen with cardiac cycle, no areas of persistent colour change are seen normally, the presence of which indicates abnormal or turbulent velocity implying the disease in the vessels. The severity of disease or stenosis in the arteries can be quantified either by velocity measurements in the area of narrowings or by direct visualisation and measurement of the stenosis.

Doppler criteria In the normal vessels, the peak velocity measurements are taken from common carotid artery about 2-3 cm below the bifurcation, from the internal carotid arteries about 2-3 cm above the bulb and from the external carotid artery about 1-2 cm above the bifurcation.

In the diseased arteries the waveforms are obtained from the areas of maximum velocity. The final position of the sample volume is determined by sound of Doppler shift as well as by the imaging on the screen. Where colour Doppler is not available it becomes necessary to reduce the size of sample volume and move it slowly around area of stenosis till maximum shift is seen as well as heard, on the speakers.

The internal carotid artery supplies the low resistance capillaries of cerebrum and therefore shows flow throughout the cardiac cycle with appreciable flow even during diastole. The external carotid artery on the other hand supplies the tissues of neck and scalp which have higher resistance and only minimal flow if at all is seen in diastole. Besides, dicrotic notch following peak systole is a rather prominent feature of the waveform.

Of the various indices used for measurements of blood flow, the most important are the peak systolic velocity, end diastolic velocity and the ratio of peak systolic velocities of the internal and the common carotid arteries. The exact normal values and those belonging to different degree of the stenoses have been quoted differently by various authors because they vary from centre-to-centre and one equipment to another and on the techniques used. Every centre should optimise values for itself, it needs to be pointed out.

The physiological variations due to heart rate (tachycardia), cardiac output, contralateral stenosis or occlusion may affect velocities potentially misdiagnosing the mistakenly pathological velocities.

In such cases velocity ratios rather thin single peak velocity should be referred to as a general increase in velocity affect flow in both internal and external carotid arteries, as against the local flow in the internal carotid artery. Otherwise peak systolic and diastolic values refer to just the internal carotid arteries and not to the external carotid and the common carotid arteries.

Very severe degree of stenosis (greater than ninety per cent) with very narrow lumen, results in weak signals and low velocities because of small blood flow through the residual lumen. Hence it is important to change the settings of the equipment to those geared to detect very low intensity, low velocity signals unless the false diagnosis of occlusion instead of stenosis is made, and the patient gets denied the benefit of surgery. In fact ignoring the subtotally occluded vessel and allowing it to occlude may lead to permanent risk of stenosis of 5 per cent per year.

At the point of maximal narrowing in the carotid vessel the velocity of the moving blood typically increases because of the restriction of the arterial lumen. The compensatory flow develops in collaterals from ipsilateral external carotid artery, vertebral artery or contra lateral vessels. This decreases the amount of blood being delivered to diseased artery as a function of increasing stenosis. The positive association is maintained until the stenosis is somewhere near 90-95 per cent.

At the point of maximal narrowing and for about 2 cm distally, despite increased blood velocities cohesive flow is maintained which tends to get dissipated further downwards, because of jet phenomenon. For a distance 1-2 cm therefore, it is possible to get a relatively accurate Doppler tracing in terms of velocity increase caused by stenosis. The point of maximal stenosis however is sometimes masked by calcification. Further a zone of turbulence is established 1-2 cm distal to the area of stenosis. The colour Doppler offers a good estimate of the direction of the blood flow. This is achieved by taking multiple longitudinal projections until one projection allow a velocity jet of sufficient magnitude to be measured. It is important to ensure that correct angle correction is applied for the measurement. A deficient algorithm for angle correction especially for linear array transducers leads to the over estimation of stenosis.

The waveforms obtained also depend upon conditions remote from the site of measurement of the disease at a site proximal such as aortic valve abnormmities or stenosis at carotid origin, tend to affect the waveform. The significant distal disease in carotid siphon also increases the pulsatility at proximal sites. Occlusion or severe stenosis in the contralateral carotid artery results in the increased flow velocity in the remaining carotid.

Suggested diagnostic criteria for Doppler diagnosis of various degrees of stenosis are in Table 7.1.

Criteria for assessing the severity of carotid artery stenosis (Figs 7.6a and b).

Some observers feel that taking only one velocity whether systolic or diastolic for estimating stenosis does not take into account other considerations such as cardiac output change, etc. They propose instead-Internal carotid artery to common carotid artery (at a point 2-4 cm distal to bifurcation) peak systolic velocity ratio to allow for corrections due to change in cardiac output or arrythmias. But this suffers from the limitation induced by compounding of error in the individual measurement of each velocity. The other velocity ratios proposed are end diastolic velocity in the internal carotid artery divided by and diastolic velocity in the common carotid artery (ii) peak systolic velocity in the internal carotid artery divided by end-diastolic velocity in the common carotid artery.

However few facts are to be kept note of. Common carotid artery velocities are higher by as much as 10-20 cm near the origin and decrease near the bifur-

	Suggested diagnostic criteria for Doopler diagnosis of various degrees of stenosis					
Table 7.1	*Diameter reduction*	*PSV (cm/sec)*	*PDV (cm/sec)*	*Systolic VICA/VCCA*	*Diastolic VICA/VCCA*	*% Spectral broadening*
	0	< 110	< 40	< 1.8	< 2.6	< 30
	1-39	< 110	< 40	< 1.8	< 2.6	< 40
	40-59	< 130	< 40	< 1.8	< 2.6	< 40
	60-79	> 130	> 40	> 1.8	> 2.6	> 40
	80-99	> 250	>100	> 3.7	> 5.5	> 80

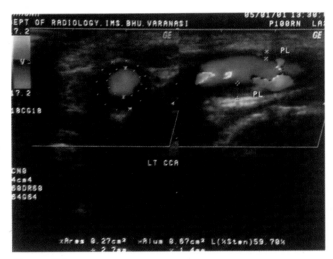

Figure 7.6a
CDFI of the common carotid artery shows approximately 60% area stenosis

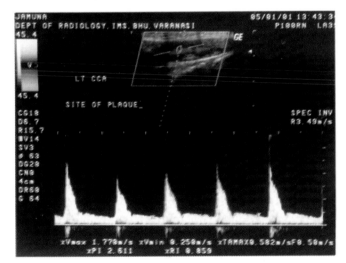

Figure 7.6b
Duplex scanning through the area of stenosis demonstrates increased peak systolic velocity, consistent with > 60% luminal narrowing (stenosis)

cation. Also, blood flow tends to be more consistent approximately 3 centimetres from the bifurcation.

Direct stenotic measurements. This can be either by the diameter reduction or area reduction method. The diameter measurement is quicker but area reduction measured in the transverse section does take into account the effect of asymmetrical plaques. A reduction of diameter by 50 per cent will corresponds to the area reduction of approximately 70 per cent and these two are not just interchangeable as such. For the purpose of measurement in the transverse image colour and power Doppler are helpful but it needs to be ensured that Doppler gain settings are set optimally

so that not only better assessment of boundries of residual lumen be made but also the distinction between peripheral poorly reflective plaque and inadequate colour filling because of subintimal gain settings be made.

The distinction between complete occlusion and severe stenosis which is important from treatment point of view can be achieved with colour Doppler. The accuracy of Doppler Ultrasound as described in the literature is quite high. As per one report Doppler had an overall sensitivity of 96 per cent specificity as high as 86 per cent and negative predictive value of 94 per cent, positive predictive value of 89 per cent for the significant stenosis (diameter less than 50 per cent).

Plaque characteristics It has been known that softer, more delicate lipid-rich plaques are more likely to fracture and dislodge than firm, more fibrotic, coherent plaques. Based on the plaque characteristics it has been suggested that symptoms relating to carotid artery disease are more common with echopoor type 1 and 2 than echo-reflective type 3 and 4.

Classification (Steffen) of plaque morphology
Type 1 : Predominantly echo poor with thin reflective cap (Fig. 7.7)
Type 2 : Substantially echo poor with small areas of increased reflectivity (Fig. 7.8)
Type 3 : Predominantly reflective lesions with areas of low reflectivity accounting for less than 25 per cent
Type 4 : Uniformly reflective types.

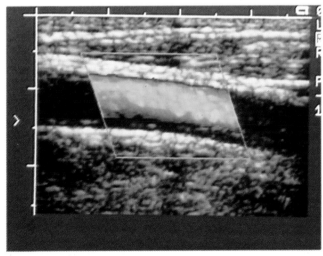

Figure 7.7
Power Doppler image of common carotid artery showing smooth, thin, homogenous plaque in the posterior wall

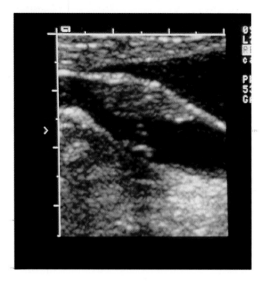

Figure 7.8
B-mode image of distal common carotid artery showing a homogenous plaque causing significant narrowing of lumen

There can be various complications which the plaques might undergo. They may undergo haemorrhage which may suddenly increase in size. The surface disruption may lead to release of plaque content in the blood stream. The thrombus may form on the ulcerated surface and may break off with distal embolisation. The results of correlating the risk of stroke with attempted ultrasound visualisation of ulcerated plaques and intra-plaque hemorrhage have not been very successful. There are a few limitations of ultrasound interpretations of surface characteristics as well. The echopoor areas in the plaque may be due to haemorrhage or due to an aggregation of lipids. The apparent ulceration on sonography may be due to a breach on the plaque surface or because of an irregular but intact surface. Further, some plaques might be visualized clearly while others may not show a clear outline. However, overall a homogenous, smoothly outlined, predominantly reflective plaque is less likely to have symptoms while a heterogenous, irregular, echo-poor lesion is more likely to have symptoms or complications.

Based on signals or echogenicity the plaques can be characterised as higher intensity, hyperechoic or isoechoic. The high intensity, hyperechoic signals are comparable to the fascial layers or, advential layer of the artery while isoechoic signals are compared to those returning from muscle of neck. Both of these represent fibrous constituents of plaque. It is helpful to differentiate them from hypoechoic signals within the plaque which by definition have echogenicity similar to blood and represent lipid, haemorrhage or smooth muscle proliferation.

The newer advances in ultrasound technology allow rendering of 3 D reconstruction of acquired images and help improve conspicuity and better define the extent of pathology. This can be used to advantage for showing complex tortousity of carotid arteries and their branches.

Contrast enhanced imaging of carotid arteries can be done by injecting US contrast agents or by altering the sensitivity of ultrasound mechine to detect signals emitted by moving blood. This can be helpful for evaluating patients with difficult anatomy. Further, contrast agents improved conspicuity of luminar interface and improve visualisation and characterisation of plaque and analyse residual lumen. Further improvement is achieved by the digital encoding scheme that increases ultrasound delivery and also increase signal intensity or reflected signals of returning echos from moving blood cell. This has the potential for mapping more accurately plaque characteristic such as ulceration.

An almost totally hypoechoic plaque or the one which is centrally hypoechoic with a rim of increased echogenicity is classified as homogenously hypoechoic. On the other hand a plaque which is homogenously echogenic is classified as homogenously hyperdense plaque. Of heterogenous plaques, the ones with greater than 5 per cent plaque elements hyperechoic are labelled as heterogenously hyperechoic while those with more than 50 per cent hypoechoic are calcified plaques may also be seen (Fig. 7.9) classified as heterogenous hypoechoic.

KEY POINTS

Carotid Doppler
- For stenosis–PSV, PDV, Systolic and diastolic pressure and % of spectral broadening should be taken into consideration.
- In plaque—symptomas related to carotid artery are more common with echopoor type 1 and 2 than echo reflector type 3 and 4.
- Contrast enhanced imaging—improve visualization and characteristics of plaque.

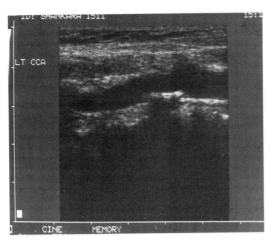

Figure 7.9
B-mode image of common carotid artery shows a densely calcified plaque in the posterior wall with posterior acoustic shadowing

Surface characters of plaque too may have some impact in patients with acute neurological symptoms. Because of extent of surface irregularity and its relation to transient ischaemic attack like symptoms. By definition an ulcer is an inter-plaque defect or excavation greater than 2 × 2 mm. Unfortunately neither gray scale ultrasound nor angiogram are very sensitive or specific in this regard. Colour Doppler may help by showing areas of flow reversal within the matrix of plaque.

A classification has been prescribed incorporating the plaque characteristics, surface outline and degree of stenosis into one. This classification (Thiele) is as given below:
1. Haemodynamic
   H_1 0-20% diameter reduction : Normal to mild
   H_2 20-60% diameter reduction : Moderate
   H_3 60-80% diameter reduction : Severe
   H_4 80-90% diameter reduction : Critical
   H_5 occluded (Fig. 7.10)
2. Morphological components
   P_1 homogenous
   P_2 heterogenous
3. Surface characteristics
   S_1 smooth
   S_2 irregular (defect < 2 mm)
   S_3 ulcerated (defect > 2 mm) (Fig. 7.11).
   A lesion classified $H_4 S_2 P_2$ as above will correspond to the 80 per cent dimeter reduction. The degree of narrowing can also be quantified in terms of area stenosis (Figs 7.12a to c).

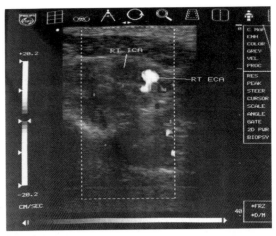

Figure 7.10
Transverse colour flow image just above the carotid bifurcation shows complete lack of colour filling of internal carotid artery suggesting thrombosis. External carotid artery shows normal flow

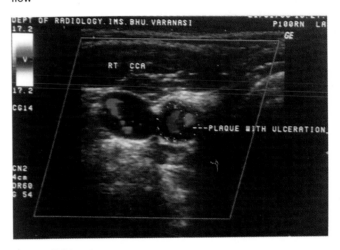

Figure 7.11
Transverse colour Doppler image of common carotid artery shows a hypoechoic plaque with area of reversed low velocity flow suggesting presence of plaque ulceration

Carotid occlusion While carotid stenosis, even the critical one may be salvagable by surgery carotid occlusion is not. Hence distinction is of clinical importance and should be made by colour Doppler, power Doppler or by the use of echo-enhancer agents. A number of pitfalls need to be avoided as small external carotid artery branches close to the occluded internal carotid artery. Another pitfall is when internal carotid artery occludes while external and common carotid artery are patent. The wave form in common carotid artery might reflect external carotid artery circulation with reduced or absent diastolic flow. On the other hand, in case of significant diversion of flow

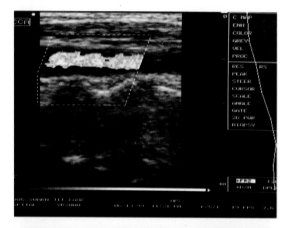

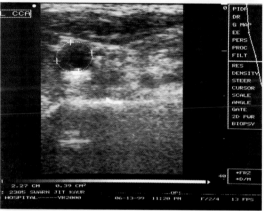

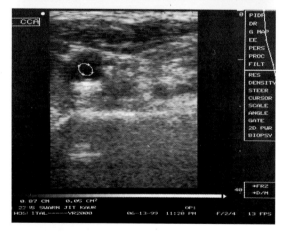

Figures 7.12a to c
(a) colour Doppler image of common carotid artery shows narrowing of lumen due to circumferential wall thickening, (b) transverse section showing circumferential wall thickening, (c) measurement of area of vessel and residual lumen by electronic calipers shows 87% area stenosis

to internal carotid circulation via ophthalmic and meningeal arteries the wave form is more like internal carotid artery with substantial diastolic flow, called the internalisation of external carotid artery. Still another situation may arise because occlusion of the common carotid artery may not always result in the occlusion of internal carotid artery. While the patency might be maintained by the retrograde collateral flow down the external carotid artery, these patients still remain at the risk of significant brain ischaemia in the distribution of the internal carotid artery.

Carotid dissection The causes can be as variable as spontaneous, because of atheroma, extension of the aortic dissection up the carotids, following hyperextension neck injury or iatrogenic during angiography. The appearances on ultrasound too may vary. There may be complete occlusion of vessels or a smoothly tapered stenosis with or without haematoma or thrombosis of false lumen might be recognisable. Alternatively, on Doppler ultrasound double lumen with variable flow pattern in two channel may be seen. Recanalisation of occluded lumen may be seen in as high as sixty per cent of the cases.

Pulsatile neck masses can be due to prominent carotid bulb, ectatic neck arteries, enlarged lymphadenopathy adjacent to carotid sheath, carotid artery aneurysm or carotid body tumours. Prominent and ectatic arteries can be easily made by Doppler ultrasound. Enlarged nodes too can be easily made out. Fixity or invasion to carotid sheath is made out by scanning while patient swallows.

Carotid aneurysms May arise because of mural degeneration, atheroma or following trauma. While aneurysm itself may be visible on ultrasound, patent lumen above carotid aneurysm may not be clearly seen. The evidence of flow in the ophthalmic artery on the same side may not indicate patency, as it may come from opposite side via circle of Willis.

Carotid body tumours Characteristically spread and separate the two arteries, the internal and external carotids. Poorly reflective and highly vascular mass is seen on ultrasound at bifurcation. The external carotid artery may show low resistance pattern.

The vertebral arteries The clinical significance of the disease in the vertebral arteries as compared with the carotid arteries is far less clear, because basilar artery and posterior circulation is supplied by two vertebrals and connected to circle of Willis allowing compensatory flow unless both vertebrals are narrowed. Failure to visualise vertebrals in the locations suggested (as above) might be due to congenital absence or hypoplasia. The altered waveform may be seen because of localised disease in the form of colour and spectral evidence in the segment being examined. Alternatively, damped waveforms may be due to involvement of proximal vertebrals or subclavian disease.

In case of proximal subclavian stenosis, phenomenon of subclavian steal may occur. Blood reaches affected arm down (instead of up) the ipsilateral vertebral artery from posterior circulation which itself gets supplied from opposite side. Thus posterior circulation get stolen. The direction of flow can be made out on Doppler.

Transcranial Doppler Ultrasound In the neonates the assessment of midline intracranial structures dates back to the days of A scan. The high quality images and Doppler studies could be obtained recently through fontanelles and thin calvarial bones recently. In 1982 Aaslid first decribed pulsed transcranial Doppler for adults. Since then techniques of pulsed transcranial Doppler have been further refined. More recently improvement in technology has allowed realtime colour transcranial Doppler, providing useful physiolgoical, pathological and pharmacological information and also including intraoperative and postoperative monitoring of endarteriology patients.

The main problem in the transcranial Doppler is attenuation and scattering of ultrasound beam by vault not only at soft tissue/bone interface but also at multiple interfaces in the skull vault. The attenuation is greater in older patients, females and the black subjects.

Anatomy The internal carotid artery as it exits up the cavernous sinus at the base of brain in the region of basal cisterns divides into three branches. The anterior cerebral artery turns forwards. Up and medially to run around corpus callosum. The middle cerebral artery passes laterally into the sylvian fissure and then posteriorly and superiorly in the fissure towards the parietal region. The two vertebral arteries enter the skull through foramen magnum and form the basilar artery at the base of tbe brain at the lower border of pons. The basilar artery runs anterior to pons to divide at its upper border into two posterior cerebral arteries. The posterior cerebral arteries pass around cerebral peduncles supply the occipital lobe.

The complete, classic circle of Willis is seen only in 50-60 per cent of cases, the most common variation is absence or hypoplasia of anterior cerebral artery, (20%) the supply being maintained by the opposite anterior cerebral artery through anterior communicating artery. Similarly proximal posterior cerebral artery may be absent, the supply coming from the psilateral internal carotid artery via posterior communicating artery (30%).

Examinations technique The three main access portals are transtemporal, suboccipital and transorbital window.

The trans temporal window renders visualisation of circle of Willis and all it's major branches. The transorbital window provides alternative access for internal carotid arteries, anterior cerebral artery and ophthalmic artery. The low frequency (2 MHz) is used with maximum possible sensitivity settings and maximum possible power for adult except in transorbital window to avoid excessive insolation and damage to lens. For neonates, lowest possible power output is to be maintained regardless of the window to be used.

Transtemporal window The side of this window is quite big and search is to be made for the thinner segment. The generous application of gel is required to avoid air-pockets trapped between hair of patient. The transducer is to be placed above and in front of external auditory meatus and a transverse (axial) section is taken. Failure to visualise the cerebral peduncle, third ventricles and perisellar region constitutes inadequate visualisation. Good visualisation of brain ensures proper and successful Doppler scan of blood vessels unless pathological. In 10 per cent of cases (elderly) completely impenetrable temporal bone is present precluding visualisation. Ipsilateral middle cerebral artery (MCA) can be traced back to the region of the circle of Willis and to subsequent branches with some cranial caudad angling of the probe. It may not be possible to get full circle of Willis on one scan and the communicating arteries may not be seen at all because of their small size or congenital abscence. The direction of flow is to be noted particularly in the proximal anterior cerebral arteries (ACAs), as they are the major source of collateral pathways. Spectral Doppler gives this information rather than power Doppler which is more sensitive for locating the flow. The use of echo enhancer agents improves visualisation considerably above either of these. The proximal and distal segments of PCA are visible around the peduncles to the inferior aspect of occipital lobe. The termination of basilar artery is seen in 56 per cent of cases more often with power Doppler.

The internal carotid artery (ICA) is examined by angling probe interiorly lying as it is in the region of the foramen lacerum and then angling it progressively more superiorly. The ICA termination is also visualised by turning transducer through 90 per cent and scanning medial side of middle cranial fossa, requiring several planes because of the curves of carotid siphon.

The suboccipital window The location is midline posteriorly at the level of hairline and directing probe upwards towards the foramen magnum. The visualisation is improved by scanning just to the side of midline to avoid dense midline ligaments. The third part of vertebral artery is seen running upwards towards foramen magnum. The junction of vertebral arteries to from basilar artery may be seen if it lies low enough.

The transorbital window The beam is directed upwards and medially towards the apex of orbit. The structures visualised are ophthalmic artery, carotid siphon and the contralateral ACA. With power output reduced to minimum, transducer is put over closed eyelid using sterile aqueous gel instead of ultrasound gel. The colour transducers being heavy and bulky find limitation with this approach but need to do so is reduced as ACA's are well-visualised by transtemporal approach.

The flow in the ophthalmic artery should be assessed close to the orbit rather than just behind the eye as the flow in the retinal artery is towards the eye. There is collateral circulation in the mid and posterior orbit between orbital branches of external carotid artery and ophthalmic artery to supply circle of Willis in case of ipsilateral ICA blockade.

Transcranial pulsed Doppler The ordinary transcranial Doppler has a role to play when colour Doppler equipment is not available or cannot be used example in theatres where the space at the side of patient head is insufficient.

Using the transtemporal window the bifurcation can usually be detected at a depth of 65 mm and the flow in MCA is towards the probe while that in the ACA is away from it. Both arteries are then followed by adjusting the greater and lesser depth. The MCA is located at a shallow depth of 35 mm while ACA is located between 65-75 mm and angulating more anteriorly. The patency of ACA can be confirmed by the flow reversal in response to compression of ipsilateral carotid in the neck, but is to be avoided.

The PCA is located by angulating the probe posteriorly, at a depth of 55 mm as it curves round brainstem. The signal direction is towards that of probe normally. Further down as PCA is tracked medially to termination of BA at a depth of >5 mm signal is biphasic. Small changes in probe angle are required to trace the path of the arteries.

The carotid siphon is identified at 55-70 mm through transorbital approach. The direction of flow obviously varying as per anatomy. (Towards the probe in lower part and away from the probe in the upper part). The vertebral arteries are located through suboccipital approach at 40-70 mm. The origin of basilar artery 15 mm deeper at 70-80 mm and passes anterior to brainstem still deeper at 100 mm.

The highest velocities are seen in the MCA followed by ACA, PCA, BA and the ICA in the last. All velocities decline with age. The peak or mean MCA velocities should not vary by more than 20 per cent.

	Peak velocities (Age 40-60 years)		Mean velocities	
	Mean	Range	Mean	Range
MCA	91	57-125	58	35-81
ACA	86	46-127	53	32-74
PCA	60	19-101	37	17-56

Applications of colour and pulsed TCD are:
1. Identification of occluded/stenosed arteries and collateral pathways
2. Investigation in the setting of vasospasm complicating SAH
3. Investigation of brain death
4. Assessing the venous system
5. During carotid surgery and neuro-intensive care
6. Emboli detection
7. Estimating the cerebral perfusion reserve
8. Detection of intracranial aneurysms and identifying large feeders to AVM's.

Indications vary from institution to institution and also depend upon the logistic involved. Colour Doppler systems are more bulky. Hence for ICU, theatre or immobile ward patient, smaller pulsed system is used though colour Doppler gives better waveform and velocity information. Pulsed Doppler system are better for monitoring cerebral purfusion reserve and emboli counting.

Cerebral purfusion reserve Prior to carotid endarterectomy the ability of cerebral vessels to dilate in response to breath-holding, CO_2 rebreathing or acetazolamide challenge is noted. Some vascular surgeons do not find this useful. They think adequacy of patency of anterior and posterior communicating arteries (collateral pathways) is enough.

Emboli counting It is done by identifying characteristic embolic noise correctly. It requires sensitive equipment, time (minimum 20 minute recording, optimally 60 minute), quality control and rigorous training. Emboli are more frequent with tight stenosis, before starting aspirin therapy. They might also be present with heart valves, though that remains unproven a related application of embolus detection is identifying patent form a men ovale.

Patient monitoring By pulsed, TCD is done when prolonged monitoring is required e.g. neuro-intensive care, during neurosurgical operations or carotid arterial operations. The MCA is insolated with probe fixed to temporal region with a head band. A fall in diastolic velocity and increase in pulsatility give indirect measure of cerebral flow and rising ICP.

TCD is used by some surgeons during carotid endarterectomy for monitoring. The effect of clamping carotid is monitored to assess the need for shunting. Also during shunt insertion and removal tiny air embolisms is a part of procedure through showers of multiple and recurrent embolism is a cause for concern. Particulate emboli produce coarser sound.

Postoperatively, cerebral blood flow is to be monitored.

Ischaemic stroke Colour TCD is better for this purpose. It is useful for monitoring the revascularisation therapy or to detect intracranial stenosis which might be the cause for TIA's in patients in whom no disease in the neck is present.

Subrachnoid haemorrhage To diagnose ischaemic neurological deficit. The intra- cranial velocities always rise following SAH and if severe enough can result in neurological defect or deterioration of consciousness. The diagnosis includes excluding other causes of neurological deterioration and by finding markedly elevated velocities (e.g. >150 cm/sec) in MCA. The velocities may be elevated in all or one artery. It may not be consistently predicted which patient will develop vasospasm, based on velocity measurements.

Aneurysms and AV malformations Though initial results have shown promise it is early to say whether ruptured or unruptured aneurysms can be reliably shown.

Cerebral venous thrombosis TCD can be used to assess the intracranial veins and venous sinuses. In sup. sagittal sinus blockage venous flow is increased in veins running parallel to MCA to the cavernous sinus this bypassing blocked sagittal sinus. A variety of abnormal drainage patterns may be identified though reliability of this is being questioned.

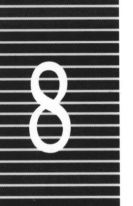

Transcranial Doppler Sonography

Vipul Gupta

INTRODUCTION

Transcranial Doppler sonography (TCD) is an emerging technique in which a hand held transducer is used to measure velocities within the circle of Willis and vertebrobasilar system through regions of calvarial thinning, orbits or foramen magnum. This technique is very useful in certain clinical conditions to assess the intracranial vasculature, because it is a non-invasive, non-ionizing and a portable technique that is safe for serial or prolonged studies. However, variations in arteries and lack of a good temporal window can be source of error or incomplete studies. Therefore, for proper use of TCD, understanding of its limitations, knowledge of cerebral haemodynamics and vascular anatomy as well as correlation with clinical situation is necessary.

Basic Instrumentation

For TCD, excellent signal-to-noise ratio is necessary. Therefore, the available TCD machines have a lower bandwidth and secondarily a larger and less well-defined sample volume than most other pulse Doppler instruments. TCD is performed using low frequency transducer (2-3 MHz), sensitive to Doppler frequencies upto 10 kHz without aliasing and adjustable levels of transmitted sound energy ranging from 10 mW/cm^2 to the currently recommended maximal level of 100 mW/cm^2. Commercially available TCD scanners with colour capability have recently been introduced (Fig. 8.1). Transcranial colour Duplex sonography technique allows correction of angle of insonation resulting in more accurate estimation of flow velocities. It is also more reproducible and shortens the examination time.[1]

Recently, TCD machines with dual monitoring capability have become available in which two transducers are used to monitor two arteries

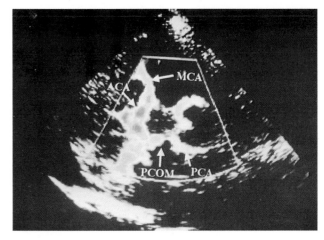

Figure 8.1
Colour Duplex TCD image (transtemporal window) shows circle of Willis including middle cerebral artery (MCA), anterior cerebral artery (ACA), posterior cerebral artery (PCA) and posterior communicating artery (PCOM)

simultaneously. These probes are synchronized to insonate during the silent period of the other probe. This dual monitoring capability gives better assessment in monitoring during carotid or cardiac surgery. They are also useful to distinguish carotid or cardiac source of emboli and shorten the examination time in emboli detection techniques. Special high frequency transducers (20 MHz) are also available to directly assess the intracranial arteries during surgery.[1]

Technique and Normal Parameters

Before starting the intracranial vascular examination, the examiner should ascertain the status of extracranial arteries, because changes in the extracranial system will reflect on intracranial vessels.

The preferred position for the examiner is at the head end of the bed. The patient's head should face forward or, to the side during the insonation. The patient should be resting comfortably to avoid major fluctuations of PCO_2 (alteration in arterial PCO_2 will alter intracranial flow) and movement artifacts.

Ultrasonic Windows

The transmission of ultrasound through the cranium is a significant problem. Experiments have shown that loss of ultrasound energy depends upon the thickness of the skull. Therefore loss of transmission varies greatly in different parts of the skull in the same patient, and from patient to patient. The temporal window is an attractive area for ultrasound evaluation because of absence of bony specula and is generally

the most useful site of the examination.[2] The other useful TCD approaches are transorbital, suboccipital, and submandibular approaches.[1,2]

Another important concept to understand is regarding the vessel identification. Most of the TCD machines used worldwide do not have the colour imaging capability. Therefore, instead of direct visual identification, other criteria are described for vessel identification as listed in Table 8.1.[1]

Criteria for vessel identification
Table 8.1 Cranial window used Depth of sample volume Direction of blood flow Distance over which the vessel can be traced (traceability) Relationship to TICA-MCA-ACA junction Angle of transducer Relative blood velocity (MCA > ACA > PCA = BA = VA) Response to compression maneuvers
Note: **ACA**-Anterior cerebral artery, **BA**-Basilar artery, **MCA**-Middle cerebral artery, **PCA**-Posterior cerebral artery, **TICA**-Terminal internal carotid artery, **VA**-Vertebral artery

Transtemporal Window

The gel-coated transducer is placed just anterior to the external auditory canal. At the depth of approximately 65 mm, flow can be detected towards the transducer, which is due to middle cerebral artery (Fig. 8.2). By decreasing the depth in approximately 5 mm

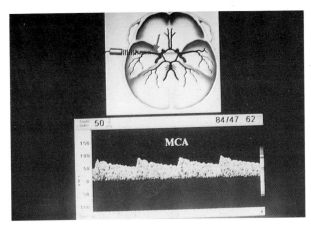

Figure 8.2
Middle cerebral artery: Picture depicting middle cerebral artery insonation through transtemporal approach and spectral waveform from the artery showing low resistance waveform with flow towards the transducer

increments, the artery can be traced, confirming that it is middle cerebral artery. After this the bifurcation of the terminal internal carotid artery is identified at depth of 60 to 65 mm by its bi-directional flow (Fig. 8.3). Terminal internal carotid artery shows bi-directional flow because sample volume generally includes origin of both middle and anterior cerebral arteries. Anterior cerebral artery can be insonated at depth of 75 mm by tilting the transducer antero-superiorly (Fig. 8.4). It shows the flow away from the transducer. After returning to the bifurcation of terminal internal carotid artery and tilting the transducer inferiorly, the examiner can obtain a tracing

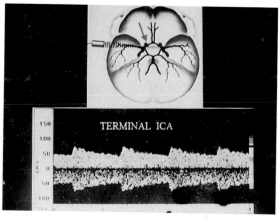

Figure 8.3
Internal carotid artery (terminal portion): Picture depicting terminal carotid artery insonation through transtemporal approach and spectral waveform from the artery showing typical bi-directional flow

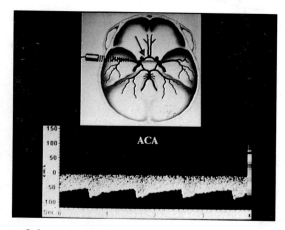

Figure 8.4
Anterior cerebral artery: Picture depicting anterior cerebral artery insonation through transtemporal approach and spectral waveform from the artery showing low resistance waveform with flow away from the transducer

of the terminal portion of the internal carotid artery. It characteristically exhibits the lowest velocity of the anterior vessels because of the large angle of insonation necessary for localization. Finally, the posterior cerebral artery (PCA) can be insonated at depth of 60 to 75 mm by tilting the transducer posteroinferiorly. The posterior cerebral artery can than be tracked to the basilar artery (BA) at approximately 75 mm depth and from there to the contralateral posterior cerebral artery (80 to 85 mm). The display of bilateral blood flow at the junction with the BA and the change in flow direction within the contralateral posterior cerebral artery can be useful features to identify the posterior cerebral artery.

Transorbital Window

Gel coated transducer is gently applied on the closed eyelid and lowest acoustic intensity (10 mW/cm^2) is used to minimize the risk of eye damage.[3] Ophthalmic artery is usually insonated at depth of 45 to 60 mm by scanning in the axial plane with slight medial angulation. By tilting the transducer slightly superiorly and inferiorly, the carotid artery is insonated at depth of 60 to 75 mm. Ophthalmic artery shows pulsatile (triphasic) flow, while internal carotid artery shows less pulsatile (biphasic) flow. Parasellar portion of the internal carotid artery shows flow towards the transducer, whereas flow in the genu portion is bi-directional and away from the transducer in the supraclinoid portion.[1]

Transforaminal (Suboccipital) Window

The transforaminal window is optimally accessed with patient seated and head flexed slightly forwards. The transducer is placed between the posterior margin of the foramen magnum and the posterior arch of the first cervical vertebra. This approach is useful to insonate the vertebral and the basilar arteries. By aiming the transducer at the nasal angle with slight lateral angulation, vertebral arteries can be localized at depth of 65 to 85 mm with the blood flow away from the transducer. If the transducer is angulated relatively inferiorly and the depth is decreased, the extracranial portion of the vertebral arteries can be localized. Basilar artery can be scanned at depth of 90 to 120 mm by scanning directly in the midline and can be tracked from the vertebral artery junction onwards.[1,2]

Submandibular Approach

By this approach the retromandibular and more distal extradural portion of the internal carotid artery can be evaluated. Transducer is placed in submandibular portion and angled superiorly and posteriorly near the angle of mandible and internal carotid artery can be tracked upto the depth of 80 to 85 mm where it bends to form the carotid siphon.[4]

The typical insonation depths and flow velocities are shown in Table 8.2.

In many individuals compression tests may be necessary to identify certain arterial segments unequivocally. These maneuvers are particularly valuable in assessing the collateral pathways. Compression tests during TCD examinations can be performed on the carotid arteries, low in the neck with two fingers, or on the vertebral arteries at the mastoid slope.[2] There is a slight risk of causing an embolism from plaques during the compression tests. Therefore, they should be performed by experienced investigators after performing a B-mode examination of the carotid arteries. The possible effects of compression manoeuvers on intracranial flow are listed in Table 8.3.

Subarachnoid Haemorrhage and Vasospasm

Most common cause of subarachnoid haemorrhage is the rupture of intracranial aneurysm into the subarachnoid space. It can also occur due to vascular malformations, vasculitis or trauma. In a significant percentage of patients, no definite cause is found. After the haemorrhage, focal or diffuse spasm of intracranial vessels can occur. This spasm peaks between 11 and 17 days after the bleed and then gradually subsidises.[5-7] In a significant percentage of patients, ischaemic deficits occur due to the vasospasm and it remains a significant clinical problem. TCD has been used to detect vasospasm based on increased flow velocities in these arteries due to decreased cross sectional area of the vessel (Fig. 8.5). Bedside TCD monitoring can accurately document the development and resolution of

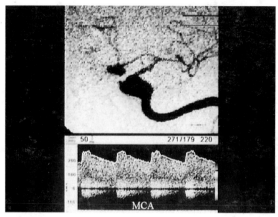

Figure 8.5

Subarachnoid haemorrhage-vasospasm: IADSA image in a case with subarachnoid haemorrhage showing aneurysm arising from anterior communicating artery with marked spasm of internal carotid, middle cerebral and anterior cerebral arteries. Spectral waveform from middle cerebral artery shows increased velocities (220 cm/s) and spectral broadening, diagnostic of spasm

Table 8.2							

Summary of vessels identification criteria

Artery	Window	Depth (mm)	Direction of flow (relative to transducer)	Relation to TICA-MCA-ACA Junction	Velocity (cm/sec)	Response to carotid Compression
MCA (M1)	Transtemporal	45-65	Towards	At	46-86	↓, 0
MCA-ACA bifurcation	Transtemporal	60-65	Bi-directional	At	—	↓, 0
ACA	Transtemporal	60-75	Away	Anterosuperior	41-76	↓, 0, r
PCA (P1)	Transtemporal	60-75	Toward	Posteroinferior	33-64	0, ↓ (foetal origin: ↓, 0)
PCA (P2)	Transtemporal	60-75	Away	Posteroinferior	33-64	0, (fetal origin: ↓, 0)
TICA	Transtemporal	60-65	Toward	Inferior	30-48	0, r
Ophthalmic artery	Transorbital	45-60	Toward	—	21-49	0
CS, Supraclinoid	Transorbital	60-75	Away	—	50-60	0, r
CS, Genu	Transorbital	60-75	Bi-directional	—	—	0, r
CS, Parasellar	Transorbital	60-75	Toward	—	50-60	0, r
Vertebral artery	Transtemporal	65-85	Away	—	27-55	—
Basilar artery	Transtemporal	90-120	Away	—	30-57	—

Note: Anterior and posterior communicating arteries are detectable only with transcranial Doppler sonography if they act as collateral routes of circulation (i.e. exhibiting increased blood flow).

Abbreviations: **ACA**– Anterior cerebral artery; **CS**–Carotid siphon: **MCA**–Middle cerebral artery; **PCA**–Posterior cerebral artery: **r**–Reversal of flow; **TICA**–Terminal internal carotid artery; ↓–decreased flow

Table 8.3 Effect of compression tests of the common carotidarteries on various vessels segments and their diagnostic meanings

Insonated vessels segment	Findings at rest	Effect of ipsilateral CCA compression test	Effect of contralateral CCA compression test	Functional meaning of compression test
MCA (M1/M2)	Normal flow velocity, flow toward probe	↓ Or ↓↓ or [STOP]	0 or [↓]	Confirmation of vessel identity
ACA (A1)	Normal flow velocity flow away from probe	[↓↓] or [STOP] or with D	[0] or ↑ or ↑↑ with or without D	Confirmation of vessel identity, presence or absence of potential anterior collateral pathway
ACoA	No signal available	[↑↑ with D and flow toward probe]	↑↑ With D and flow away from the probe	Confirmation of existence of ACoA
	Indistinguishable from contralateral ACA	0 or ↑ or ↑↑	[↓↓] or [STOP] or with D	See ACA
	Indistinguishable from ipsilateral ACA	See ACA	0 or ↑ or ↑↑	See ACA
PCA (P1)	Normal flow signal, flow toward probe	0 or ↑ or ↑↑	0 or ↑	Confirmation of vessel identity and presence or absence of potential collateral pathway
PCA (P2)	Normal flow signal, flow away from probe	0 or ↑, or ↓↓ or [STOP] if ICA supplied	0 or [↓]	Confirmation of vessel identity and type of PCA supply differentiation of basilar and/or ICA blood supply
PCoA (transtemporal or transorbital)	No signal available Indistinguishable from PCA or AMCA branches without compression maneuvers Alternating flow	In nonembryonal type: With D or ↑↑ With D With flow toward probe in vicinity of PCA With flow toward probe during transorbital insolation In embryonal type" ↓ or ↓↓ or *↓ or # ↓	No reaction thus far	Confirmation of existence of PCoA differentiation of posterior and anterior collateral pathway, differentiation of basilar or ICA blood supply
DVA	Normal flow signal away from probe	0 or ↑	0 or ↑	Confirmation of existence of vessel
BA conclusive insonation	Normal flow signal away from probe	0 or ↑ or [↑↑]	0 or ↑ or [↑↑]	Confirmation of existence of posterior collateral pathway differentiation from carotid vascular tree within large depth
ICA, C2-C4 segments of collateral siphon, (transorbital approach)	Normal flow toward probe away from probe, or bi-directional	[STOP] or ↓↓ and/or [with D]*	0 or ↑	Exclusion of silent ICA occlusion, analysis of potential pathways
ICA-C1, (transtemporal approach)	Low-frequency flow toward probe Indistinguishable from MCA (M1)	[STOP] or ↓↓	0 or ↑	Analysis of potential collateral pathways differentiation from MCA often possible

CCA–common carotid artery; MCA–middle cerebral artery; ACA–anterior cerebral artery; ↓–slight decrease of flow velocity; [ ]–very rare event; 0–no effect; ACA–anterior cerebral artery; #↓–reversal of flow towards or away from transducer; D–local distortion of blood flow due to relative stenosis; ↑–slight increase of flow velocity; ↑↑–strong increase of flow velocity; ACoA–anterior communicating artery; PCA–posterior cerebral artery; P1–precommunicating part of PCA; P2–postcommunicating part of PCA; ICA–internal carotid artery; *↓–alternating flow; DVA–distal vertebral artery; BA–basilar artery. This list reflects our present experience but may not be complete. It refers to findings in normal subjects.

*Due to jet of PCoA collateral channel, overlap of ↓↓ and ↓↓ signals is possible.

vasospasm, aiding in assessment of risk of ischaemic neurological complications. It is also useful to time the surgery or to take decisions regarding therapies such as induced hypervolemia and hypertension, calcium channel blockers, transluminal angioplasty or intra-arterial papaverine treatment.[1]

TCD is most accurate in detecting vasospasm in the middle cerebral artery as compared to other intracranial arteries. The relatively superficial and predictable location of middle cerebral artery, compared to other arteries of the circle of Willis, allows easier localization. Also, unlike the anterior cerebral arteries and other arteries, middle cerebral artery rarely acts as a route for collateral circulation.[1, 5-7] Therefore, accelerated blood flow in the middle cerebral artery is typically due to vasoconstriction rather than increased blood flow. TCD sensitivity and specificity to detect vasospasm have been reported in range of 84 to 94 per cent and 89 to 90 per cent, respectively, in two large studies.[8,9] Statistically significant correlation between flow velocities and stenosis has also been demonstrated for terminal internal carotid artery, posterior cerebral artery, vertebral artery and basilar artery.[10, 11] The relative lack of accuracy in anterior cerebral artery can be due to anatomic variations (atretic A1 segments), or aberrant course (with suboptimal angle of insonation) or because anterior cerebral artery may frequently act as collateral route of blood supply.[10]

In general, mean middle cerebral artery flow velocities upto 120 cm/s correlate with mild angiographic vasospasm. Mean middle cerebral artery flow velocities between 120 cm/s and 200 cm/s correlate with moderate angiographic vasospasm (25 % to 50% diameter narrowing), whereas flow velocities more than 200 cm/s imply severe angiographic vasospasm (greater than 50% narrowing).[12]

In addition, the rate of rise of velocities can predict the site of vasospasm induced ischaemia. A rise of more than 25 per cent over previous day and greater than 200 cm/s often occur 2 days before onset of clinical vasospasm and infarction in the middle cerebral artery territory[13] (Fig. 8.6). To exclude the possibility that increased flow velocity in middle cerebral artery relates to vasospasm rather than increased flow, the middle cerebral artery to internal carotid artery velocity ratio can be determined. Normally, the ratio is 1.7 ± 0.4; a ratio above 3 indicates middle cerebral artery vasospasm that would be

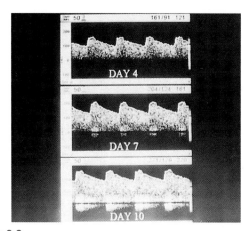

Figure 8.6
Subarachoid haemorrhage with vasospasm- serial studies: Spectral waveforms from left middle cerebral artery in a case with subarachnoid haemorrhage shows mildly increased velocity (121 cm/s) at day 4 (a). Progressive increase in velocity (161 cm/s) seen at day 7 (b) and day 10 (220 cm/s). This patient developed ipsilateral middle cerebral artery infarct. Therefore, evolution of vasospasm can be observed by TCD and rapid rise in flow velocities can be a warning signal for significant vasospasm and subsequent infarction

visible angiographically, whereas ratio over 6 suggests severe vasospasm with attendant risk of infarction.[5]

However, it is important to be aware that some studies have demonstrated lack of correlation between flow velocities, clinical grade, change in blood flow and neurological deficit.[10] Errors may arise because of arterial variations or different resting diameters in different population groups. Coexisting proximal haemodynamically significant lesion (due to preexisting extra or intracranial disease or due to vasospasm of proximal intracranial internal carotid artery) may also result in false negative studies. Increased intracranial pressure in cases with subarachnoid haemorrhage may also change cerebral perfusion pressure and result in change in flow velocities. Change in blood pressure, volume status or PCO_2 variations may also give rise to change in flow velocities with resultant difficulty in interpretation. Therapeutic interventions may also result in change in flow velocity and the sonographers should be aware of any of these factors before making a diagnosis. The sonographer and clinician must carefully consider the patient's clinical findings, the flow velocities from all vessels in their likelihood of reflecting vasospasm, the limitations of TCD technique, and, in some cases correlation with CBF and neuro imaging data.[10] Analysis of all available data may then permit optimal interpretation and use of TCD results.

Arterial Stenosis and Occlusion

Although, middle cerebral artery or carotid siphon stenosis are responsible in only a small percentage of ischaemic strokes, a timely diagnosis may be crucial in preventing a major ischaemic event. This is important because in Asian populations, intracranial vascular diseases are two or three times more common than European populations.[14] Previously, these clinical conditions went undiagnosed because angiography which was used to study intracranial arteries, is an invasive investigation with potential complications. Non-invasive means to investigate intracranial stenosis such as TCD have radically changed the situation. If intracranial stenosis is detected, appropriate medical therapy can be started or in selected cases intracranial angioplasty can be done.

Middle Cerebral Artery Stenosis/Occlusion

Middle cerebral artery is a common site for intracranial stenosis. TCD can diagnose middle cerebral artery stenosis with high reliability with reported sensitivity for stenosis/occlusion 94.1/85.7 per cent and specificity for stenosis/occlusion 96.7/100 per cent.[15] Most important finding to diagnose middle cerebral artery stenosis is a "focal" segment with increased velocities (Fig. 8.7), other various features are also described as listed in the Table 8.4.[15]

Velocities exceeding the corresponding site of the contralateral artery by 30 cm/s and unassociated with turbulence or low-frequency noise indicate a moderate

Criteria for diagnosis of stenosis in the main stem of the middle cererbal artery
Table 8.4 **Acceleration of flow**
Flow velocity change must be "circumscribed"
Flow velocity becomes damped distal to the stenosis
Side-to-side difference of mean flow velocity of at least 30 cm/s
Circumscribed, disturbed flow
Spectral broadening
Increased low-frequency components (during systole in low grade stenosis, during the entire cycle in high grade stenosis)
Arterial wall covibrations
Non harmonic low frequency noise
Musical murmurs

stenosis with a diameter narrowing of approximately 40 to 50 per cent. High-grade stenosis (more than 50 per cent diameter narrowing) produces all the abnormalities listed in Table 8.4. Very high-grade stenosis (90% or more) result in velocities of 200 cm/s or more.

Acute middle cerebral artery occlusion may not produce any signal. To exclude technical factors for lack of insonation, ipsilateral anterior cerebral artery and posterior cerebral artery should at least be insonated. Increased velocities in anterior cerebral artery and posterior cerebral artery may indicate collateral flow through leptomeningeal anastomosis and further supports the diagnosis of middle cerebral artery occlusion.[16, 17] Limitations of middle cerebral artery stenosis diagnosis on TCD include inability to distinguish it from very distal carotid siphon stenosis and difficulty in diagnosing stenosis beyond M1 segment.

Carotid Siphon Stenosis

The ultrasonic features of carotid siphon stenosis are similar to those of middle cerebral artery stenosis. Typical findings in a case of siphon occlusion include markedly reduced flow velocities in proximal ICA and the common carotid artery. The flow signal is characterized by reverberating systolic low flow within the blind stump and by absence of any flow during the diastole. In patients with intact circle of Willis with carotid occlusion reversal of flow in the ipsilateral A1 segment of anterior cerebral artery may also be demonstrated.

Unpredictable topography of carotid siphon and the osseous openings within the orbits may cause difficulty in evaluation of carotid siphon stenosis. In addition, ipsilateral posterior communicating artery, when

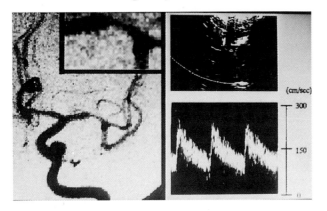

Figure 8.7
Middle cerebral artery stenosis: IADSA image in a patient with transient ischaemic attacks in left middle cerebral artery shows significant stenosis of middle cerebral artery. Special waveform (shown on the left side) had shown significantly increased velocities (200 cm/s) in this artery

it functions as a collateral channel may have increased flow velocities and it may be misdiagnosed as carotid stenosis due to its proximity to the carotid artery.

Moya-moya disease is a progressive cerebrovascular disorder with bilateral occlusion of the basal circulation and development of collateral blood supply. This disease may be diagnosed by TCD (Figs 8.8a to h).[18,19] Intracranial internal carotid and middle cerebral arteries may show high or low velocities depending upon the stage of disease. Increased flow velocities are seen in the earlier stage while decreased flow velocities in these arteries are seen in the later stage. Increased flow velocities may also be seen in posterior cerebral and ophthalmic arteries because of the collateral flow.

Posterior Circulation

The distal vertebral artery can be a site for atherosclerotic disease or dissection. Significant stenosis of verte-

bral or basilar artery may be diagnosed by occipital approach. However, TCD evaluation of these vessels is difficult and requires considerable expertise. Ultrasonic features of stenosis or occlusion are similar to describe above. Dolicoectasia of all or portion of the vertebrobasilar system may suggested by TCD when

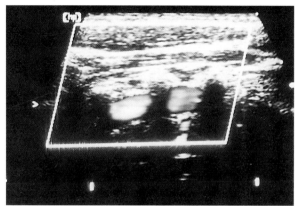

c

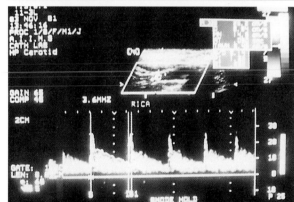

d

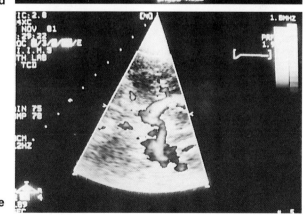

e

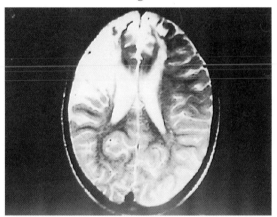

a

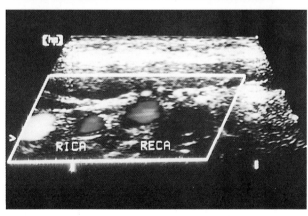

b

Figures 8.8a and b
Moya-moya disease: Axial T2-weighted image (a) in a child with repeated strokes show multiple infarcts. Colour Doppler image (b) in neck region shows internal carotid artery is smaller than external carotid artery

Figures 8.8c to e
Moya-moya disease: Vertebral artery is dilated (c) spectral waveform from cervical internal carotid artery (d) shows decreased flow velocity (23 cm/s), due to decreased flow. Colour TCD image (e) shows dilated posterior cerebral arteries in contrast to poorly visualized middle and anterior cerebral arteries

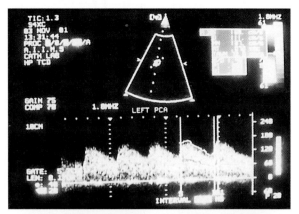

f

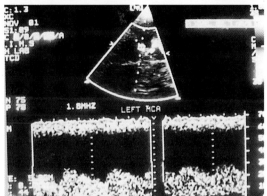

g

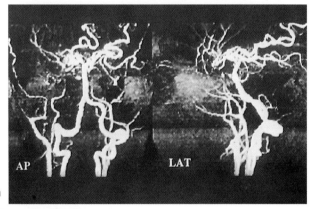

h

Figures 8.8f to h

Moya-moya disease: Spectral waveform from posterior cerebral artery (f) shows increase flow velocities (160 cm/s) because it is providing collateral flow while middle cerebral artery (g) shows decreased flow velocity (28 cm/s) because of the proximal obstruction. These findings considered together are consistent with B/L intracranial internal carotid artery stenosis/occlusion (Moya-moya pattern). MRA (h) confirms the diagnosis. This case illustrates the need to evaluate the extracranial arteries for proper interpretation of TCD findings

a significantly lower than normal flow velocities are demonstrated, particularly on patients with clinical evidence of brainstem ischaemia or cranial nerve

deficits.[20] TCD has also been used to prove that decrease in blood flow due to neck rotation or hyperextension and concomitant vertebral artery narrowing is the cause of symptoms in positional vertebrobasilar ischaemia[21] and the adolescent stretch syndrome.[22]

Assessment of Effects of Extracranial Occlusive Disease

Carotid Stenosis or Occlusion

Extracranial carotid Duplex sonography is a sensitive and specific investigation to detect stenosis of proximal internal carotid artery due to atherosclerotic disease or dissection. TCD is a useful adjunct to this investigation because it can be used to evaluate the effect of such lesions on cerebral haemodynamics by measuring intracranial flow velocities (Figs 8.9a to c), demonstrating the presence or absence of collateral routes of circulation, and testing autoregulation.[23-26] It can also be used to demonstrate embolic phenomenon and to depict "tandem" lesions.[23-26]

When a high-grade stenosis or occlusion of the internal carotid artery is present, TCD may demonstrate a decrease in mean blood flow velocity, with diminished pulsatility because of vasodilatation in the distal arterial circulation. Increased velocities in contralateral anterior cerebral artery, ipsilateral posterior cerebral artery, anterior communicating and posterior communicating arteries[23-26] may demonstrate presence of collateral circulation. The presence of functioning anterior communicating artery is indicated by increased velocity in contralateral anterior cerebral artery and reversal of flow in the ipsilateral anterior cerebral artery. Similar findings are shown in posterior communicating artery collateral flow from posterior cerebral artery to internal carotid artery. TCD can be used to demonstrate the presence or lack of improved intracranial blood flow after extracranial-intracranial arterial bypass surgery.[27]

Subclavian Steal Syndrome

The subclavian steal can occur when a high-grade stenosis or occlusion of a subclavian artery occurs proximal to the vertebral artery origin. Flow in basilar artery is usually not affected unless there is a high-grade stenosis in the vertebral artery supplying the steal.[28, 29] Duplex examination of vertebral artery is the primary method used to diagnose this disease. TCD can be used as adjunct and both methods can be used to suggest

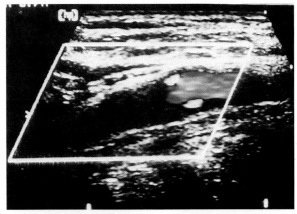

a

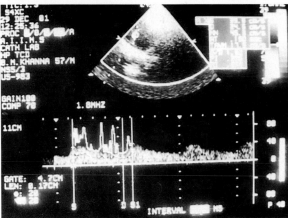

b

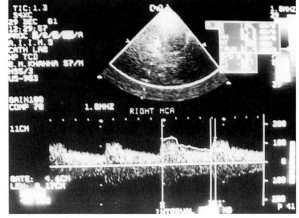

c

Figures 8.9a to c
Cervical internal carotid artery block: intracranial hemodynamic effect: Colour doppler image (a) of left cervical internal carotid artery showing block in its proximal portion. TCD examination shows decreased velocity (39 cm/s) and therefore reduced flow in left middle cerebral artery (b) as compared to the contralateral (c) middle cerebral artery (102 cm/s)

whether lesion is incomplete or complete. Incomplete steal effects cause a decrease in systolic blood flow velocity and, when more severe, alternating blood flow direction in the vertebral artery on the side of the subclavian lesion. When the complete reversal of blood flow is demonstrated, it is called as complete steal.[28, 29] Basilar artery blood flow is resistant to any critical changes resulting from the steal mechanism. In fact, it has been reported that even in symptomatic patients most vertebrobasilar symptoms are caused by cerebral microangiopathy rather than a large artery flow disturbance.[2, 30]

Emboli Detection

TCD can be used to detect microemboli in the intracranial arteries. Both solid (atheromatous material) and gaseous emboli can be detected. Microemboli can be detected because they are much larger than the red blood cells and much more sound is reflected from them, which produce a pathognomonic high amplitude "spike" (Fig. 8.10). Doppler instrumentation used for emboli detection should have a high dynamic range (in excess of 50 dB) and the receiver should enable measurement of the signal power increase caused by emboli, which may be more than 40 dB.[31,32] Gain or automatic control may further extend the dynamic range, and this is mandatory for gaseous embolus detection because these usually overload the Doppler instrumentation.

Although use of emboli detection in day to day clinical work is still not very well-defined, potential uses of embolic signal monitoring are listed in Table 8.5.[32]

Artifacts, too, may cause power increase in the Doppler spectrum and may be mistaken as emboli. They are usually due to electrical interference, fast movements of the probe, or bumping of the probe.

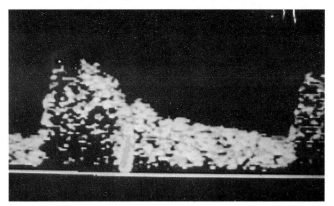

Figure 8.10
Microemboli: Detection of middle cerebral artery embolus (bright signal) in a patient with internal carotid artery plaque

Potential uses of emboli detection

Table 8.5
1. Localization of embolic source
2. Identification of at risk patients
   a. Carotid stenosis
   b. Cardiac embolism
   Prosthetic cardiac valves
   Native valve disease
   Atrial fibrillation
   Postmyocardial infarction
   Other cardiac embolic disease
3. Monitoring during procedures
   a. Cardiopulmonary bypass
   b. Carotid endarterectomy
   c. Coronary angiography
   d. Carotid angioplasty
4. Monitoring effectiveness of treatment
   Anticoagulation or antiplatelet therapy

These artifacts can be distinguished from microemboli because the signal arising due to them is bi-directional, low frequency, and coincident with transducer impacts, motion, or electrical switching transients.[31, 32]

Intraoperative and Procedural Monitoring

Carotid Endarterectomy

Intraoperative complications of carotid endarterectomy are mainly due to ischaemia during cross-clamping, hyperemic phenomenon, or embolization of atheromatous or gaseous materials. TCD has been used to assess ischaemia after cross-clamping in these patients, by monitoring the middle cerebral artery flow and status of collateral routes.[32-36] If ischaemia is suspected by this technique, a surgeon may take adequate precautions such as temporary shunt placement. Hyperemic phenomenon can occur after the surgery. It occurs because of sudden normalization of blood flow in part of brain in which autoregulation is impaired due to chronic ischaemia. This may result in cerebral oedema or haemorrhage and can be detected by TCD by demonstration of sudden and prolonged increase in flow velocities in the middle cerebral artery.[36,37] As stated before, microemboli detection during surgery by TCD is useful because it can warn the surgeon to modify the surgical technique.[32] It has been shown that significant deterioration in postoperative cognitive function may occur in patients in whom TCD detected 10 or more particulate microemboli during initial carotid detection.[38] Postoperatively, Doppler can be used to monitor the operative site in the neck and if indicated, the middle cerebral artery flow.[33-35]

Direct Intraoperative Doppler Sonography

Doppler probe may be placed directly on the intracranial vessels to evaluate them during neurosurgery. For this purpose, special transducers (upto 20 MHz) are needed which are capable of insonating the blood vessel by direct contact.[39] Velocity measurements using these systems may be inaccurate because of relatively large size of range-gated sample volume in relation to vessel size, but it is possible to determine vessel patency, direction of flow, presence of laminar or non-laminar flow, and change in flow velocity during the procedure.[39] Intraoperative Doppler sonographic technique has been used to monitor the graft during extracranial-intracranial bypass surgery.[39] It has also been used in aneurysm surgery to assess patency of the parent vessel after clip placement or to evaluate the anastomosis and distal cerebral flow during vascular bypass of unresectable aneurysms.[39]

Neuroradiologic Procedures

It has been demonstrated by TCD that large number of microemboli enter intracranial circulation during catheter angiography.[40] Most of these emboli are thought to be gaseous and occur most commonly during catheter flushing and injection of contrast medium. Although no case of transient or permanent ischaemic deficits have occurred because of these emboli TCD can be used to improve angiographic techniques and to improve catheters, guide wires and flushing systems used during these procedures. TCD has also been used during the interventional procedures such as to monitor intracranial flow during balloon occlusion, so as to determine the efficacy of collateral flow.[41] It has also been used during angioplasty, thrombolysis and arteriovenous malformations treatment.[41,42]

Cardiopulmonary Bypass

TCD enables a dynamic evaluation of cerebral blood flow during cardiopulmonary bypass as well as to detect emboli, which may occur during aortic cannulation or cardiac manipulation, or other surgical maneuvers.[32]

Brain Death

The accurate diagnosis of brain death is important, more so in view of issues that surround the transplantation of organs. TCD can be used to confirm cerebral circulatory arrest, although the diagnosis of brain death must be made by the physician on basis of clinical findings as well as result of diagnostic studies. Arrest of intracranial flow results in a characteristic pattern of to and fro blood flow which can be documented in the middle cerebral artery and other patent basal cerebral arteries.[43-45] This oscillating pattern is caused by systolic forward flow in the large basal arteries and diastolic reversal of flow produced by the microcirculatory obstruction and reflex contraction of the basal arteries.

Arteriovenous Malformations

In arteriovenous malformations, feeding arteries, nidus and draining veins display unusual haemodynamics related to increased blood flow velocity and vessel diameter, decreased arterial pressure, increased venous pressure and diminished or absent autoregulation. TCD shows increased flow velocities with reduced pulsatility in the feeder vessels.[46-48]

Maneuvers performed during TCD studies to document normal autoregulation produce no response in the vessels of arteriovenous malformations.[49] These abnormalities permit localization of arteriovenous malformation and assessment of the haemodynamic status. TCD has also been used to monitor the effects of surgical or endovascular interventions.[50] However, one should be aware that angiography remains the primary investigation for detection, assessment, and follow-up in cases of cerebral arteriovenous malformations.

Cerebral Trauma

TCD has been used to demonstrate increased intracranial pressure after trauma.[1, 51] In the early stage of increased intracranial pressure, increase in systolic velocity, a decrease in diastolic velocity, and increased pulsatility are demonstrated without an increase in the mean velocity (Fig. 8.11). With further increase in intracranial pressure, diastolic velocity approaches zero as the intracranial tissue pressure equals diastolic pressure. Finally, reversal of diastolic flow demonstrable in the late stages of increased intracranial pressure heralds compromise of intracranial circulation.[1,51]

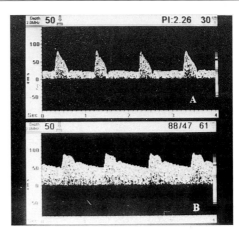

Figure 8.11
Trauma–raised intracranial pressure: Spectral waveform image of middle cerebral artery (a) in a case with significant head trauma shows decreased diastolic flow while the systolic velocities are well maintained (increased pulsatility). This finding indicates raised intracranial pressure in this clinical setting. Normal spectral waveform (b) is shown below for comparison

After severe head injury, impairment of autoregulation may occur which will allow passive increase or decrease in cerebral blood flow secondary to changes in systemic pressure. Defects in autoregulation may be specifically suggested by TCD examination.[2]

After a head injury generalized decrease in cerebral blood flow velocities often occur and typically is followed by progressive increase in velocities beginning 2 to 3 days after the injury with peak velocities by day 5 or 7.[52, 53] These velocity increases is thought to be due to vasospasm. In most cases permanent deficits due to this vasospasm are rare.

Functional Reserve Testing

The term cerebral autoregulation refers to the ability of cerebral arteries to maintain cerebral blood flow and therefore cerebral perfusion, at a relatively constant level despite fluctuation in cerebral perfusion pressure. If systemic pressure and consequently cerebral perfusion drops, dilatation of cerebral arteries occur which result in maintenance of cerebral blood flow.

TCD is an ideal test for detecting rapid changes in cerebral perfusion and cerebral autoregulation, because this technique allows observation of changes in flow velocities in realtime. Functional tests are aimed at evaluation of this reserve mechanism using various stimuli such as hypocapnia or hypercapnia, increased or decreased systemic arterial pressure.[2] A patient can be made to breathe room air followed by increasing concentrations of CO_2. Because of increased arterial PCO_2, peripheral vasodilatation, resulting in increased intracranial flow will occur. This will manifest as increased flow velocities in the cerebral arteries in TCD examination.[54] Therefore, autoregulatory response in a particular person can be assessed. Intactness of autoregulatory response implies that a drop in systemic arterial pressure can be counter balanced by vasodilatation of cerebral arteries to maintain adequate blood flow. The vasomotor response may become exhausted if the resistance vessels of brain are already maximally dilated as in cases with extracranial occlusive arterial disease.[2,55] This test can also be used in evaluating haemodynamic effects of various conditions in which reduced cerebral perfusion may occur, such as occlusive arterial diseases, migraine, hypoxia, high altitude exposure and, head trauma and in cases with arteriovenous malformation.[2]

Other Uses

TCD has also been used to assess hydrocephalus, pathophysiology of headaches, intracerebral aneurysms and cerebral veins. However, discussion of all these diseases is beyond the scope of this chapter. Readers are referred to several excellent texts covering these topics.[1,56]

CONCLUSION

TCD can be a tremendously useful investigation in many intracranial diseases such as vasospasm, stroke, and in monitoring during various operative and endovascular interventional procedures. It is also very useful to evaluate cerebral haemodynamics in various disease states for research purposes. It is an investigation, which is relatively inexpensive and free of risks. It can be repeated over the time and can be easily performed at the bedside or wherever a procedure or surgery is being performed (Table 8.6).

However, it also suffers from many inherent difficulties, few of which are common to Doppler examination elsewhere in the body, but some are particular to TCD evaluation as listed in Table 8.7.[4] It is operator dependent, and the examiner should be aware of anatomy and physiology of cerebral vascular system. To properly interpret the information, clinical correlation and as well as the status of extracranial arteries should be known and the examiner should be well aware of the limitations of this examination technique.

REFERENCES

1. Lupetin AR, Beckman I, Asturi R *et al:* Transcranial Doppler sonography. In Orrison WW Jr (Ed): *Neuroimaging:* Philadelphia WB Saunders, 411-43, 1998.

Clinical applications of transcranial Doppler

Table 8.6 • Diagnosis of intracranial occlusive disease (individual and epidemiological aspects)
• Auxiliary test for extracranial occlusive disease in inconclusive extracranial test
• Evaluation of haemodynamic effects of extracranial occlusive disease of intracranial blood flow (e.g. internal carotid artery occlusion, subclavian steal)
• Detection and identification of feeders of arteriovenous malformations
• Preoperative compression tests for evaluation of collateralizing capacities of circle of Willis
• Detection of right to left shunts in the heart (e.g. patent foramen ovale) and paradoxical embolism
• Intermittent monitoring and follow-up of:
  – Vasospasm in subarachnoid haemorrhage and migraine
  – Spontaneous or therapeutically induced recanalization of occluded vessels
  – Establishment of collateral pathway after occluding interventions
  – Occlusive disease during anticoagulative or fibrinolytic therapy
• Continuous monitoring during:
  – Neuroradiologic interventions (e.g. balloon occlusion, embolization)
  – Short-term pharamacologic trials of vasoactive drugs and anaesthetics
  – Carotid endarterectomy (shunt)
  – Cardiac surgery (ischaemic encephalopathy, Embolism)
  – Increasing intra-anterior cerebral artery pressure
  – Evolution of brain death
• Functional test:
  – Stimulation of cerebral vasomotors with CO_2 or other vasoactive drugs (e.g. acetazolamide)
• Neuropsychologic tasks for hemispheric dominance (with simultaneous bilateral and TCD recording)

Table 8.7 Common sources of error and trouble spots

- **Anatomic**
  - Variations and incomplete circle of Willis
  - Missing or hypertrophied anterior cerebral artery
  - Posterior cerebral artery stemming directly from the internal carotid artery
  - Atretic vertebral artery
- **Technical**
  - Absent temporal windows
  - Not identifying the best temporal window
  - Small temporal window
  - Too transparent a temporal window
- **Instrumentation**
  - Large sample volume
  - Exceeds Nyquist limits
  - Improper use and adjustment of gain control
  - Unknown Doppler angle
- **Interpretive errors**
  - Misinterpretation of hyperdynamic collateral channels as stenosis
  - Displacement of arteries caused by space-occupying lesions
  - Misdiagnosis of vasospasm as stenosis
  - Poor gold standard of angiography

2. Otis SM, Ringelstein EB: Transcranial Doppler Sonography. In Zwiebel WJ (Ed): *Introduction to vascular ultrasonography* (4th Edn): Philadelphia WB Saunders, 177-201, 2000.
3. Spencer MP, Whisler D: Transorbital Doppler diagnosis of intracranial artery stenosis. *Stroke* 17: 916-21, 1986.
4. Otis SM, Ringelstein EB: The Transcranial Doppler examination: Principles and applications of Transcranial Doppler sonography. In Tegeler CH, Babikian VL, Gomez CR (Eds): *Neurosonology* Mosby: St. Louis, 113-128, 1996.
5. Sieler RW, Newell DW: Subarachnoid hemorrhage and vasospasm. In Newell DW, Aaslid R (Eds): *Transcranial Doppler* 101-07, New York: Raven, 1992.
6. Aaslid R, Huber P, Nornes H: Evaluation of cerebrovascular spasm with transcranial Doppler ultrasound. *J Neurosurg* 60: 37-41, 1984.
7. Harders AG, Gilsbach JM: Time course of blood velocity changes related to vasospasm in the circle of Willis measured by transcranial Doppler ultrasound. *J Neurosurg* 66: 718-28, 1987.
8. Lindergaard KF, Nornes H, Bakke SJ *et al:* Cerebral vasospasm diagnosis by means of angiography and blood velocity measurements. *Acta Neurochir (Wien)* 100: 12-24, 1989.
9. Creissard P, Proust F: Vasospasm diagnosis: Theoretical sensitivity of transcranial Doppler evaluated using 135 angiograms demonstrating vasospasm. *Acta Neurochir (Wien)* 131: 12-18, 1994.
10. Sloan MA: Transcranial Doppler monitoring of vasospasm after subarachnoid hemorrhage. In Tegeler CH, Babikian VL, Gomez CR (Eds): *Neurosonology* St. Louis: Mosby 156-71, 1996.
11. Sloan MA *et al:* Transcranial Doppler detection of vertebrobasilar vasospasm following subarachnoid haemorrhage. *Stroke* 25: 2187-97, 1994.
12. Newell DW: I Distribution of angiographic vasospasm after subarachnoid hemorrhage: implications for diagnosis by TCD. *Neurosurgery* 27: 574-77, 1990.
13. Seiter RW *et al:* Cerebral vasospasm evaluated by transcranial ultrasound correlated with clinical grade and CT-visualized subarachnoid hemorrhage. *J Neurosurg* 64: 594-600, 1986.
14. Caplan LR, Gorelick PB, Hier DB: Race, sex and occlusive cerebrovascular disease: A review. *Stroke* 17: 648-55, 1986.
15. Ley-pozo J, Ringlestein EB: Non-invasive detection of occlusive disease of the carotid siphon and middle cerebral artery. *Ann Neurol* 28: 640-47, 1999.
16. Biass L, Duterte DL, Mohr JP: Anterior cerebral artery velocity changes in disease of the middle cerebral artery stem. *Stroke* 20: 1737-40, 1989.
17. Zanette EM, Fieschi C, Bozzao L *et al:* Comparison of cerebral angiography and transcranial Doppler sonography in acute stroke. *Stroke* 20: 899-903, 1989.
18. Takase K, Kashihara M, Hashimoto T: Transcranial Doppler ultrasonography in patients with Moya-moya disease. *Clin Neurol Neuro Surg* 99(Suppl)2: S101-05, 1997.
19. Muttaqin Z, Ohba S, Arita K *et al:* Cerebral circulation in Moya-moya disease: A clinical study using transcranial Doppler sonography. *Surg Neurol* 40(4): 306-13, 1993.
20. Rautenberg W, Aulich A, Rotter J *et al:* Stroke and dolichoectatic intracranial arteries. *Neurol Res* 14(Suppl): 201-03, 1993.
21. Weintraub MI, Khoury A: Transcranial Doppler assessment of positional vertelsrobasilar ischaemia [Letter]. *Stroke* 26: 330-31, 1995.
22. Sturzenegger M, Newell DW, Douville CM *et al:* Transcranial Doppler and angiographic findings in adolescent stretch syncope. *J Neurol Neurosurg Psychiatry* 58: 367-70, 1995.
23. Schneider PA, Rossman ME, Torem S *et al:* Transcranial Doppler in the management of extracranial cerebrovascular disease. Implication in diagnosis and monitoring. *J Vasc Surg* 7: 223-31, 1988.
24. Cantelmo NL, Bakikian VL, Johnson WC *et al:* Correlation of transcranial Doppler and non-invasive tests with angiography in the evaluation of extracranial carotid disease. *J Vasc Surg* 11: 786-92, 1990.
25. Thiel A, Zickman B, Stutman WA *et al:* Cerebrovascular carbon dioxide reactivity in carotid artery disease–Relation to intraoperative cerebral monitoring results in 100 carotid endarterectomies. *Anesthesiology* 82: 655-61, 1995.
26. Silvestrini M, Troisi E, Cupini LM *et al:* Transcranial Doppler assessment of the function effect of carotid stenosis. *Neurology* 44: 1910-14, 1994.

27. Cooperberg EB, Rudenev IN, Lavrentev AV *et al:* Evaluation of hemodynamic effects of extracranial-intracranial arterial bypass in unilateral internal carotid artery occlusion. *Cardiovasc Surg* **1**: 704-08, 1993.

28. Von Reutern, GM, Pourcelot L: Cardiac cycle-dependent alternating flow in vertebral arteries with subclavian artery stenosis. *Stroke* **9**: 229-36, 1978.

29. Klingelhofer J, Conrad B, Benicke R *et al:* Transcranial Doppler ultrasonography of caroticobasilar collateral circulation in subclavian steal. *Stroke* **19**: 1036-42, 1988.

30. Ringlestein EB, Busker M, Buchner H: Evaluation of hemodynamic effects of subclavian steal mechanism as basilar artery blood flow with the help of transcranial Doppler sonography. Presented at the first International Conference on Doppler sonography. Rome, Italy, 1986.

31. Russell D, Brucher R: Embolus detection with Doppler sonography. Methods and Clinical Potential . In Tegeler CH, Babikian VL, Gomez CR (Eds): *Neurosonology* Mosby: St. Louis, 235-38, 1996.

32. Markus H, Russell D, Brucher R: Doppler embolus detection: Stroke treatment and prevention.In Tegeler CH, Babikian VL, Gomez CR (Eds): *Neurosonology:* St. Louis, Mosby 239-51, 1996.

33. Sundt TM, Sharbough FW, Anderson RE *et al:* Cerebral blood flow measurements and electroencephalographic changes during carotid endarterectomy. *J Neurosurg* **41**: 310-20, 1974.

34. Zuccarello M, Yeh H, Tew TM: Morbidity and mortality of carotid endoarterectomy under local anesthesia. A retrospective study. *Neurosurgery* **23**: 445-50, 1988.

35. Ferguson GG: Intraoperative monitoring and internal shunts: Are they necessary in carotid endarterectomy? *Arch Surg* **122**: 305-07, 1987.

36. Magre TR, Davies AH, Baird RN *et al:* Blood flow in the internal carotid artery and velocity in the middle cerebral artery during carotid endarterectomy. *Cardiovasc Surg* **2**: 37-40, 1994.

37. Jansen C, Springers AM, Moll FL *et al:* Prediction of intracerebral hemorrhage after carotid endarterectomy by clinical criteria and intraoperative transcranial Doppler monitoring. Results of 233 operations. *Eur J Vasc Surg* **8**: 220-25, 1994.

38. Jansen C, Ramos LMP, van Heesewijk JPM *et al:* Impact of microembolism and hemodynamic changes in the brain during carotid endarterectomy. *Stroke* **35**: 992-97, 1994.

39. Gilsbach JM: Intraoperative Doppler sonography in *Neurosurgery* New York: Springer-Verlag, 1-88, 1983.

40. Dagirmanjian A, Davis BA, Rothfus WE *et al:* Silent cerebral microemboli occurring during carotid angiography: Frequency as determined with Doppler sonography *AJR* **161**: 1037-40, 1993.

41. Giller CA, Sterg P, Batjer HH *et al:* Transcranial Doppler ultrasound as a guide to graded therapeutic occlusion of the carotid artery. *Neurosurgery* **20**: 307-11, 1990.

42. Giller CA, Purdy P, Giller A *et al:* Elevated transcranial Doppler ultrasound velocities following therapeutic arterial dilatation. *Stroke* **26**: 123-27, 1995.

43. President's Commission: Guidelines for the determination of brain death. *JAMA* **246**: 2184-87, 1981.

44. Powers AD, Graeberg MC, Smith RR: Transcranial Doppler ultrasonography in the determination of brain death. *Neurosurgery* **24**: 884-89, 1989.

45. Petty GW, Mohr JP, Pedley TA *et al:* The role of transcranial Doppler in confirming brain death. Sensitivity, specificity and suggestions for performance and interpretation. *Neurology* **41**: 300-03, 1990.

46. Lindegaard KF, Grolimund P, Aaslid R *et al:* Evaluation of cerebral AVM's using transcranial Doppler ultrasound. *J Neurosurg* **65**: 335-44, 1987.

47. Hassler W, Steinmetz H: Cerebral hemodynamics in angioma patients: An intraoperative study. *J Neurosurg* **67**: 822-31, 1987.

48. Hassler W: Hemodynamic aspects of cerebral angiomas. *Acta Neurochir* **37 (Suppl)**: 1-136, 1986.

49. Hassler W, Burger R: Arteriovenous malformations. In Newell DW, Aaslid R (Eds): *Transcranial Doppler* New York: Raven, 123-35, 1992.

50. Petty GW, Massaro AR, Tatimichi TK *et al:* Transcranial Doppler ultrasonographic changes after treatment for arteriovenous malformations. *Stroke* **21**: 260-66, 1990.

51. Hassler W, Steimetz H, Gawlowski J: Transcranial Doppler ultrasonography in raised intracranial pressure and in intracranial circulatory arrest. *J Neurosurg* **68**: 745-51, 1988.

52. Steiger HJ, Aaslid R, Stooss R *et al:* Trans-cranial Doppler monitoring of head injury. Relations between type of injury, flow velocities, vasoreactivity and outcome. *Neurosurgery* **34**: 79-85, 1994.

53. Compton JS, Teddy PJ: Cerebral artery vasospasm following severe head injury: A transcranial Doppler study. *Br J Neurosurg* **1**: 435-39, 1987.

54. Markwalder TM, Grolimund P, Seiler RW *et al:* Dependancy of blood flow velocity in the middle cerebral artery on the end-tidal carbon dioxide partial pressure–a transcranial ultrasound Doppler study. *J Cereb Blood Flow Metab* **4**: 368, 1984.

55. Bullock R, Mandelow AD, Bone I *et al:* Cerebral blood flow and CO_2 responsiveness as an indicator of collateral reserve capacity in patients with carotid arterial disease. *Br J Surg* **72**: 348, 1985.

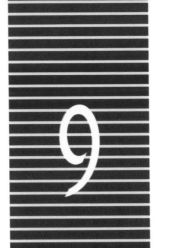

Doppler in Liver

Suchi Bhatt
Poonam Narang
Shalini Verma
Shashank Jain

Liver

Sonography is considered to be the most effective primary investigation of choice is elucidation of liver pathology. Colour Doppler sonography is a superb, non-invasive alternative to anteriography and phlebography.

The hepatic artery and portal veins are best interrogated by Doppler ultrasound of the porta hepatis using oblique intercostal scans.

Technique

The abdominal vessels are insonated using established techniques. The Doppler sample volume is adjusted to encompass but not exceed the diameter of the vessel studied. The pulse-repetition frequency (PRF) is adjusted manually when aliasing occurs. Low PRF and lowest available filter of Doppler receiver are used. A low frequency (3 MHz) is chosen for examination of deep vessels and for detection of high velocities and a high frequency (5-7.5 MHz) transducer is used for the examination of superficial vessels, studies of children or detection of low blood flow velocities.

The portal vein is the most readily accessible vessel in the portal system. The entire length of the portal vein can be examined from an entire abdominal subcostal approach, using a right paramedian, slightly oblique plane.

The splenic vein is examined at the splenic hilum by angling the transducer to follow the long axis of the vessel.

The superior mesenteric vein is examined through a longitudinal right paramedian upper abdominal approach.

The hepatic veins usually are explored easily through an oblique, subcostal or intercostal approach, yielding excellent Doppler signals. The inferior vena cava is insonated along its visible length noting any localised increase in calibre and/or flow velocity.

The hepatic artery is insonated at its origin at the coeliac axis and where it crosses the portal vein. Intrahepatic branches are examined adjacent to portal venous branches. The splenic artery was examined concomitantly with the vein, at the splenic hilum and within the spleen.[1]

Normal Patterns

Portal Veins

Approximately 25 per cent of the flow into the liver is supplied by hepatic artery, the remainder by the portal vein. Normal portal venous flow is hepatopetal and is usually monophasic with some fluctuation due to respiration and cardiac activity

(Figs 9.1a and b). Thus when colour flow is being used to assess the portal vein, flow into the liver will conventionally appear red.

Hepatic Artery

The hepatic artery can be identified in most patients at porta hepatis lying between the portal vein and common bile duct. In a small percentage of patients, this anatomy may be altered and the hepatic artery may lie anterior to the bile duct. Colour flow imaging allows rapid differentiation of bile duct from hepatic artery. The hepatic artery waveform characteristically has a high diastolic phase due to the low resistance of the hepatic vascular bed.

Hepatic Veins

The hepatic veins characteristically have a triphasic waveform which reflects right atrial and inferior vena cava pressures (Fig. 9.2). This results in flow in the hepatic veins being predominantly coded blue, i.e. away from the probe on the colour Doppler.[2]

Physiological Variations

1. *Respiratory variations* Calibre variations of vessels of the portal venous system during deep inspiration are easily observed with realtime equipment. A significant calibre increase is noted

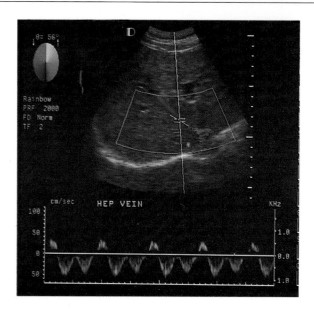

Figure 9.2
Pulsed Doppler tracing of Rt hepatic vein in a normal subject showing the characteristic three-phase profile according to the phases of the cardiac cycle

during inspiration in normal patients. This increase (50-100%) is particularly clear at the level of the splenic and superior mesenteric veins. During expiration, the calibre of the splenic and superior mesenteric veins always rapidly decreased. Calibre variations in the portal trunk were either very slight or completely absent.[3]

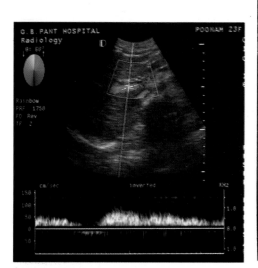

Figure 9.1a
Duplex Doppler showing normal portal venous waveform

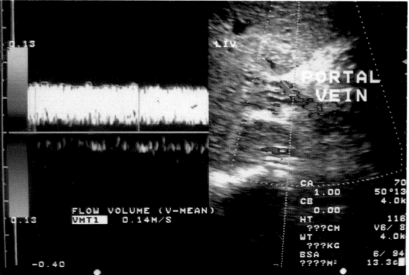

Figure 9.1b
Duplex Doppler evaluation of portal vein showing portal venous flow pattern. Loss of phasic variation is noted

2. *Variations due to posture* In normal patients, shift from supine to sitting position significantly decrease portal venous velocity, cross sectional area of portal vein and portal venous flow. This effect of posture is attributed to absence of values in the splanchnic venous system.[4]

3. *Variations due to physical exercise* During physical exercise, vasodilation in the muscular vessels takes blood away from the splanchnic system. Hence immediately after exercise, the cross-sectional area of the portal vein and portal venous flow were significantly decreased. After ten minutes post-exercise, portal venous velocity, the cross sectional area of the portal vein and portal venous flow seen to return to the basal pre-exercise values.[4]

4. *Post-prandial variations* Studies show that eating causes vasodilatation and flow increase in the splanchnic system. An increase in the diameter of portal vein and increase flow in both splanchnic arteries and veins has been reported. This is attributed to increase in mean flow velocity caused mostly by the increase in the diastolic component of the mesenteric arterial flow.[5]

5. *Humoral variations* Significant increase in portal velocity and flow has been noted after glucagon and secretin administration.[6]

PORTAL HYPERTENSION

Realtime sonography has become increasingly useful in the examination of patients with long standing liver disease and/or portal hypertension.

Portal hypertension develops when increased resistance to portal flow and/or increased portal blood flow occur. Recent evidence suggests that both the mechanisms are involved in the maintenance of chronic portal hypertension they result in enlargement of the extrahepatic portal vessels, the development of spontaneous porto-systemic collaterals and slow portal vein flow.

Sonographic Findings in Portal HT

Portal vein diameter is measured in basal conditions (quiet respiration, supine and fasting). In patients with advanced cirrhosis and portal hypertension, a threshold of 13 mm is used. Dilatation of portal vein to over 13 mm occured in 56 per cent of patients (Figs 9.3 and 9.4). Some authors have demonstrated that presence of oesophageal varies is correlated with

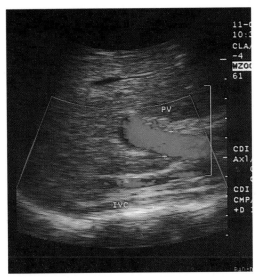

Figure 9.3
Dilated portal vein in a case of portal hypertension

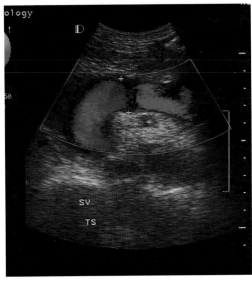

Figure 9.4
Grossly dilated splenoportal axis with normal direction of flow

dilatation of portal vein, a calibre over 17 mm is 100 per cent predictive for large varices. A normal calibre of portal vein does not, however, exclude portal hypertension. The main intrahepatic portal branches are normally also dilated.

Varying degrees of dilatation of splenic and superior mesenteric veins also occur in portal hypertension. The upper limit of normal splenic and superior mesenteric veins range from 10-12 mm. Splenomegaly is usually associated with dilatation of splenic vein (Fig. 9.5), possible because of increased splenic blood flow. Ascites, hepatomegaly with altered liver architecture

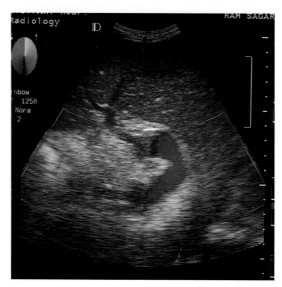

Figure 9.5
Dilated and tortuous splenic vein with splenomegaly

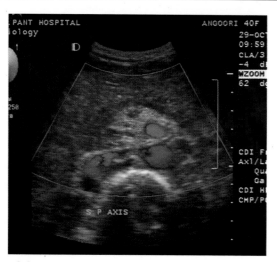

Figure 9.6
Chronically thrombosed splenoportal axis showing thin lumen with no flow

are indicators of steatosis and cirrhosis. Opening up of vessels between high pressure portal venous system and low pressure systemic circulation is usually seen with portal hypertension. Occasionally collaterals may be seen in gallbladder wall. Direct visualisation of oesophageal varices is often difficult or impossible, though their presence may be inferred by demonstrating thickening of the oesophageal wall, irregularity of the lumen and variation of of oesophageal wall thickness with respiration.

Doppler Findings in Portal Hypertension

The clinical applications of Doppler studies of the splanchnic vessels include the assessment of the presence, direction and characteristics of blood flow. The haemodynamic parameters provided by Doppler ultrasound (US) can be classified as qualitative, semiquantitative, and quantitative. The qualitative data include evaluation of the presence, the direction and the characteristics of the blood flow and their alterations. Semiquantitative measurements include vascular impedance which is calculated by means of pulsatility and resistance indices. Quantitative data includes calculation of the maximum and mean flow velocity and of the flow volume in larger diameter veins.

QUALITATIVE FINDINGS

Portal System Thrombosis

Establishing the presence of blood flow within the portal veins is the simplest Doppler finding and is

usually easy to perform. Colour Doppler directly shows the blood flow inside the vein, distinguishing the portal vein from other channel like structures such as dilated biliary ducts at porta hepatis.

In cases of chronic portal thrombosis, when ultrasound shows the portal vein to be small and hyperechogenic, (Fig. 9.6) Doppler flowmetry at porta hepatis shows no blood flow. An indirect sign of thrombosis of the portal vein consists of presence of high frequency arterial signals in both porta hepatis and the intrahepatic branches, due to the increase in arterial circulation in the attempt to compensate for portal thrombosis. When cavernous transformation takes place, colour Doppler shows turbulent flow inside the small serpentine vessels which cross the thrombosed veins (Fig. 9.7a).

Partial thrombus appears as an absence of colour signal and this can equally be identified when the thrombus is anechoeic. Neovascularisation within the thrombus, a pathognomic sign of tumour thrombus, may be identified as arterial signals within the thrombus (Fig. 9.7b). Given its reliability, sensitively and non-invasiveness, Doppler is considered as the most suitable technique to assess the prevalence of portal thrombosis in cirrhosis.

Directions of Blood Flow

Flow direction is another unequivocal qualitative finding provided by Doppler ultrasound. Kawasaki *et al* reported a prevalence of spontaneous hepatofugal flow of 6.1 per cent in liver cirrhosis.[7] Hepatofugal

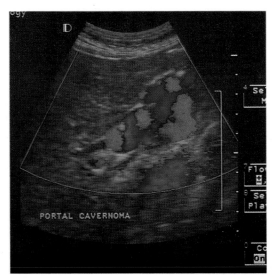

Figure 9.7a
Portal cavernoma formation in main portal vein thrombosis

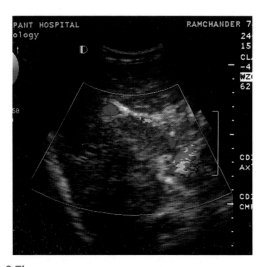

Figure 9.7b
Colour Doppler flow image shows and echogenic tumour thrombus partially occluding the portal vein. The thrombus is contiguous with a heterogenous mass lesion in the adjacent color flow is also seen within the tumour thrombus

portal flow is associated with a decreased risk of variceal bleeding, while it does not predict survival.[8] Reversed portal flow is generally associated with a significant reduction in the diameter of the portal vein. A close correlation was demonstrated between hepatofugal flow of the splenic vein and hepatic encephalopathy, probably in relation to the drainage of a great deal of blood in the large splenorenal collaterals. Colour Doppler clearly shows flow inversion which show the colour opposite to that of the arterial branches, in which the blood flow increases to compensate for the inversion of portal flow. These intrahepatic flow inversions are probably determined by arterioportal shunts where the signal becomes turbulent and rapid.[9]

Porto-systemic Collaterals

The diagnosis of portal hypertension must include search for collateral beds. Realtime US and Doppler can explore the paraumbilical veins and the splenorenal collaterals and those of left gastric vein and of the gastro-oesophageal plexus. Doppler flowmetry though cannot provide precise measurement of the collateral bed flow rate, however, contributes to provide an approximate idea of the haemodynamic importance of collateral vascular bed.

Paraumbilical veins are generally quite large and run in a straight line towards the umbilical region (Figs 9.8a and b). On other occasions, the paraumbilical vascular bed appears as one or more irregular vessels

which cross hepatic parenchyma. The presence of a high velocity venous flow makes it possible to differentiate between these beds and peripheral portal branches in which the venous flow is much slower, the paraumbilical bed flow is rarely hepatopetal.

The collateral vascular beds of the left gastric vein are often difficult to study due to obesity, especially in patients in whom the left lobe of the liver is not greatly enlarged. Moreover, the origins and the course of the left gastric vein is variable hence makes it difficult to study. These may be seen as dilated and tortuous vessels in epigastrium or left gastric vein may be visualised at its origins, running towards the diaphragms with hepatofugal flow (Figs 9.9 and 9.10).

At level of lower splenic pole, the splenorenal collaterals (Fig. 9.11) appear as tortuous vessels with a high velocity Doppler signal and a broad spectrum of frequencies due to tubulence. Their presence is often associated with flow reversal in the splenic vein.

Other collateral vessels may occasionally be identified at the level of the gastric fundus, in the pancreatic region or in the pericholecystic area (Figs 9.12 to 9.14).

Flow Characteristics

The characteristics of the tracing and of the spectral distribution of the frequencies are directly consequent to the vessel haemodynamics. Each vessel has its own characteristic tracing which leads to its recognition.

Hepatic veins in normal conditions show a three-phase tracing dependent on the cardiac cycle and

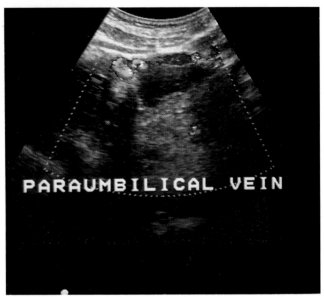

Figure 9.8a
Patent paraumbilical vein in a case of advanced cirrhosis

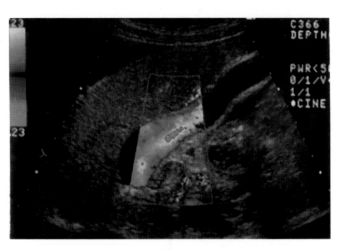

Figure 9.8b
Colour Doppler imaging in patient with advanced cirrhosis. Enlarged para-umbilical vein flow gradients, increased parenchymal vascularity and turbulent hepatic arterial flow are all present

particularly on the pressure variations in the right atrium. This phasic fluctuation of the flow is either notably reduced or completely abolished in case of liver cirrhosis with portal hypertension.

The impedance changes in the splanchnic vessels have been studied in the three main arterial beds: the superior mesenteric, splenic and hepatic.

The superior mesenteric artery supplies a large part of the intestine and subsequently the portal system. Elevated sinusoidal pressure triggers a reduction of mesenteric arterial resistance leading to a hyper-dynamic splanchnic circulation. Thus the portal vein

flow is increased and this contributes to the main-tenance of portal hypertension.[10] This dilatation of intestinal arterioles decrease the impedance indices in the superior mesenteric artery.[11] A decrease in pulsatility index is seen to accompany worsening liver function and development of oesophageal varices.

Doppler impedance indices measured in the intra-parenchymal branches of the splenic artery were found to be increased in patients with cirrhosis, and they correlate closely with splenoportal vascular resistance.[12]

Hepatic arterial impedance indexes are increased in patients with liver cirrhosis. This increase becomes

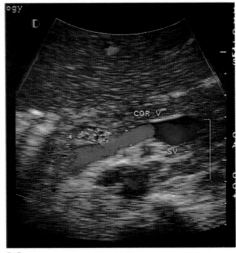

Figure 9.9
Dilated coronary vein in a patient of portal hypertension with history of repeated variceal bleeding

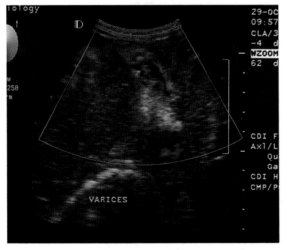

Figure 9.10
Tortuous varices at gastro-oesophageal junction

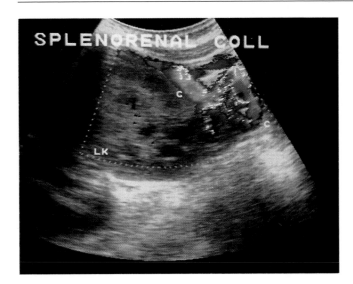

Figure 9.11
Splenorenal collaterals

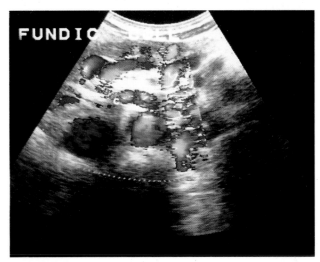

Figure 9.12
Voluminous collaterals at gastro-oesophageal junction and at fundus of stomach

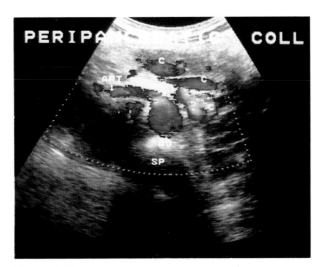

Figure 9.13
Peripancreatic collaterals

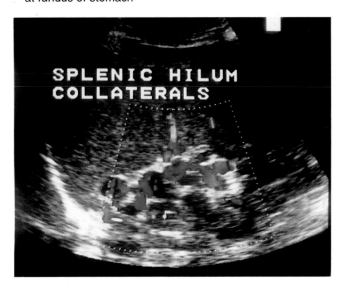

Figure 9.14
Splenic hilar collaterals

even more pronounced if portal vein thrombosis occurs.[13]

SEMIQUANTITATIVE FINDINGS

Evaluation of the flow alteration can also be performed by semiquantitative methods based on the analysis of the velocity profile and on calculation of the relations between maximum, minimum and mean spectrum frequency. Numerous indices have been proposed to describe the characteristics of arterial flow:

$$\text{Pulsatility index (PI)} = \frac{A - B}{\text{mean}}$$

A = Peak systolic velocity
B = Peak diastolic velocity

Mean = Mean of velocity in a set interval of time

$$\text{Resistance index (RI)} = \frac{A - B}{A}$$

PI of the superior mesenteric artery was significantly reduced in patients affected by liver cirrhosis.

QUANTITATIVE FINDINGS

A complete haemodynamic evaluation of the portal venous system in portal hypertension should include measurements of:

a. The volume of portal venous flow (Qpv).

b. The portal perfusion pressure (pressure gradients between the portal vein and the hepatic veins (Ppv – Phv)

c. The portal vascular resistance (Pvr)[14]

$$Pvr = Ppv–Phv/Qpv.$$

Non-invasive measurements using Doppler ultrasound presupposes uniform insonation in which the entire volume of blood in a cross section of the vessel is exposed to a uniform ultrasonic beams. The time-averaged mean velocity (V), calculated from the mean Doppler shift, is multiplied by the cross sectional area (A) of the vessel to give the volume flow (Q)

$$Q = VA$$

Sources of error include the non-uniform insonation, measurement of the cross sectional area of the vessel and the assessment of the beam angle.[15]

A further critical point is the calculation of the mean velocity. Both direct calculation by the software of the instrument and its estimation as a fixed fractions of the maximal velocity may be inaccurate. Estimates of the average peak velocity have been found to be reasonably reproducible, particularly after a preliminary training programme standardise methodology[16] (Table 9.1).

Ultrasound cannot directly measure portal pressure, however, an indirect assessment can be made using the 'congestion index'. The 'congestion index' is the ratio between the cross-sectional area and the mean flow velocity of the portal trunk. It takes into account the fact that in portal hypertension the portal vein tends to dilate and the blood velocity to decrease, so that higher values are found in patients with more severe portal resistance, pressure and larger varices.[17]

For the portal vein, its straight course for 3-4 cm, relatively long diameter and the oblique course with respect to the abdominal wall are factors which make the Doppler study easy to perform. Measurement of the flow velocity should be made according to the reported guidelines (*See* Table 8.1).

Quantitative measurements of the portal flow can provide a contributors not only to the diagnosis of portal hypertension but also the evaluation of haemorrhage risk and the efficacy of pharmacological therapy and surgical porto-systemic anastomosis.

Evaluation of Medical Treatment in Portal Hypertension

Many drugs which are effective on the systemic circulation also influences the splanchnic haemodynamics and have been proposed for the treatment of portal hypertension. Doppler flowmetry is a reliable method of evaluating flow changes after the administration of these drugs.

Bru *et al* reported a net reduction in portal flow and portal pressure as a consequence of IV administration of vasopressin.[18] Trans-oesophageal Doppler probe showed a reduction of 55 per cent in portal flow and 15 per cent in azygos vein flow.[19]

Using realtime US and Doppler flowmetry to determine the diameter, the velocity and flow volume in the portal vein after administration of propranolol, a significant reduction in flow velocity and volume was found.[20]

Evaluation of Porto-systemic Surgical Shunts

Ultrasonography is a useful method in the follow-up of patients after porto-systemic shunt surgery, allowing assessment of patency in 75 per cent of cases. The shunt is deemed patent when a direct confluence between portal vein and IVC or between the splenic and left renal vein is demonstrated (Fig. 9.15).

Guidelines for Doppler measurements of Portal vein (from Sabba *et al* 1995[16])
Table 9.1

1. Measure in suspended normal respiration
2. Longitudinal scan of the portal vein
3. Sample volume in the centre of the vessel, at the level of the hepatic artery, covering 50 per cent of the vessel diameter
4. Doppler angle of 55° or less
5. Pulse repititions frequency (PRF) = 4 kHz, wall filter = 100 Hz
6. Doppler and B-mode tracings recorded simultaneously
7. Average maximum velocity obtained by manual tracing of the envelope of the Doppler waveform
8. Doppler waveform calculation obtained by covering two cardiac cycles between three arterial wall artefact
9. Portal vein diameter measured from the inner anterior to the inner posterior wall
10. Values result from the mean of three consistent measurements.

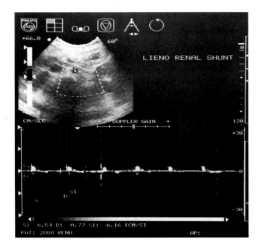

Figure 9.15
Duplex Doppler of lienorenal shunt showing low velocity turbulent flow

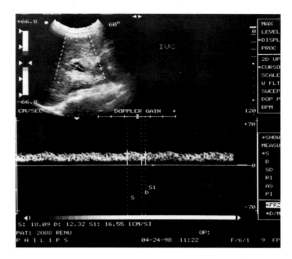

Figure 9.16
Right portal vein branch demonstrates hepatofugal flow in the same patient

When the shunt itself is not displayed, indirect signs of patency may be used. In porto-caval shunts, a decrease in calibre of the portal vein and widening of the IVC above the level of anastomosis is a useful sign of patency.[21] Dilatation of the left renal vein is consistent with a patent distal splenorenal shunt, while reversed flow in the superior mesenteric vein indicates a patent mesocaval shunt.

Doppler has proved useful in preoperative evaluation of patients as well as postoperative follow-up. Provided pre-operative baseline studies have been performed, it is possible within certain limits to assess flow through the shunt and to gauge changes in portal perfusion.

Indirect signs of patency can be found in patients by examining the direction of flow in the portal vein or characteristics of flow towards the shunt. Presence of hepatofugal flow in the intrahepatic portal branches is side-to-side portocaval shunt is a reliable indicator of patency of the shunt.[22] Conversely, hepatopetal portal flow detected is a late postoperative study raises the suspicion of thrombosis of the shunt, especially if flow was hepatofugal at a previous examination.

In end-to-side portocaval shunts, portal flow is usually absent or hepatofugal in the intrahepatic branches. Demonstration of reversal of flow in the splenic and sometimes portal veins is proof of patency of a conventional splenorenal shunt (Fig. 9.16). Distal splenorenal shunts which are performed to decompress gastroesophageal varices while maintaining hepatopetal flow in the mesoportal venous bed are not always visualised on realtime ultrasound.

However, splenic vein displays phasic flow synchronous with caval pulsatility indicating shunt patency.[23]

Transjugular Intrahepatic Porto-systemic Shunt (TIPS)

A minimally invasive option for complications of portal hypertension including variceal bleeding and refractory ascites has been developed: positioning a metallic stent between a hepatic vein and an intrahepatic portal vein branch (usually the right) by a percutaneous transjugular approach. This avoids open surgery and is safe for patients with severe liver failure. A major problem of TIPS is stenosis or occlusion of the shunt. While occlusion is irreversible, early diagnosis of stent stenosis allows angioplasty. Follow up by repeated venography is the most reliable approach but is an expensive and invasive procedure. Routine follow-up is therefore by repeated sequential Doppler examinations.

Immediately after TIPS placement, both portal vein diameter and velocity have been reported to increase resulting in a marked increase in portal vein flow volume.[24]

Blood flow in the main portal vein is hepatopetal but flows towards the shunt in the intrahepatic segments in patient with well functioning TIPS. Flow in other collaterals such as left gastric, paraumbilical veins may decrease, cease or reverse. Mean flow velocity in the shunt is high after TIPS placement.[25]

Duplex Doppler is accepted as a reliable technique in the long-term surveillance for complications such as stent thrombosis or stenosis and hepatic vein stenosis. The absence of detectable flow within a stent by Doppler sonography has proved to be sensitive and specific for occlusion.[26] A stent velocity less than 50 cm/s achieved a sensitivity of 100 per cent and a specificity of 93 per cent in the diagnosis of hepatic vein stenosis. Other diagnostic criteria are progressive reduction of peak velocity in the stent and a stent velocity less than 60 cm/s.[27] Localised acceleration of flow suggests stent stenosis while high flow velocity throughout the stent simply represents high volume flow without pathological significance. contrast enhanced power Doppler sonography has been reported to improve sensitivity and specificity in the diagnosis of stent dysfunction.[28]

Endoscopic Doppler Ultrasound

The recent introduction of endocavitary Duplex transducers has opened new perspectives for haemodynamic investigation. More recently, endocavitary Duplex transducers have been connected with fibreoptic endoscopes and are capable of providing an endoscopic visualization at the same time as the realtime imaging and Doppler flowmetry. This has made it possible to obtain haemodynamic data for the oesophageal and gastric varices, the perioesophageal vascular beds and the azygos vein with a relatively non-invasive and innovative method.[29]

The instruments currently available for endocavitary Doppler flowmetry are based on 7.5 MHz convex transducers with a 100° visual angle, incorpo-

rated longitudinally in an optical fibre endoscope. The sonographic scanning direction is longitudinal along the greater axis of the oesophagus. The perioesophageal collateral vascular bed are visualised as echopoor channel like structures with a longitudinal course, often tortuous and irregular the study of the azygos vein is performed by using the reference points provided by the US images obtained when the transducer is in contact with the oesophageal wall.

Budd-Chiari Syndrome (BCS)

It is a syndrome with clinical features of ascites, abdominal pain, hepatomegaly and jaundice that follows obstruction of the hepatic veins. If the inferior vena cava is also involved, distended superficial veins and oedema of the lower extremities may be present.[30]

The Budd-Chiari syndrome includes hepatic venoocclusive diseases, hepatic veins thrombosis, secondary obstruction of the inferior vena cava and the hepatic veins due to tumour or trauma (secondary Budd-Chiari syndrome) and primary membranous or segmental obstruction of the hepatic portion of the inferior vena cava (primary Budd-Chiari syndrome).[31]

The cause, clinical features and treatment depend on the site of the hepatic vein obstruction, at level of the small centrilobular veins, major hepatic veins or IVC.

Obstruction at the level of the central and sublobular veins may be due to toxins, particularly only pyrrolidine alkaloids. These effects are potentiated by protein-deficient diets.[32]

Obstruction of the major hepatic veins occurs most frequently in patients with coagulation abnormalities particularly polycythemia rubra vera and paroxysmal nocturnal haemoglobinuria.[33] It is also seen in Egyptian children from poor rural areas.[34] It may also be secondary to obstruction at the level of the hepatic venous ostia or within the IVC. The treatment of hepatic venous thrombosis is anticoagulant medication.[35]

Obstruction of the IVC which can extend into the orifice of the hepatic veins may be due to thrombosis, tumour extension, external compression, displacement or an obstructing membrane.

The necessity for an initial, often extensive radiologic evaluation is not surprising given the broad spectrum of anatomic abnormalities associated with Budd-Chiari syndrome.[36] After the diagnosis is established, most patients with Budd-Chiari syndrome require a decompressive shunt which is constructed to divert blood away from a congested liver via the

---

KEY POINTS

- Normal portal vein—hepatopetal, monophasic flow with some fluctuations.
- In PHT
  - dilated spleno portal axis, hepatofugal flow.
  - Porto systemic collaterals, high velocity signals with broad spectrum of frequencies.
  - Cirrhosis with PHT—phasic variation of hepatic vein is reduced or absent.
  - SMA shows, decrease pulsatility index.
  - Doppler flowmetry evaluates success of medical and surgical treatment.

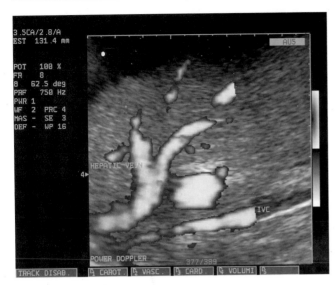

Figure 9.17
Power Doppler image: Hepatic veins draining into inferior vena cava (IVC)

portal vein. The frequency of complications in these complex decompressive shunts is relatively high and adds further to the overall radiographic procedures.[37]

Since the 1950s, angiography has been the mainstay of diagnosis in patients with Budd-Chiari syndrome, both before and after surgery. Angiography in fact, remains the definitive technique. Unfortunately, angiography is invasive and frequently the hepatic veins cannot be opacified beyond their ostia. Numerous less-invasive technique, including nuclear medicine, sonography and more recently MR imaging have had various degrees of success in characterising the underlying vascular lesions in Budd-Chiari syndrome.[38]

Doppler imaging is an appealing technique in patients with Budd-Chiari syndrome. Duplex sonography can be used to assess the presence direction and characteristics of flow within the hepatic veins and the IVC. Figure 9.17 shows power Doppler image of the normal hepatic veins confluence with the IVC.

Doppler Findings in Budd-Chiari Syndrome

1. Hepatic veins: Colour Doppler images showed absence of flow in the hepatic veins. Direction of flow, if present and areas of occlusion can be clearly visualised. Reversed flow can be detected in the hepatic veins. A flat hepatic vein waveform lacking normal phasic fluctuation indicates distal compression and supports diagnosis of BCS.[39]

2. Intrahepatic collaterals: Intrahepatic venous collaterals typical of Budd-Chiari syndrome are either intrahepatic veins that communicate or collateral vessels that shunted blood from occluded veins to non-occluded veins or to enlarged inferior right hepatic veins or caudate lobe veins.

3. Portal vein: Evaluation of portal vein is essential in patients with Budd-Chiari syndrome because portal vein thrombosis precludes decompression of liver via a porto-systemic shunt.

4. Inferior vena cava: The diagnosis of Budd-Chiari syndrome is based on an analysis of the flow direction and of the wave profile in the IVC. Abnormalities seen in IVC include no flow, reversed flow, very slow flow, visualisation of echogenic thrombus, compressions by caudate lobe, long segment narrowing without associated enlargement of caudate lobe and localised marked narrowing consistent with a web.[40]

Obstruction of the IVC at the opening of the hepatic veins is seen as a reversed and flat flow in the lower section of the IVC. In cases of partial obstruction, the tracing of IVC loses its phasic oscillations and become turbulent with high velocity.

This flat wave profile was found in all the intrahepatic vessels resembling the hepatic veins. This aspect has been defined as a major criteria for the diagnosis of Budd-Chiari syndrome with Doppler US.[41]

Role of Colour Doppler in Decompressive Shunts

Colour-flow Doppler with either 5.0 or 3.0 MHz transducer showed the patency of the shunts dramatically. The anastomosis with the native vessel is visualised clearly in patients with patent graft. Duplex scanning with a 5 MHz transducer clearly showed appropriately directed flow in all cases. Spectral analysis showed a triphasic pattern in all of the shunts which is a reflection of right atrial contractility.[42]

COLOUR DOPPLER IN HEPATIC LESIONS

The detection of a primary or metastatic liver tumour is a common clinical problem in which sonography, computerised sonography and magnetic resonance imaging are used for optimal detection. Benign pathological processes occur frequently in the liver and need to be differentiated from malignant tumours. Colour flow and Duplex Doppler can help in this

KEY POINTS

– BCS
  • HV—absent or reversed flow lacking phasic variation
  • IVC—No flow, reversed flat flow, very slow flow, or in partial obstruction-turbulent high velocity flow without phasic variation.

Intrahepatic collaterals present
  – Focal liver lesions

regard.[43] The incidental finding of a liver mass may result in a major dilemma of patient management.[44]

Echogenic focal areas of the liver are found in focal fatty infiltration, haemangiomas and a number of rare benign or tumour like conditions such as liver cell adenoma or focal nodular hyperplasia as well in malignant tumours. Commonly encountered echogenic malignant tumours include a primary hepatocellular carcinoma as well as common metastases such as those from gastrointestinal primaries, particularly from colonic primaries.

A vessel passing through an echogenic area without deviation suggests that the parenchymal abnormality is due to focal fatty infiltration, this condition should be considered especially in diabetes or alcoholics. Focal fatty infiltration may change rapidly with time.

Focal nodular hyperplasia (FNH) is a benign tumour of the liver. It is characterised pathologically by a cholangiolar proliferations associated with hyperplastic hepatocytes, blood vessels and fibrosis.[45] The favoured pathogenetic concept for FNH is that it develops from a focal excess of arterial blood flow from a pre-existing arterial malformation. Sonography is a reliable noninvasive method for evaluating focal liver lesions. Gray scale sonography has failed to distinguish between benign and malignant liver lesions. In this respect, a halo sign, i.e. a hypoechoic rim around lesions is usually considered to be a sonographic sign suggestive of malignancy.[46] However recent studies have shown this interpretation to be misleading because the halo sign is frequently detectable in benign liver lesions such as in FNH, benign liver adenoma, liver abscess or atypical haemangioma. Colour Doppler sonography has shown to be a reliable noninvasive method for evaluation of blood flow in liver lesions. In 71 per cent of patients with FNH blood

flow was detected within the halo zone (hypoechoic rim), spectral analysis of the blood flow indicated that the blood flow was arterial in all patients.[47] However, comparable blood flow in hypoechoic rim is also mentioned even in HCC by some investigators.[48] There findings indicate that colour Doppler sonography is not helpful in distinguishing FNH from HCC. In cases of risk factors for HCC or liver metastases, malignancy has to be ruled out by other investigations. Demonstration of blood flow in a hypoechoic rim of a focal liver lesion in patients without clinical suspicion of HCC or metastases suggest the diagnosis of FNH.

Haemangiomas are essentially large sinusoidal spaces which are full of slowly moving red cells. The Doppler frequency shift is small and is generally too low to be detected by Doppler systems utilising conventional wall filters of 100 Hz or less. Thus haemangiomas are well circumscribed echogenic focal masses which demonstrate little or no detectable flow. A 'spot pattern' is considered to the indication towards haemiangioma and is seen in about 50 per cent cases.[48] Colour Doppler and Duplex sonography are also very useful in characterisation of solid liver lesions. Several studies using vascular distribution criteria with colour Doppler have attempted to make a histological characterization of liver lesions with different results. In a study conducted by M Gonzalez-Anon et al, it was postulated that the intratumoral venous colour and pulsed Doppler signal regardless of other Doppler findings, is very suggestive of benignancy, with 70 per cent sensitivity and 89 per cent specificity. All lesions were benign when the only finding was venous colour intratumoral Doppler Duplex signal (specificity 100%).[50]

The occurrence of detour venous pattern has been reported in metastases by Nino-Muncia et al[49] and Tanaka et al.[48] Although it shows low sensitivity it is of great importance to objectify this vascular pattern because its specificity for malignancy in metastatic lesions is very high.

The simultaneous occurrence of both intra and peritumoral arterial flow in the same lesion strongly suggests malignancy.[50]

Tanaka et al described four patterns of vascularity in focal liver lesions on CDFI. A basket pattern of peritumoral flow and a 'vessel-in-tumour' pattern was regarded as being very specific for hepatocellular carcinomas as seen in 75 and 65 per cent of HCC respectively, while a spot pattern and a detour pattern were described for haemangiomas and metastases respectively.[51] The colour pattern of the lesion is recorded as basket when a fine blood flow network surrounding the tumour is seen, VT (vessel within tumour) when blood flow entering into and branching within the tumour, Detour when a dilated portal vein is seen meandering around the tumour, or spot when colour stained dots or patches seen in the central region of the tumour. HCC are seen to have a basket or VT pattern and hence colour flow patterns can help in distinguishing them from metastases and haemangioma. Patients with lesions measuring less than 3 cm with detectable Doppler signals are likely to have HCC. Peak-systolic shifts greater than 3 kHz were found in few patients with HCC greater than 4 cm.[51] The use of highly sensitive colour flow demonstrates neovascularisations in virtually all hepatocellular carcinomas. Utilising transducer insonating to optimise the Doppler shift, a Doppler shift greater than 2.5 kHz (at an insonating frequency of 3 MHz) or with an angle-corrected velocity greater than the main hepatic artery is highly suggestive of malignancy. These patients usually have elevated alpha-foetoprotein (AFP) levels.[52]

Power Doppler sonography is thought to be three to five times more sensitive than colour Doppler sonography. The advantages of power Doppler sonography are that it detects lower velocity flows than colour Doppler sonography, it decreases the noise background, it does not produce aliasing and it is independent of angle. Detection of the colour signals in HCC was significantly more sensitive with power Doppler sonography than with colour Doppler sonography. Power Doppler sonography however does not reveal the flow speed or direction of the colour signals. Another disadvantage of power Doppler sonography is that it is sensitive to motion.[53]

Role of Contrast Enhanced Colour Doppler Sonography in Liver Tumours

Duplex sonography and colour Doppler imaging of liver tumours have shown characteristic vascular patterns that reflect the vascular anatomy of specific types of hepatic lesions. Although colour Doppler sonography has opened up new diagnostic possibilities, it is limited in its ability to evaluate low velocity blood flow is very small intratumoral vessels particularly in small hepatic lesions and lesions located deep within the liver parenchyma because of the low intensity of Doppler signals or an insufficient Doppler shift. The use of ultrasound contrast agents has received increasing attention. Intravascular contrast agents improve the detection of low velocity blood flow because they increase the signal-to-noise ratio, allowing a more complete display of the vascular pattern of the tumour. In a study by D Strobel *et al*, sonographic contrast medium used was SHu 508A (Levovist; Schering, Berlin, Germany) a suspension of galactose based microbubbles.[54] The study demonstrated that the use of a galactose-based contrast agent improves the detection of intratumoral vascularity. An improvement of 20 to 86 per cent was seen in the detection rate of intratumoral vascularity using a contrast agent in HCCs by Tanaka *et al*.[55] Contrast enhanced colour Doppler sonography demonstrated intratumoral vascularity in 71 per cent of metastases compared to 35 per cent using conventional colour Doppler sonography.

Colour and pulsed Doppler sonography also has a role in detecting transient flow disturbance in early stage of hepatic abscesses. Chinami *et al*[56] observed transient reversal of portal flow at the periphery of the abscesses during the active stage, which normalized after treatment (Figs 9.18 and 9.19). Analysis of Doppler signal shows a decrease in RI and an increase in flow velocity in the hepatic artery followed by a decrease in the flow velocity and an increase in RI after normalisation of flow in the branch of portal vein running parellel to it. The reversal of portal flow is usually seen in abscesses measuring more than 6 cm.[57] However, a study in our institution showed this phenomenon in abscesses measuring more than 10 cm.[58] Thus a differential diagnosis of hepatic tumours with reversal of portal flow should also include early stage hepatic abscesses.

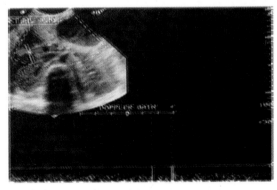

Figure 9.18
Duplex Doppler US in a case of hepatic abscess before treatment showing reversal of portal flow in the anterior branch of the right portal vein

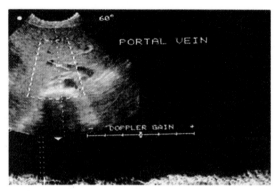

Figure 9.19
Duplex Doppler US of the same case after treatment showing normalization of portal flow

Gallbladder Carcinoma

Gallbladder carcinoma is a common gastrointestinal tumour and is three times more common in women than in men. It occurs most often in elderly patients. The lesion on gray scale sonography is imaged as (a) a solid mass occupying the whole gallbladder, (b) a focal polypoid mass or (c) diffuse wall thickening. Type a and b constitute the majority of cases and in these cases differentiation between gallbladder carcinoma and tumefactive biliary sludge is needed. It is important diagnostic problem because former should be treated surgically and the latter should be managed medically. Conventional gray scale US provide very little if any useful informations for differentiation. The addition of colour Doppler sonography offers a definite advantage for this purpose. Blood flow signals are seen in majority of cases of gallbladder carcinoma (Fig. 9.20).

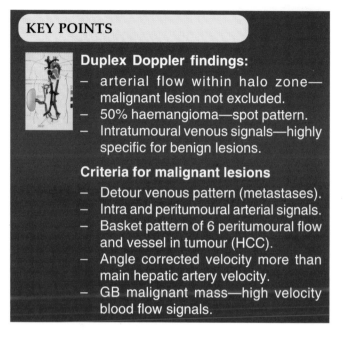

KEY POINTS

Duplex Doppler findings:
- arterial flow within halo zone—malignant lesion not excluded.
- 50% haemangioma—spot pattern.
- Intratumoural venous signals—highly specific for benign lesions.

Criteria for malignant lesions
- Detour venous pattern (metastases).
- Intra and peritumoural arterial signals.
- Basket pattern of 6 peritumoural flow and vessel in tumour (HCC).
- Angle corrected velocity more than main hepatic artery velocity.
- GB malignant mass—high velocity blood flow signals.

However no significant correlation is seen between the tumour and the maximal flow velocity. Cystic artery can also be visualised in few of the tumours. In the tumefactive biliary sludge group, colour Doppler sonography detected no blood signals in the mass. High velocity flow is considered to be an important sign suggestive of malignant nature of the tumour. Although benign tumours show a lower rate of detection of blood signals compared with gallbladder carcinoma and the presence of or absence of blood flow signals seem to be a useful sign for differentiating benign from malignant tumours.

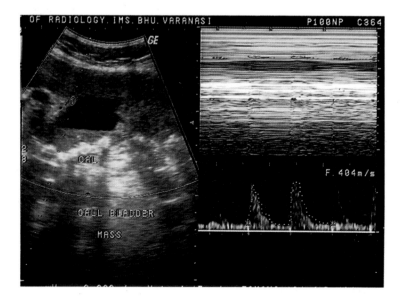

Figure 9.20
Colour Doppler flow mapping in a case of cholelithiasis associated with carcinoma of gallbladder: Poorly defined anatomical boundary of GB. Multiple calculi in the lumen associated with mass lesion in fundus and body of GB. Anterior wall is irregularly thickened due to neoplasia and vascular study show pulsatility and Resistive Index 2.153 and 0.865 respectively; suggestive of increased neovascularisation

LIVER TRANSPLANTATION

Since the first hepatic transplant was performed in 1963, this procedure has become an acceptped method of treatment for fulminant and subfulminant hepatic failure, cirrhosis, Budd-Chiari syndrome, biliary atresia and tumour. Successful transplantation requires careful selection of recipients to avoid conditions that would significantly reduce the success of the procedure. After transplantation, careful monitoring of the recipient is required to identify complications of the procedure and adverse effects of immunosuppression required to prevent rejection. Diagnostic ultrasound augmented with Duplex and colour Doppler plays an important role in both preoperative and postoperative evaluation of the patient undergoing hepatic transplantation.

Preoperative Assessment

Prior to hepatic transplantation, significant hepatic parenchymal and vascular abnormalities must be identified to aid the surgeon in planning the operation. Ultrasound, aided by Doppler, is used to document the anatomy, and patency of the inferior vena cava, hepatic veins and portal vein. In children with biliary atresia, anatomic mapping is of particular importance because approximately 25 per cent of patients with biliary atresia have portal vein or inferior vena cava anomalies. If transplantation is being performed for treatment of hepatic malignancy, ultrasound may aid in defining the extent of the tumour and determining the presence of vascular invasion or biliary obstruction.

Portal Vein Patency

Successful liver transplantation depends upon several factors, but among the most important are successful vascular anastomoses. Portal vein occlusion is a recognised sequel of long-standing liver disease and causes rapid hepatic decompensation, it is therefore important for the status of portal vein to be assessed pre-operatively. Patency of portal vein is an essential prerequisite for liver transplantation.

The extrahepatic components of the portal venous system can be assessed via subcostal scans, combination of imaging and colour flow Doppler usually rapidly confirms their patency.

Both imaging and colour Doppler studies of the intrahepatic portal venous system are best achieved via right lateral intercostal scans, which allow visualisation of the main and right portal veins even in the smallest of livers. Flow within the intrahepatic portal vein does not necessarily imply patency of the extrahepatic venous system. Low velocity forward intrahepatic flow can occur in patients in whom splenic and superior mesenteric venous occlusion have been proved. Both components of the portal system must be examined. If colour flow and power Doppler studies fail to detect flow within the portal vein the equipment control settings must be optimised to detect low velocity flow. In addition, the Doppler shift frequency must be optimised by minimising the beam/vessel angle, particularly by using lateral intercostal scans. If no flow is found, the examination should be repeated after an interval or after a meal. If doubt persists after a second or subsequent examination, the use of ultrasound contrast agents may be helpful by increasing the signal intensity from any blood within the portal vein.[59]

If little or no flow is detected in the intrahepatic portal veins, and if there is imaging evidence of either fresh or old thrombosis in the intrahepatic portal system. The superior mesenteric vein must be assessed. If the superior mesenteric vein remains patent at the level of the splenic vein confluence the surgeon may be able to use this as a source of portal supply to the grafted liver.

A further source of error in the diagnosis of portal vein occlusion is cavernous transformation of the portal vein which develops as a long-term sequel to portal vein thrombosis. Imaging alone may suggest the diagnosis by detecting numerous serpiginous channels replacing the portal veins at the porta hepatis. In the majority of patients with cavernous transformation, the intrahepatic portal vein branches are either abnormally small or absent and therefore the assessment should include both the intra and extrahepatic components of the portal vein.

The final component of portal assessment is the detection of paraportal collaterals.

It is customary to measure the maximum diameter of the spleen when assessing patients with liver disease, this should always be recorded prior to liver transplantation. Progressive splenic enlargement in the postoperative period may be the first indication of portal vein stenosis or occlusion, recurrent liver disease or rejection. A preoperative baseline measurement is therefore important.

Preoperative Donor Assessment

Usually a relative, mother, father, uncle or aunt is used as the donor. Prior to removal of the segments it is important to exclude the presence of liver disease is the donor and to assess the presence of any vascular anomalies.

Preoperative Scanning

Intraoperative ultrasound is not an accepted technique and may fulfil a number of notes in the transplant patient.

Prehepatectomy intraoperative ultrasound may be helpful to confirm the number and extent of neoplasms and to assess vascular invasion.

After successful transplantation intraoperative Doppler studies are invaluable in confirming good flow through the vascular anastomoses.[60]

Postoperative Scanning

The role of ultrasound in postoperative period varies according to the time lapsed since the operation. If circumstances permit, it is probably ideal to perform routine examinations on days 1, 3, 5 and 7, and weekly thereafter, unless otherwise indicated by clinical or biochemical findings.[61]

Before undertaking postoperative examinations it is important to be conversant with the surgical details. Detailed information concerning the hepatic artery, portal vein, IVC and biliary anastomosis is important. The operator should follow a predetermined protocol to ensure that all aspects of the transplant anatomy are carefully assessed and that all possible sites for fluid collections are evaluated.

Hepatic Artery

Problems related to hepatic artery anastomosis are the most common vascular complications after liver transplantation.[62] In adults early arterial occlusion occurs in 1-3 per cent of patients but is more common in paediatric age group, especially in patients under one year of age. Early arterial occlusion is almost always a catastrophic event, with rapid and irreversible liver cell death.

Postoperative occlusion of the hepatic artery most commonly occurs at the site of the vascular anastomosis but may occur elsewhere in the main vessel. Ideally all segments including the extrahepatic and intrahepatic main hepatic artery and right and left intrahepatic branches should be studied. A spectral trace from the hepatic artery must be obtained before its patency can be confirmed.[63] The flow velocity waveform obtained from the hepatic artery in the acute posttransplant phase is variable. However, if the velocity is formed to be extremely low or the waveforms very damped, this strongly raises the suspicion of a significant stenosis. If the Doppler studies show a progressive reduction in arterial velocity or a fall-off in diastolic flow in the absence of obvious parenchymal abnormality, the possibility of a progressive arterial obstructive lesions should be considered and angiography must be advised.[64] Doppler studies of the hepatic artery are important but in any patient in whom the Doppler findings do not concur with the clinical context angiography must be performed.

A further complication of hepatic artery occlusion is the increased risk of intrahepatic abscess formation. The whole volume of liver must be scanned in patient with known or suspected arterial occlusions.

If the arterial stenosis is treated by transluminal angioplasty serial Doppler studies are invaluable for confirming improvements in the arterial flow and for monitoring the patients subsequent progress.

Portal Vein

Early postoperative occlusion of the portal vein is rare in adults and uncommon in children. However, early occlusion may have catastrophic consequences with early graft dysfunction or variceal bleeding. Colour flow imaging is almost always sufficient for confirmation of patency. Patients with Budd-Chiari syndrome, abnormal portal vein anatomy, portal vein conduit or who have had an operative thrombectomy are all at increased risk or portal vein thrombosis.

The flow characteristics within the transplanted portal vein are often abnormal. There may be severe flow disturbances beyond the anastomoses and a relatively high velocity jet may be found at the anastomosis. Spectral Doppler studies should be attempted using colour flow imaging to detect the highest velocity, and a peak velocity estimate must be performed. If this is more than 100 cm/s, the anastomosis is likely to be unacceptably tight and patient must be carefully monitored for portal stenosis and evidence of extrahepatic portal hypertension.

Late stenosis of the portal vein is an uncommon but serious complication[65] and can usually be predicted by detecting a narrow anastomosis on the early postoperative scan.[66] In these patients serial measurements of the jet velocity permit the detection of a progressive stenosis and the spleen is seen to enlarge if the lesions becomes haemodynamically significant.

Late the sudden portal vein occlusion is rare and usually presents with a sudden deterioration in liver function tests, the onset of resistant ascites and rapidly increasing splenomegaly. Any patient with these symptoms should undergo full Doppler assessment.

Hepatic Veins and IVC

Early hepatic veins thrombosis is almost always unheard of except in patients who have been transplanted for Budd-Chiari syndrome. The clinical relevance of hepatic vein Doppler studies in liver transplantation remains uncertain.

Stenosis of IVC is extremely rare and generally presents with ascites and lower limb oedema. The diagnosis is established by demonstration of a dilated and pulseless vena cava below the level of the stenosis,[67] but contrast cavography is the definitive diagnostic test (Figs 9.21a and b).

REFERENCES

1. Heidi Partiquin, Miche Lofortun, Peter N *et al:* Duplex Doppler Exam in Portal HT: Technique and anatomy. *AJR* **149**: 171-76, 1987.
2. David Sutton: The liver and spleen. Robert Dick, Julic FC (Eds): *Textbook of Radiology and Imaging* (6th edn) Edinburgh Churchill Livingstone.
3. Bolondi L, Gandolfi L, Arienti V *et al:* Ultrasonography in the diagnosis of portal HT: diminished response of portal vessels to respiration. *Radiology* **142**: 167-72, 1982.

4. Ohnishi K, Saito M, Nakayama T *et al:* Portal venous hemodynamic is chronic liver disease: effect of posture change and exercise. *Radiology* **155**: 757-61, 1985.
5. Jacger K, Bollinger A, Valli C *et al:* Measurement of mesenteric blood flow by duplex scanning. *J Vasc Surg* **3**: 46-51, 1986.
6. Okazaki K, Miyaraki M, Onishi S *et al:* Effect of food intake and various extrinsic hormones on portal blood flow in patients with liver cirrhosis demonstrated by pulsed Doppler with Octoron. *Scand J Gastroenterol* **21**: 1029-34, 1986.
7. Kawasaki T, Moriyasu F, Nishida O *et al:* Analysis of hepatofugal flow in portal venous system using ultrasonic Doppler duplex system. *Am J Gastroenteral* **84**: 937-41, 1989.
8. Gaiani S, Bolondi L, Li Bassi S *et al:* Prevalence of spontaneous hepatofungal portal flow in liver cirrhosis. Clinical and endoscopic correlations in 228 patients. *Gastroenterology* **100**: 160-67, 1991.
9. Nakayama T, Hiyamma Y, Ohniski K *et al:* Arterioportal shunts on dynamic computed tomography. *AJR* **140**: 953, 1983.

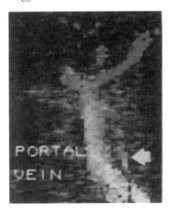 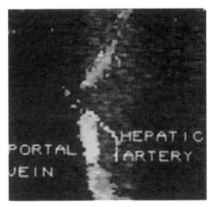

Figures 9.21a and b
Severe acute hepatic transplant rejection (a) five days after transplant. There is a hepatopetal flow in the portal vein and hepatic artery (⇐). The arterial flow velocity waveform appeared normal and (b) seven days after transplant. There is hepatofugal flow in the portal vein. Increased slow flow sensitivity Doppler signal explain the lighter colour hue in both arteries and veins. Pathology demonstrated severe rejection with centrilobular necrosis and periportal inflammation

10. Schrier RW, Arroyo V, Bernandi M, Epstein M, Henriksen JH, Rades J: Peripheral vasodilatation hypothesis: a proposal for the initiation of renal sodium and water retention in cirrhosis. *Hepatology* 8: 1151-57, 1988.

11. Piscaglia F, Gaiani S, Gramantieri L *et al:* Superior merenteric artery impedance in chronic liver diseases : relationshiop with disease severity and portal circulation. *Am J Gastro enterol* 93(10): 1798-99, 1998.

12. Bolognesi M, Sacerdoti D, Merkel C *et al:* Splenic Doppler impedance indices: influences of different portal haemodynamic conditions. *Hepatology* 23: 1035-40, 1996.

13. Sacerdote D, Merkel C, Bolognesi M *et al:* Hepatic arterial resistance indexes in cirrhosis without and with portal vein thrombosis relationships with portal haemo-dynamics. *Gastroenterology* 108: 1152-58, 1995.

14. Moriyasu F, Nishida O, Bass N *et al:* Measurement of portal vascular resistance in patients with portal hypertension. *Gastroenterology* 90: 710-16, 1986.

15. Burns PN: Interpretation and analysis of Doppler Signals. In Taylor KJW, Burns PN, Wells PNT (Eds): Clinical appli-cation of Doppler ultrasound. New York: Reven, 1988.

16. Sabba C, Mrkel C, Zoli M *et al:* Interobserver and interequipment variablity of echo Doppler examination of the portal vein: effect of a cooperative training pro-gramme. *Hepatology* 21: 428-33 1995.

17. Moriyasu F, Bass N, Nishida O *et al:* 'Congestions index' of the portal vein. *AJR* 146: 735-39, 1985.

18. Bru C, Bosch J, Navasa M *et al:* Pulsed Doppler measure-ments of portal blood flow in man: applications in the non invasive evaluationof the pharmacological therapy of portal hypertension. In Bondestam S, Alanen A, Joupplila P (Eds): Proccedings of the 6th congress of the European Federation of the societies for ultrasound in Medicine and Biology 14-18 June 1987. Finland, Helsinki, 66 1987.

19. Kinura T, Moryiasu F, Kawasaki T *et al:* Changes in the azygos venous flow evaluated using transesophageal Doppler ultrasound after vasopressin infusions in portal hypertension. *Hepatology* 10: A42 1989.

20. Zoli M, Marchesini G, Brunori A *et al:* Portal venous flow in response to acute beta-blocker and vasodilatatory treat-ment in patients with liver cirrhosis. *Hepatology* 6: 1248 1986.

21. Holmin T, Alwmark A, Forsberg L: The ultrasonic demon-stration of portacaval and interpositions mesocaval shunt. *Br J Surg* 69: 673-75 1982.

22. Lafortune M, Patriquin H, Pomier G *et al:* Haemodynamic changes in portal circulation after portosystemic shunts: use of Duplex sonography in 43 patients. *AJR* 149: 701-06, 1987.

23. Balondi L, Gaiani S, Mazziotti A *et al:* Morphological and haemodynamic changes from distal splenorenal shunt: an ultrasound and pulsed Doppler study. *Hepatology* 8: 652-57 1988.

24. Lafortune Martenet JP, Denys A *et al:* Short and long term hemodynamic effects of transjugular intra hepatic porto systemic shunts: a Doppler/manometric correlative study. *AJR* 164: 997-1002, 1995.

25. Feldstein VA, Patel MD, LaBergē JM: Transjugular intrahepatic portosystemic shunts: accuracy of Doppler US in determination of patency and detection of stenoses. *Radiology* 200: 141-47, 1996.

26. Chong WK, Malioch TA, Marer MJ *et al:* Transjugular intrahepatic portosystemic shunt: US assessment with maximum flow velocity. *Radiology* 189: 789-93, 1993.

27. Foshager MC, Ferral H, Nazarian GK *et al:* Duplex sonography after transjugular intrahepatic portosystemic shunts (TIPS): normal haemodynamic findings and efficacy in predicting shunt patency and stenosis. *AJR* 165: 1-7, 1993.

28. Uggowitren MM, Kugler C, Machan L *et al:* Value of echo enhanced Doppler sonography in evaluation of transjugular intrahepatic portosystemic shunts. *AJR* 170: 1041-46, 1998.

29. Sukigara M, Komarali T, Yamaraki T *et al:* Colour flow mapping of the esophageal varices and vessels in and around the liver with real time two-dimensional Doppler echography. *Clin Radiol* 1987.

30. Parker RGF: Occlusion of the hepatic veins in man. *Medicine* 38: 369-402, 1959.

31. Masatoshi Makuuchi, Hishoshi Hasegava, Suoumu Yamazaki *et al:* Primary Budd-Chiari syndrome: Ultrasonic demonstration. *Radiology* 152: 775, 1984.

32. Philip Stanley: Budd-Chiari syndrome. *Radiology* 170: 625-27, 1989.

33. Mitchell MC, Boitnott JK, Kaufman S *et al:* Budd-Chiari syndrome: etiology, diagnosis and management. *Medicine* 61: 199-218, 1982.

34. Safouh M, Shehata AH: Hepatic vein occlusion disease of Egyptian children. *J Pediatr* 67: 415-22, 1965.

35. Campbell DA Jr, Rolles K, Jamieson *et al:* Hepatic trans-plantation with perioperative and long term antico-agulation as treatment for Budd-Chiari syndrome. *Surg Gynecol Obstet* 166: 511-18, 1988.

36. Scissors IW: Membranous obstruction of the infection vena cava and hepatocellular carcinoma in South Africa. *Gastroenterology* 82: 171-78, 1982.

37. Longer B, Stone RM, Colapinto RF *et al:* Clinical spectrum of the Budd-Chiari syndrome and its surgical manage-ments. *Am J Surg* 129: 137-45, 1975.

38. Stark DD, Hahn PF, Trey C *et al:* MRI of the Budd-Chiari syndrome. *AJR* 146: 1141-48, 1986.

39. Philip W Rallo, Meade B Johnson, D Randall Radin *et al:* Budd-Chiari syndrome: Detection with colour Doppler sonography. *AJR* 159: 113-16, 1992.

40. Peter Millener, Edward G Grant, Steven Rose *et al:* Colour Doppler imaging findings in patients with Budd-Chiari syndrome: correlation with venographic findings. *AJR* 161: 307-12, 1993.

41. Horoki T, Kuroda C, Tokunaga K *et al:* Hepatic venous outflow obstruction: evaluation with pulsed Doppler sonography. *Radiology* 170: 733, 1989.

42. Edward G Grant, Rita Parrella, Franklin N Tessler *et al:* Budd-Chiari syndrome: the results of duplex and colour Doppler imaging. *AJR* 152: 377-81, 1989.

43. Onishi K, Nomura F: Ultrasonic Doppler studies of hepatocellular carcinoma and comparison with other hepatic focal lesions. *Gastroenterology* 97:1489-97, 1989.

44. Taylor CR, Taylor KJW: Imaging techniques. An incidental hemangioma of the liver: the dilemma of patient management. *J Clin Gastroenterol* 3: 93-97, 1981.

45. Wanless IR, Mawdsley C, Adams R: On the pathogenesis of focal nodular hyperplasia of the liver. *Hepatology* 5: 1194-1200, 1985.

46. Yoshida T, Matuse H, Okazaki N *et al:* Ultrasonographic differentiation of hepatocellular carcinoma from metastatic liver cancer. *J Clin Ultrasound* 15: 431-37, 1987.

47. Herbay A, Frieling T, Niederau C *et al:* Solitary hepatic lesions with a hypoechoic rim: value of colour Doppler sonography. *AJR* 169: 1539-41, 1997.

48. Tanaka S, Kitamura T, Fujita M *et al:* Colour Doppler flow imaging of liver tumours. *AJR* 154: 509-14, 1990.

49. Nino-Murcia M, Ralls PW, Jeffrey RB *et al:* Colour flow Doppler characterisation of focal liver lesions. *AJR* 159: 1195-97, 1992.

50. M Gonzalez-Anon *et al:* Characterisation of solid liver lesions with colour and pulsed Doppler imaging 24: 137-43, 1999.

51. DN Srivastava, Amit Mahajan, M Berry *et al:* Colour Doppler flow imaging of focal hepatic lesions. *Australasian Radiology* 44: 285-89, 2000.

52. Ebara M, Ohto M, Shiragawa T *et al:* Natural history of minute hepatocellular carcinoma smaller than 3 cm complicating cirrhosis. *Gastroenterology* 90: 289-98, 1986.

53. Rubin JM, Bude RO, Carson PL *et al:* Power Doppler US: a potentially useful alternative to mean frequency-based colour Doppler US. *Radiology* 190: 853-56, 1994.

54. Deike Strobel, Udo Krodel, Peter Martus *et al:* Clinical evaluation of contrast-enhanced colour Doppler sonography in the differential diagnosis of liver tumours. *J Clin Ultrasound* 28: 1-13, 2000.

55. Tanaka S, Kitamra T, Yoshioka F *et al:* Effectiveness of galactose based intravenous contrast medium on colour Doppler sonography of deeply located hepatocellular carcinoma. *Ultrasound Med Biol* 21: 157, 1995.

56. Chinami: Liver abscess with reversal of portal flow. *Ultrasound International* 3: 135-38, 1997.

57. Linzy, Wang JH, Wang LY: Changes in intrahepatic portal hemodynamics in early stage hepatic abscesses. *J Ultrasound Med* 8: 595-98, 1996.

58. Mehrotra P, Bhargava SK: Reversal of Portal flow in liver abscesses. Ind J Radiol Imag 10: 21-23, 2000.

59. Teefey SA, Middleton WD, Crowe TM *et al:* Doppler sonographic evaluation of the portal vein: effects of intravenous dodecafluoropentane. *J Ultrasound Med* 16: 641-45, 1997.

60. Waldman DL, Lee DE, Bronsther O *et al:* Use of intraoperative ultrasonography during hepatic transplantation. *J Ultrasound Med* 17: 1-6, 1998.

61. Hellinger A, Roll C, Stracke A *et al:* Impact of colour Doppler sonography on detection of thrombus of the hepatic artery and the portal vein after liver transplantation. *Langenbecks Arch Chir* 381: 182-85, 1996.

62. Wozeney P, Zajko AB, Bron KM: Vascular complications after liver transplantation: a five year experience. *AJR* 147: 657-63, 1986.

63. Flint EW, Sunkin JH, Zajko AB: Duplex sonography of hepatic artery thrombosis after liver transplantation. *AJR* 147: 481-83, 1988.

64. Marnjo WC, Langnas AN, Wood RP *et al:* Vascular complications following orthotopic liver transplantation: outcome and the role of urgent revascularisation. *Transplant Proc* 23: 1484-86, 1991.

65. Malassagne B, Soubrane O, Dousser B *et al:* Extrahepatic portal hypertension following liver transplantation: a rare but challenging problem. *HPB Surg* 10: 357-63, 1998.

66. Lee J, Ben-Ami T, Yousefzadeh D *et al:* Extrahepatic portal vein stenosis in recipients of living-donor allografts: Doppler sonography. *AJR* 167: 85-90, 1996.

67. Brouwers MA, de Jong KP, Peeters PM *et al:* Inferior vena cava obstruction after orthotopic liver transplantation. *Clin Transplantation* 8: 19-22, 1994.

Suchi Bhatt

Poonam Narang

Shalini Verma

Shashank Jain

Role of Colour Doppler in Splenic Lesions

Portal Hypertension

Portal hypertension results in changes in various vessels along with development of multiple portosystemic collaterals.

Along with dilatation of portal vein, varying degrees of dilatation of splenic and superior mesenteric veins also occur in portal hypertension. A calibre of splenic vein over 12 mm should be regarded as suspicious whereas splenic vein over 20 mm diameter or greater should be considered a specific sign of portal hypertension. Splenomegaly, usually associated with portal hypertension, is also responsible for dilatation of splenic vein possibly because of increased splenic blood flow (Fig. 10.1).

Dilatation of splenic artery was also found to accompany splenomegaly which is required to supply a more extensive capillary bed. Splenic artery dilatation was also found to occur more frequently in cirrhosis caused by chronic viral hepatitis than in alcohol abuse. A ratio between the diameter of the hepatic and splenic arteries above 0.9, measured at 1.5-3 cm from their origins, suggests an alcoholic cause for cirrhosis, whereas a lower ratio is indicative of an infectious cause.

Another important sign of portal hypertension is the lack of variations in calibre with respiration in the splenic and superior mesenteric veins (Fig. 10.2).

Along with hepatofugal portal flow, splenic vein also shows hepatofugal flow which has proved to be closely correlated with hepatic encephalopathy.

At level of lower splenic pole, splenorenal collaterals appear as tortuous vessels with a high velocity Doppler signal and a broad spectrum of frequencies due to turbulence (Fig. 10.3). Their presence is often associated with flow reversal in the splenic vein.

Splenic Infarction

Splenic infarcts occur in patients with myeloproliferative syndromes, haemolytic anaemias and sepsis especially in sepsis associated with

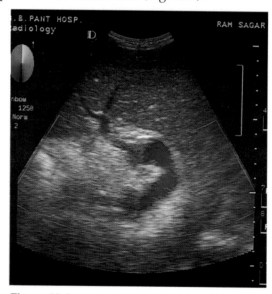

Figure 10.1
Dilated and tortuous splenic vein with splenomegaly

endocarditis. The striking clinical feature is sudden onset of pain in the upper left abdomen, occasionally associated with a painful restriction of the respiratory excursion or local pain on palpation. However, clinical diagnosis can be difficult because pain can be associated with almost all cases of splenomegaly and infarct may be silent.

Splenic infarcts can be visualised at ultrasound scanning and B-mode pulsed Doppler US can identify infarct related complications.

For the imaging diagnosis of splenic infarction, a wide range of ultrasound appearances have been observed. About 24 hours after therapeutic embolization of the splenic artery for treatment of portal hypertension, splenic infarcts appear as wedge shaped, hypoechoic and well-damarcated lesions at sonography. This is the typical US appearance of acute stage without complications. Scar stage of infarction may be seen as in homogeneity of splenic texture months later.

Severe infarct related complications might develop in the course of disease that can be detected by follow-up US and Doppler scanning. The findings that require surgical intervention are the following:

1. Increasing subcapsular haemorrhage
2. Extravasation of blood into peritoneal cavity
3. Flow phenomena in the area of infarction as seen at B-mode pulsed Doppler US.

In patients demonstrating arterial signals within the infarction area, histological examination revealed superinfection of the splenic infarcts. The present of arterial signals and increasing subcapuslar haemor-

Characteristics and complications of splenic infarction

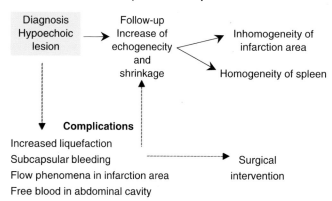

rhage were signs of occurrence of spontaneous splenic rupture. Hence with clear sonographic signs of life-threatening splenic rupture, splenectomy should be recommended.

Intrasplenic Pseudoaneurysms

Post-traumatic pseudoaneurysms involving splanchnic arteries are very rare in the paediatric age group and effect mostly the splenic artery or intrasplenic arterial branches. Because of the potential for life-threatening complications, intrasplenic pseudoaneurysms must be diagnosed and treated immediately. Although the trend in the management of blunt splenic injuries has been towards conservative treatment, formation of a pseudoaneurysm at the site of a splenic hematoma may cause delayed splenic rupture requiring splenectomy. This has necessitated routine follow-up of blunt splenic injuries by colour Doppler sonography or CT

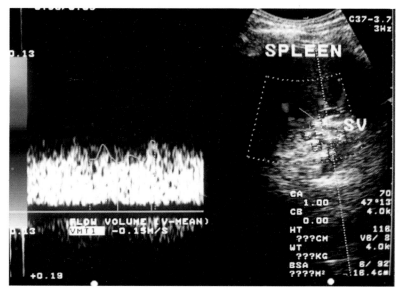

Figure 10.2
Splenic venous flow pattern in a portal hypertensive

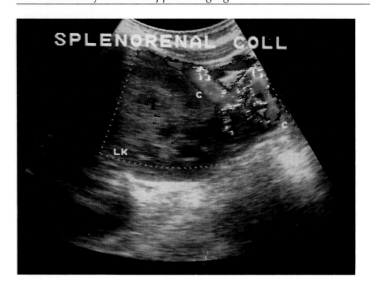

Figure 10.3
Voluminous splenorenal collaterals

to detect pseudoaneurysms at an early stage when selective embolization might prevent expansions of the haematoma and rupture of the spleen.

Intrasplenic pseudoaneurysms are formed by active bleeding from injured intrasplenic arterial branches. Although spontaneous thrombosis is possible the usual evolution of the lesions is gradual expansion of the haematoma with eventual rupture of the splenic capsule. This unpredictable ominous complications necessitates a meticulous search for there lesions in all cases of blunt splenic trauma.

Initial scanning in patients who have experienced blunt splenic trauma may be performed with colour Doppler sonography or contrast enhanced CT. Intrasplenic pseudoaneurysms appear on gray scale sonography as nonspecific anechoic lesions. Their aneurysmal nature can be revealed by the demonstration of arterial flow on colour Doppler sonography. Turbulent arterial flow within the lesion suggests a diagnosis of pseudoaneurysms. Not all intrasplenic pseudoaneurysms develop at the time of initial trauma. Some lesions develop in a delayed fashions presumably

because of gradual lysis of the clot sealing the injured arterial wall. Thus conservative management of blunt splenic trauma should include periodic follow-up with colour Doppler sonography or CT even if admission scans are negative. Coil embolization of splenic artery is the preferred method for haemostasis of intrasplenic pseudoaneurysms.

KEY POINTS

Spleen
– PHT
  • Dilated splenic vein (>12 mm), lack respiratory variation, hepatofugal flow splenorenal collaterals.
– Complications of splenic infarction.
  • Doppler detects—arterial signals in infarct—super infection.
  • Arterial signals in infarct and increasing subcapsular haemorrhage suggests possibility of spontaneous splenic rupture.

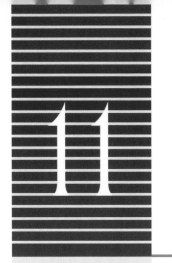

Colour Doppler in Pancreas

Suchi Bhatt
Poonam Narang
Shalini Verma
Shashank Jain

Colour Doppler sonography displays blood flow information on the morphologic data obtained from the gray scale sonogram and becomes a useful imaging modality for the evaluation of patients with abdominal tumours.[1]

Although the use of angiography and computed tomography (CT) in the preoperative evaluation of pancreatic tumours has been well-documented, it is highly desirable to obtain the most accurate diagnostic information possible with more non-invasive and cost-effective technique such as colour Doppler sonography. Colour Doppler sonography has been found to be more sensitive than angiography in depicting vascular involvement of carcinoma. Hence a preoperative assessment in suspected pancreatic carcinoma patients with initial colour Doppler sonography helps in improved patient management.

To look for vascular involvement in patients with pancreatic carcinoma, all the peripancreatic mesenteric vessels, i.e. coeliac artery, superior mesenteric artery, hepatic artery, splenic artery, splenic vein, superior mesenteric vein and main portal vein are to be examined. Colour Doppler sonographic criteria used for staging vascular involvement are normal (no contact between tumour and vessel), abutment (tumour adjacent to vessel and no clear in growth), encasement (circumferential narrowing of the vessel lumen) and occlusion (sudden interruption of the vessel). A vessel if normal or showed abutment favoured resectability whereas encasement or occlusions of vessel favour non-resectability. This is important because pancreatic carcinoma is one of the leading cause of adult cancer death.[2]

Only patients whose tumours are completely resected can expect to survive. Unnecessary surgical exploration may result in increased post operative morbidity and a prolonged recovery. Hence precise preoperative staging is rapidly increasing. Patients showing signs of peripancreatic vessel involvement are considered to be unresectable.[3]

In a study conducted by H Ishida *et al*, accuracy of colour Doppler sonography in the staging of 26 patients with pancreatic carcinoma and compared with accuracy of angiography. The study showed that colour Doppler sonography was more sensitive than angiography in the diagnosis of vascular involvement. This tendency was more obvious in the arteries than in the veins. Hence, it was concluded that in predicting the unresectability of pancreatic carcinoma rarely requiring additional confirmatory studies. In contrast in prediction of resectability, it is sometimes inaccurate and additional examinations are needed for more accurately unresectable pancreatic carcinoma patients.[4]

Pancreatic Transplantation

First segmental pancreatic transplant was performed in 1966. It has now become an increasingly important option for the management of type I diabetes mellitus.

Technical features and graft rejection were the major causes of high graft failure rates and recipients' mortality. With recent technical success and improvements in immunosuppression, there has been an increase in the number of patients undergoing pancreatic transplant. With improvement in immunosuppression causing better control of graft rejection, the major cause of transplant failure in early post-transplant period is graft ischaemia due to arterial or venous thrombosis or stenosis. As in other organ transplants, arterial and venous integrity is critical in pancreatic transplantation. Colour and Duplex Doppler are commonly used to monitor blood flow postoperatively to the pancreas.[5]

Procedure

The transplanted pancreas is superficially located and is easily accessible for examinations with ultrasound imaging with high-frequency transducers (5-7.5 MHz) is possible and major vessels can be readily examined with Duplex or colour Doppler interrogation. The arterial supply of the pancreatic allograft is from the coeliac and superior mesenteric arteries. These vessels are anastomosed to the iliac artery. The portal veins are anastomosed to the external iliac vein to provide venous drainage. Pancreatic secretions are drained by a variety of procedures, frequently by duodeno-cystostomy.

Complications

Common complications of pancreatic transplantation are vascular thrombosis, intra-abdominal infections, rejection, anastomotic leaks and pancreatitis. Imaging techniques include ultrasound, Doppler ultrasonography, CT and radionuclide imaging. Sonography with Doppler is the procedure of choice in detecting fluid collections and identifying pancreatitis, vascular thrombosis and rejection to some extent.

Postoperative Evaluation

Postoperative evaluation of the pancreas transplant should include careful inspection of the pancreas, the surrounding structures and the transplant vessels. The normal pancreatic transplant appears sonographically as a homogenous structure of low to moderate echogenecity lying medial to iliac vessels. The normal anteroposterior dimension of the pancreatic allograft ranges

from 1.5-2.0 cm. Pancreatic enlargement though non-specific, may accompany infarction, pancreatitis and rejection.[6] Peritransplant fluid collections indicating pseudocyst, abscess, haematoma, serum or lymphocoele can be seen in over 50 per cent of patients with transplantation.[7]

With Doppler ultrasound, arterial flow to the transplant is characterised by a low-resistance waveform with flow continuing throughout the diastole. Duplex and colour Doppler ultrasound aid in the early identification of mechanical problems with arterial and venous anastomosis and are important in transplant evaluation.[8]

Confirmation of flow within the body of the pancreas is easily performed with visualisation of the splenic artery and vein along the posterior aspect of the allograft. The iliac artery and vein are examined to identify the anastomosis of the coeliac and superior mesenteric arteries and portal vein. Thrombosis of the veins draining the pancreatic transplant is a particularly important for the graft loss.[9]

Venous thrombosis is most common during first week following transplantation, if untreated. Duplex Doppler findings associated with venous thrombosis include absence of demonstrable flow in the transplant veins and abnormalities in the transplant coeliac and splenic arteries with a blunted systolic peak and reversal of flow in diastole. This waveform is indicative of high vascular resistance and when present should suggest the possibility of venous outflow obstruction.

The role of Doppler in transplant rejection is non-specific. Some studies have suggested relation of transplant arterial resistive index (RI) with signs of rejection. A RI of more than 0.70 per cent was a pointer towards rejection.[10] However, the utility of RI measurements in predicting rejections is not confirmed. However, when rejection is suspected, biopsy is usually necessary. Biopsy guidance with ultrasound and colour Doppler can be done and reduces the possibility of inadvertent vascular damage during biopsy.

REFERENCES

1. Mrerton DA, Golberg BB: Abdominal applications of colour flow imaging. In Goldberg BB, Merton DA, Deane Cr (Eds): *An atlas of ultrasound colour flow imaging.* London: Martin Dunitz, 67-142, 1997.
2. Weill FS: Pancreatic tumours and overview of pancreatic disease. In Weill FS (Ed): *Ultrasound dignosis of diagestive disease.* New York: Springer, 481-510, 1996.

KEY POINTS

Pancreas
- Colour Doppler sensitive than angiography—detecting vascular involvement by pancreatic carcinomas, Encasement/occlusion—nonresectibility.
- Pancreatic transplant postoperative evaluation
  - A low resistance arterial waveform with forward diastolic flow.
  - 1st week-venous thrombosis m/c complication—R1 > 0.7-pointer towards rejection.

3. Raijman I, Levin B: Exocrine tumours of the pancreas. In Haubrich WS, Schaffner F, Berk JFB (Eds): *Gastroenterology.* Philadelphia: WB Saunders, 3002-04, 1995.

4. H. Ishida, K Konno, Y Hamashina *et al:* Assessment of resectability of pancreatic carcinoma by colour Doppler sonography. *Abdom Imaging* **24**: 295-98, 1999.

5. Yang HC, Neumyer MM, Thicle BL *et al:* Evaluation of pancreatic allograft circulation using colour Doppler ultrasonography. *Transplant Proc* 22: 609-11, 1990.

6. Letourneau JG, Maile CW, Sutherland DE *et al:* Ultrasound and computed tomography in the evaluation of pancreatic transplantation. *Radiol Clin North Am* **25**: 345-55, 1987.

7. Patel BK, Garsim PJ, Aridge DL *et al:* Fluid collections developing after pancreatic transplantation: radiologic evaluation and intervention. *Radiology* **181**: 215-20, 1991.

8. Kubota K, Billin H, Kelter U *et al:* Duplex-Doppler ultrasonography for evaluating pancreatic grafts. *Transplant Proc* **22**: 183, 1990.

9. Hanto DW, Sutherland DER: Pancreatic transplantation: clinical consideration. *Radiol Clin North Am* **25**: 333-43, 1987.

10. Patel B, Wolverson MK, Mahanta B: Pancreatic transplant rejection: assessment with duplex US. *Radiology* **173**: 131-35, 1989.

12

Role of Colour Doppler in Urinary System

Suchi Bhatt
Shefali Gupta
Satish K Bhargava
Shashank Jain

KIDNEYS

Gray scale ultrasound has greatly increased the morphologic detail that could be displayed within the kidney. Further the addition of pulsed Doppler allowed arterial and venous perfusion to be assessed both qualitatively and quantitatively. Recent addition to colour flow and power Doppler imaging now allow superb demonstration of the entire renovascular tree from the main renal arteries and their fine terminal branches (Figs 12.1a and b).

Technique

The main renal arteries arise from the lateral aspect of aorta just inferior to the superior mesenteric artery and left renal vein. Using these vessels as landmarks, the origin and proximal portion of the main renal arteries are best examined with the patients supine using a 3 MHz transducer and a transverse midline approach. Patients should ideally fast for at least 8 hours prior to examination. In larger patients decubitus positioning with intercostal scanning may be more helpful.

Approximately 20 per cent of patients will have accessory renal arteries.[1] Visualization of the entire course of the main renal arteries is incomplete in over 30 per cent of adult patients.

The normal waveform (Fig. 12.2) of the main renal artery demonstrates a low impedance pattern with continuous forward diastolic flow reflecting the low resistance of blood flow to the native kidney. When the origins of the main renal arteries can be identified angle corrected velocity estimates can be made. Peak systolic velocity is usually less than 100 cm/sec. The resistive index should be less than 0.7.[2,3]

The segmental renal branches which lie within the renal hilum as well as

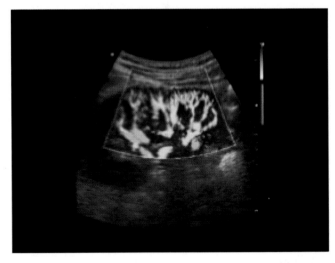

Figure 12.1a
Colour Doppler image of native kidney demonstrates intraparenchymal renal arteries and veins

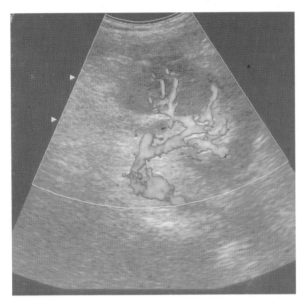

Figure 12.1b
Power Doppler image of native kidney. Blood flow is coded yellow on this colour map

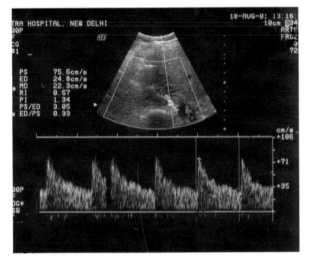

Figure 12.2
Duplex Doppler image of normal renal artery showing low impedance pattern with continuous forward diastolic flow

the more distal interlobar and arcuate vessels within the renal cortex are readily identified on colour or pulse Doppler examination. Renal parenchymal vessels are best examined from a lateral intercostal approach. Decubitus positioning may be helpful. Most patients can be imaged with a 3 to 5 MHz transducer. The Doppler sample volume should be kept small (2-5 mm) and the wall filter should be set as low as possible (< 50 Hz). In order to minimize the relative error the Doppler tracing should be maximized by

using minimum frequency range (pulse repetition frequency) possible before aliasing occurs. With this technique the deflection of the Doppler spectrum from the baseline is maximised, thus filling as much of the scale as possible. The larger the spectrum the smaller will be the relative error produced by any fault when positioning cursors or placing calipers. A spectrum is considered optimal if three to five consecutive similar appearing waveforms are noted. Both kidneys are always examined even if renal disease in unilateral.

Pulsed Doppler interrogation of the intrarenal vessel reveals a low resistance waveform with a decreasing peak systolic velocities as the vessels are traced distally (Fig. 12.3). To characterise intrarenal Doppler waveform, most investigators have used the resistive index (RI). This parameter is defined as peak systolic shift-minimum diastolic shift/peak systolic shift. Increases in downstream resistance result in a relative reduction is diastolic flow compared with systolic. Hence RI can be used as an estimates of state of renal arterial resistance.

The RI of intrarenal vessels is normal adult kidney has been reported to range from 0.58 to 0.64 + 0.05,[2,3] and an intrarenal RI of 0.7.

Children and neonates will have RI's of higher value. In premature infants, neonates and toddlers an RI 0.7-1.0 may be normal. The RI in children decreases with age and after age 4-5 years it stablises in the adult-range.[4,5]

Doppler signals from parenchyma or main renal veins demonstrates continuous flow in the opposite direction that of arterial flow. Respiratory and cardiac variation are typically present.

Intrarenal Duplex Doppler Sonography of the Dilated Collection System

Conventional sonography is indeed quite sensitive for diagnosing renal obstruction by detecting dilatation of the collection system. However the converse is not true, as pyelocaliectasis identified by sonography is

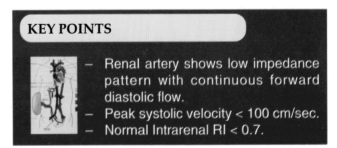

KEY POINTS

- Renal artery shows low impedance pattern with continuous forward diastolic flow.
- Peak systolic velocity < 100 cm/sec.
- Normal Intrarenal RI < 0.7.

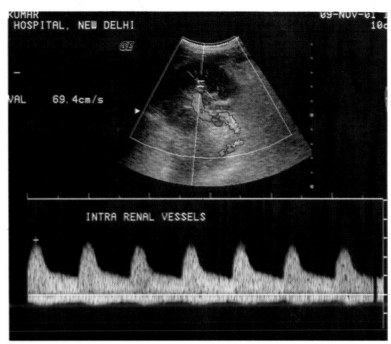

Figure 12.3
Normal pulse Doppler waveform of intrarenal artery showing low resistance pattern with continuous forward diastolic flow

certainly not synonymous with true obstruction.[6] This clinically important distinction of true renal obstruction from non-obstructive dilatation cannot be resolved by gray scale sonography and often requires the use of invasive procedures and tests. Intrarenal Doppler has a great potential value in identifying true renal obstruction.

The non-obstructive causes of a dilated collecting system include a distended urinary bladder, overhydration, mediation, diabetes insipidus, congenital megacalyes, postobstructive dilatation, chronic reflux and acute pyelonephritis.

Complete or Nearly Complete Obstruction

The haemodynamic changes that occur with renal obstruction must be understood to explain the observed Doppler changes. Most studies have described a triphasic renal vascular and ureteral pressure response to obstruction.[7]

The initial phase occurring in the first 1-2 hours after obstruction is characterised by a transient rise in renal blood flow and prostaglandin mediated vasodilation.[7] Although this very stage would rarely be relevant in the clinical setting, one would except a normal RI immediately after the onset of obstruction.

The second phase begins after 2 hours of obstruction and last approximately 3 hours. This phase is characterised by elevated postglomerular renovascular resistance decreased renal blood flow and elevated ureteral pressure. This is the only stage in which renal vascular resistance and ureteral pressure one both elevating at the same time.

The third phase, beginning after 5 hours of obstruction is characterised by decreasing and often normalised ureteral pressure at a time when renal vascular resistance is markedly rising.[7]

This phase is characterised by an elevation in preglomerular resistance with ureteral pressure appearing to be less important. In this phase marked elevation of renal vascular resistance and hence RI elevation would be expected.

Currently many researchers believe that renal vascular resistance changes observed with obstruction may be due to locally acting circulating vasoactive factors and hormones.[8]

Recently investigators have evaluated the ability of Doppler to detect these renal vascular changes.[2,3,9] These studies have defined a resonably discriminatory RI value of 0.7 to differentiate obstructive from non-obstructive pyelocaliectasis. That is, in a kidney with a dilated collecting system an RI value of 0.70 or more is suggestive of obstruction, while RI values less than 0.70 are suggestive of non-obstructive dilatation.

Acute Renal Obstruction

Although conventional US is sensitive though not specific in detection of the collecting system dilatation that accompanies established obstruction, previous researchers have shown conflicting results in evaluation of the suspected but early renal obstruction.[55, 56] These studies demonstrated a key limitation of conventional US. Acutely obstructed kidneys may demonstrate only mild pyelocaliectasis or none. Laing *et al*[55] in a previous study found that 35 per cent of acutely obstructed kidneys exhibited no pyelocaliectasis. Previous animal research indicates that acute obstruction elevates renal arterial resistance within a few hours[7,8] Platt *et al*[56] found an elevated mean RI of 0.77 is acutely obstructed kidney. Elevation of RI occurs after as few as 6 hours of clinical obstruction.[56] Kidneys obstructed for a somewhat longer period of time (12-36 hours) did not have significantly higher RI than those with shorter duration < 12 hours. One potential limitation of Doppler analysis is the patient with intermittent very acute renal colic. If the obstruction is present for a few hours only and then is relieved theoretical considerations would suggest that the RI may not increase even of this pattern of intermittent obstruction and relief persists for days.

In conclusion analysis with intra renal duplex Doppler US is a valuable addition to the standard sonographic examination in patients with acute renal colic. The Doppler study enables detection of marked elevation in renal arterial resistance by 6 hours of clinical obstruction at a time when conventional US often reveals little pyelocaliectasis or none. Because obstruction of less than 6 hours duration or pyelosinus extravasation may cause normal RI in obstruction a knowledge of clinical history and identification of perirenal fluid on real time US scan are crucial.

Release of Significant Obstruction

Animal data indicates that duration of obstruction prior to relief is crucial for predicting what types of vascular changes will be observed.[10]

If obstruction is relieved within the first two phases (by 5 hours) if obstruction is relieved within to normal renal vascular resistance and hence RI. However is obstructive is prevent for at least 18-24 hours the normalisation of renal vascular resistance may not be immediate and may take days or even weeks to return to baseline levels. This continued elevation in RI is presumably due to renal vasoconstriction caused by persisting local factors such as thrombaxane.[10]

Partial or Mild Obstruction

Unlike significant obstruction, which appears mediated by vasoconstriction such as TXA_2, mild partial obstruction is characterised by prostaglandin mediated vasodilation.[10,11] Studies[11] also have found that the presence or degree of pyelocaliectasis does not predict or correlate with renal atrophy and nephron loss. Clearly the use of pyelocaliectasis as the gold standard for significant partial obstruction is not correct. Renal vascular resistance should only be elevated in partial obstruction significant enough to result in renal vasoconstriction. Milder degree of partial obstruction mediated by renal vasodilators produce no elevation in renal vascular resistance and a normal RI would be expected.

Partial obstruction highlights the fact that Doppler analysis attempts to provide physiologic rather than anatomic information while a normal RI argues against significant physiologic obstruction it does not imply that a ureter is free of any mild region of narrowing or structures, the renal Doppler examination alone does not suffice if precise anatomic information is required. The clinical utility of an elevated RI value in a child with a dilated urinary tract is less well defined. In a child over age 5 years an RI ≥ 0.70 is suggestive of obstruction. However RI values that are elevated by adult standards are frequently observed in children under age 5 years. When there is unilateral collecting system dilatation a resistive index ratio RIR, which is defined as the RI of the dilated kidney divided by RI of the contralateral nonobstructive kidney of 1.1 or greater is suggestive of obstruction.[57] However, an RIR between 1.0 and 1.1 may be found in children with obstructive dilatation if the child is not hydrated. Therefore, a fluid and/or diuretic challenges may be needed to unmask the obstruction. Nonetheless the lasix renogram remains the gold standard for evaluation of renal obstruction is children and relative glomerular filtration rates are very helpful when deciding if a child needs surgical repair.

Pitfalls in Resistive Index Analysis of Obstruction

A few potential pitfalls in Doppler evaluation of the dilated collecting system are useful to consider.

One potential pitfall that generally can be avoided is very acute obstruction of less than 8 hours in which the RI may not have had sufficient time to reach 0.70.

However in these early obstructed cases the difference in RI between the obstructed and the contralateral normal kidney is 0.10 or more. Therefore the accuracy of the RI discriminator value (0.70) can be improved by evaluation of contralateral kidney.

A theoretical limitation of RI analysis is severe chronic obstruction with marked parenchymal loss. It is possible that interstitial infiltrate thought to lead to circulating renal vasoconstrictors is lost in these cases with less elevation of renal vascular resistance (RI). Such cases of end stage obstruction will generally not be clinically problematic as the presence of obstruction will be known.

One very important potential limitation in the case of Doppler in the evaluation of obstruction is in imaging children. Elevated RI values (by adult standards) are commonly observed in children. Available animal data suggest the altered renal blood flow with obstruction involves the outer portions (cortex) of the kidney to a greater degree than the medulla, so the vessels interrogated may be an important factor especially in children.[7,8]

One of unavoidable limitation of Doppler analysis of possible obstruction is that RI is a non-specific parameter. Obstruction is not the only cause of an elevated RI.[3,12] Therefore in the setting of known renal medical disease (RMD) and pyelocaliectasis an elevated RI could be due either to true obstruction or to renal medical disease with coexistent nonobstructive dilatation. If the dilatation is unilateral, the examines can study the contralateral non-dilated kidney and look for significant difference in RI (> 0.1) to suggest obstruction superimposed on renal medical disease. The specific setting where Doppler imaging is truly limited is in the patient with bilateral pyelocaliectasis known and usually severe renal medical disease and an elevated RI.

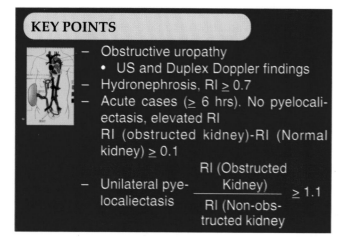

KEY POINTS

- Obstructive uropathy
  - US and Duplex Doppler findings
- Hydronephrosis, $RI \geq 0.7$
- Acute cases (≥ 6 hrs). No pyelocaliectasis, elevated RI
  RI (obstructed kidney)-RI (Normal kidney) ≥ 0.1
- Unilateral pyelocaliectasis $\dfrac{RI \ (Obstructed \ Kidney)}{RI \ (Non\text{-}obstructed \ kidney)} \geq 1.1$

Colour Doppler of Vesicoureteric Junction

Colour Doppler evaluation of ureteric jets within the bladder may also be useful is diagnosing ureteric obstruction. Colour Doppler examination of the bladder demonstrate ureteric jet. If a ureteric jet is not seen after 15 minutes of continuous observation the ureter is obstructed.

Haemolytic Uremic Syndrome

The haemolytic uremic syndrome comprised of the clinical triad of hemolytic anaemia, thrombocytopenia and renal failure, most frequently presents is children less than two years of age following a bout of gastroenteritis. The associated renal microangiopathy is characterised by endothelial swelling and thrombus formation. In children vascular obstruction typically occurs at the level of the glomerulus whereas in adults, arteries or arteriols are primarily involved.

Decreased arterial renal parenchymal blood flow has been documented on renal scintigraphy. The resultant oliguria or anuria frequently requires dialysis. A diuretic phase generally precedes recovery which typically occurs within 1-2 week. Recovery is more common in children than in adults. Using pulse Doppler in children aged 1-7 years Patriquin[13] have demonstrated abnormal renal parenchymal arterial waveform characterised by abnormal diastolic flow (absent, reversed or markedly reduced) and elevated intrarenal $RI \geq 0.9$ during the oliguric phase. These Doppler changes reflect increased arteriolar resistance most likely as a direct result of narrowing of arteriolar lumen or loss of arteriolar elasticity due to endothelial swelling and intraluminal thrombus formation. Furthermore in their series the reappearance of normal diastole blood flow and drop of RI normal (0.65-0.70) in children accurately predicted recovery of renal function and urine output allowing dialysis to be terminated. Improved end diastolic flow or decreased RI usually preceded the diuretics phase by 24-48 hours.[13] The authors hypothesize that if normal Doppler signal are present in the oliguric patient with haemolytic uraemic syndrome, the disease will have a mild course and dialysis will not be required.

Hepatorenal Syndrome

It is defined as unexplained kidney failure in a patient with liver disease who does not have clinical laboratory or anatomic evidence of other known cause of kidney failure. The progressive kidney dysfunction that accomapanies liver disease is generally considered to be functional because consistent pathologic changes are absent because the kidney failure can be reversed with liver transplantation and because kidneys in patients with hepatorenal syndrome can be successfully transplanted into patients with normal liver.[17]

Renal haemodynamic changes begin early in the course of liver disease related functional kidney failure even before changes in serum creatinine concentration are detectable. The hallmark change is intrarenal vasoconstriction.[18]

Duplex Doppler sonography can be used to assess vascular resistance in small renal intraparenchymal vessels by measuring RI. An elevated RI reflecting intrarenal vasoconstriction has been observed in various condition associated with elevated renal vascular resistance such as kidney obstruction, acute tubular necrosis, renal vein thrombosis and haemolytic uraemic syndrome and should be detectable in liver disease related functional kidney failure Patt *et al*[19] have found renal RI to be useful new non-invasive predictor of subsequent kidney states in non-azotomic patients will liver disease. An abnormal renal RI predicts an increased chances for development of hepatorenal syndrome by presumably detecting renal vasoconstriction. When an elevated RI is obtained, a formal evaluation for hepatorenal syndrome. Including fluid challenge should be considered. A normal renal Doppler study would indicate that hepatorenal syndrome is very unlikely. Doppler will be useful for prognosis and in the management of liver disease whenever they require paracentesis, diuretic therapy potentially nephrotoxic medicine or radiographic contrast examination.[19]

Renal Masses

The most common use of ultrasound in the evaluation of renal mass is to differentiate a cyst from a solid neoplasm.

Pulse and colour Doppler examination can be useful for further evaluation of solid renal masses. Most renal cell carcinomas are hypervascular and contain numerous arteriovenous shunts. Increased vascularity can be readily demonstrated on colour Doppler imaging. On pulse Doppler imaging arteriovenous shunting will lead to high peak systolic frequency shifts secondary to the rapid drop in pressure gradient across the anastomosis. Several authors have demonstrated significantly elevated peak systolic frequency shift on pulse Doppler in renal cell carcinoma.[14,15] Kier[14] in their series reported that

83 per cent of untreated renal cell carcinoma demonstrated peak systolic frequency shifts greater than 2.5 KHz and above those in the main renal artery. Renal cell carcinoma have a propensity to invade renal veins (20-30% of cases) and the tumour thrombus may extend into IVC (5-10%) occasionally growing into right atrium. Accurate diagnosis of venous extension is important both for prognosis and patient management. The presence and extent of tumor thrombus within these veins can be easily detected by colour Doppler examination as a filling defect within distended veins. Tumour thrombosis is typically isoechoic with the primary neoplasm and the renal vein is often distended. In addition unlike haemorrhagic thrombus, tumor thrombus will demonstrate neovascularity which can be detected on Doppler examination. Even if main renal vein cannot be visualised pulse Doppler examination may suggest renal vein thrombosis. In three patients with renal cell carcinoma and angiographically confirmed renal vein extension Dubbins and Wills[16] documented high impedance intrarenal arterial waveforms characterised by little or no forward flow in end diastole (Figs 12.4 and 12.5a to c).

Renal Vein Thrombosis

Acute renal vein thrombosis (RVT) most often presents in adults with flank pain, macroscopic haematuria and deteriorating renal function characterised by proteinuria.

In adults, acute, RVT occurs most frequently as a result of dehydration, vascular congestion, hypercoagulopathies, malignancy or trauma. Patients usually improve following thrombolytic therapy.

In neonates and children, the mortality rate is higher and acute RVT occurs most commonly in the clinical setting of severe dehydration secondary to diarrhoea, sepsis, birth trauma, maternal diabetes or maternal hypertension.

Conventional sonographic findings of altered renal size and echogenicity are nonspecific. Duplex Doppler sonography of the kidney with the study of the main renal vein is often used in the non-invasive evaluation of this condition. Typical findings include the presence of thrombosis and the absence of a Doppler signal in the renal vein. Because thrombus often is not seen and because lack of renal venous signal can be due to technical consideration (e.g. the patient's condition or body habitus) rather than true renal venous

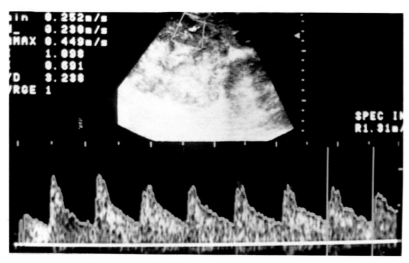

Figure 12.4
Duplex Doppler showing high velocity flow signals in Wilm's tumor

thrombosis, ancillary sonographic sign are useful. Prior experience in transplanted kidneys suggests than absent or reversed end diastolic flow in intraparenchymal arteries is highly suggestive of renal vein thrombosis.[20]

Acute RVT may result in increased renal vascular impedance secondary either to compromise of venous drainage or to intrarenal oedema. Increased renal vascular impedance will result is diminished or reversed diastolic flow and elevation of RI.[23] Laplarte et al[24] have recently reported that intrarenal venous flow may often be present in children with renal vein thrombosis due to collateral circulation. They note however that the normally transmitted cardiac pulsatility may be absent in these collateral vein and that the RI of segmental arteries may be 10% higher than in contralateral normal kidney.

However in a study by Platt et al[32] intrarenal arterial Doppler analysis is neither sensitive nor specific for renal vein thrombosis in native kidneys. This is probably secondary to the development of venous collaterals in the native kidneys which allows a decrease in renal resistance and normalisation of arterial RI. Extensive venous collaterals can develop in native kidney but not in transplanted kidneys which lack capsular venous anastomosis.[22]

Chronic RVT is more difficult to diagnosis both clinically and radiographically. Patients with nephrotic syndrome have an increased incidence of RVT. Criteria are same as for

diagnosis of acute RVT. However the kidney may not be enlarged, renal vein may not be dilated. Development of venous collateral which is more common in chronic DVT than in acute DVT may reduce renal impedance such that secondary sign of RVT namely diminished diastolic arterial flow and increased RI will not be present.

Renal Artery Stenosis

Hypertension is a significant risk factor for the development of cardiovascular disease, renal failure and stroke and renovascular hypertension is the most common surgically curable cause of hypertension. Estimates of prevalence of renovascular hypertension among the general hypertensive population range from 0.5 to 5 per cent.[25]

Figure 12.5a
Renal cell carcinoma: Gray scale sonography showing well-defined heterogenous mass with cystic areas

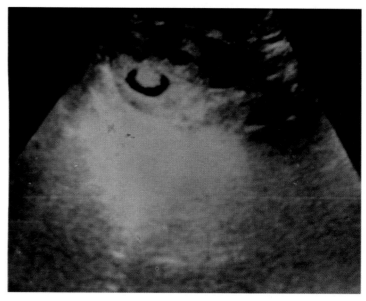

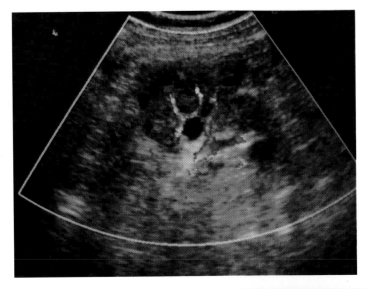

Figure 12.5b
Renal cell carcinoma: Colour Doppler showing moderate vascular signals

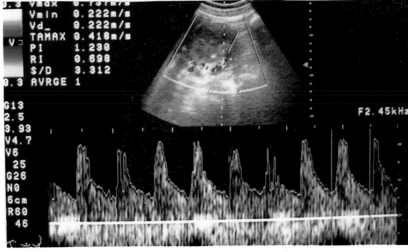

Figure 12.5c
Renal cell carcinoma: Duplex Doppler in another patient showing high velocity low resistance waveform

Because renovascular hypertension has such a low prevalence in the large hypertensive population, effective low cost screening for the disease remains a problem, clinicians have relied on the clinical history and on new or changing physical findings to identify patients at higher risk for RVH. Atherosclerotic RAS as a cause of RVH should he suspected under the following circumstances:

1. Onset of hypertension is a patient over 60 years of age.
2. Worsening hypertension that is difficult to control.
3. Associated peripheral vascular disease, coronary, artery disease or cerebrovascular disease.
4. Cigarette smoking more than 25 pack years.
5. Abdominal bruit
6. of White race.

7. Concomitant renal dysfunction is a patient with new hypertension. Atherosclerosis tends to involve the proximal 1 cm of the main renal artery or branch points (Figs 12.6 and 12.7).

One should suspect the fibromuscular group of abnormalities as cause for hypertension in women under 30 years of age and in young patients with abdominal bruit. Typically the disease involves middle of the main renal artery and other arteries including carotid are involved. Once patients are suspected of having RVH the question of how to proceed with their evaluation becomes somewhat controversial. The imaging modalities that have had the greatest clinical impact in recent years include intravenous and intra-arterial digital subtraction angiography and captopril renal scintigraphy. The newer modalities including MR angiography and colour Doppler sonography

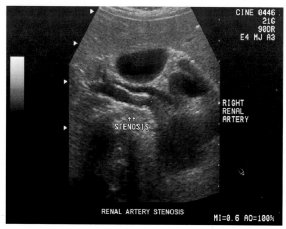

Figure 12.6
Gray scale sonogram shows a plaque at the origin of right renal artery

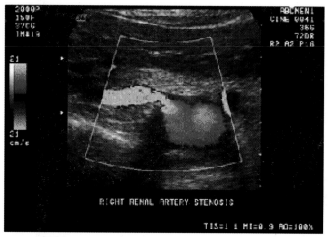

Figure 12.7
Colour Doppler flow image in another patient showing narrowing of right renal artery at its origin

continue to be investigated as to their role in RVH. Angiography is the gold standard for diagnosis RAS. However there are several factors which limit the use of angiography as a screening technique. Angiography is costly and invasive. As many patients with renovascular hypertension have borderline or frankly impaired renal function, the use of potentially nephrotoxic intravenous contrast is to be avoided if possible.

Further the demonstration of an anastomotic stenosis is a patient with atherosclerotic disease does not necessarily establish a causal relationship with hypertension.

Therefore, an imaging modality providing physiologic data and/or anatomic detail would be a more ideal screening technique IVP and nuclear medicine renal scans have been abandoned as screening test for RVH due to their low sensitivity (74 to 86%) and specificity (86% or less).[25,26]

Recently captopril scintigraphy has been demonstrated to have a very high sensitivity (91%) and specificity (93%) for diagnosis renovascular hypertension.[27] This physiologic study roughly measures the glomerular filtration rate which will decrease when the kidney is ischaemic. However no anatomic detail other than renal size is provided by captopril renogram.

During the 1980's the potential of pulse Doppler US as a screening method for diagnosing RAS was explored at numerous institutions. As a screening method pulse Doppler US has many attractive features. It is noninvasive and relatively inexpensive. There is no nephrotoxicity. Further more analysis of the pulse Doppler waveform has the ability to suggest physiological information whereas realtime US provides anatomic detail often identifying the stenotic lesion.

There are two basic approaches to the Doppler US diagnosis of RAS. The first depends on the ability of both realtime and Doppler US to identify a focal area of increased peak systolic velocity (PSV) at the anatomic site of stenosis and the second involves demonstrating a decrease in the rate of systolic acceleration distal to a stenosis. A haemodynamically significant arterial stenosis leads to a focal increase in peak systolic velocity at the anatomic site of stenosis (Fig. 12.8). Compensation for individual variation in cardiac output can be made by comparing the PSV of main renal artery to the PSV of the aorta at the level of renal artery.

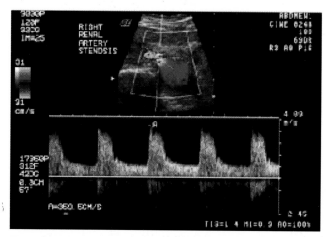

Figure 12.8
Pulse Doppler tracing at the point of narrowing shows high peak systolic velocity in renal artery

Studies have suggested that a PSV > 100 cm/sec and or RAR > 3.5 (ratio of peak systolic renal artery velocity to peak systolic aortic velocity) have sensitivities of 79-91 per cent and specificities of 73 to 92 per cent for haemodynamically significant RAS (>50-60% diameter reduction).[28,29]

However, despite initial enthusiasm experiences has shown that pulse Doppler evaluation of the main renal arteries has limited practical application as a screening technique.

The examination is very operator dependent and time consuming often requiring 1.2 hour or repeat examinations. It may be impossible to visualise the main renal arteries completely in upto 42 per cent of patients due to presence of bowel gas, obesity, surgically incision and/or aortic calcification.[30]

Tortuosity of the main renal artery may make it impossible to obtain accurate angle corrected velocity calculations. In addition accessory renal arteries have been reported in upto 14-26 per cent of patients[30] but the detection rate by US for accessory renal arteries is very low near zero. Detection of renal artery occlusion may be difficult because collateral vessels may be inadvertently sampled. Finally it is also unlikely that stenosis in branches of the main renal artery would be detected via this technique.

Virtually all these technical limitations result from the need to visualise the main (plus accessory) renal arteries along their entire course in order to document a focal increase in peak systolic velocity at the exact site of an anatomic stenosis.

However, on the basis of high technical success rate, high sensitivity and specificity and short examination time waveform analysis of the segmental renal arteries has been recommended as an alternative to direct examination of the main renal arteries for evaluation of RAS by various studies.[31,32]

Haemodynamically significant arterial stenosis cause changes is velocity waveworms that can be detected with Duplex sonography in distal contiguous arteries. Kotval reported such changes in peripheral arteries and called them tardus and parvus.[33]

Tardus refers to delayed or prolonged early acceleration and parvus to the diminished amplitude and rounding of the systolic peak. In continuation the two changes cause prolonged acceleration time (AT) and diminished acceleration index (AI).

The AI is the systolic slope of the time velocity waveform per unit time adjusted for the transmitted frequency [systolic frequency MHz after 1 sec/transmitted US frequency (MHz)]. The AI is the length of time in second from onset of systolic to peak systoles.[32]

RAS induced AT and AI abnormalities are detectable with Duplex sonography in the distal main renal artery and segmental renal arterial branches.[32] RAS may also cause an additional morphologic abnormality of velocity waveforms obtained from these arteries loss of normal early systolic compliance peak/reflective wave complex ESP.

In their study Handa *et al*[32] an AI of < 3.78 had an accuracy of 95 per cent, sensitivity of 100 per cent and specificity of 93 per cent for RAS defined as a 50 per cent diameter reduction by angiography. An AT of > 0.07 seconds had an overall accuracy of 87 per cent a sensitivity of 100 per cent and a specificity of 83 per cent for diagnosing RAS. Furthermore because these measurements were made in segmental renal arteries within the renal hilum is distal to stenosis. Doppler interrogation could be performed via the translumbar approach with a technical success rate of 98 per cent Starves *et al*[31] in their study have reported that while an AT of 0.07 seconds or longer and an AI less than 3.0 m/sec or less were each effective simple pattern recognition for loss of early systolic peak (ESP) had better sensitivity (95%) and specificity (97%) than either of the semi-quantitative parameter. The normal wave form morphology in 0 to 59 per cent RAS is shown in Figure 12.9a. AT and AR are measured from beginning of early systolic rise to the ESP. The normal ESP is defined as follows: (a) The leading edge is continuous with and has the same slope as early systole, (b) The peak has an acute angle and rises above the second part of systole (c) It is completed by angle less than 180° between it and the second part of systole. Figure 12.9b waveform corresponding to 60 to 79 per cent RAS. An abrupt change in slope still exists between early systole and middle systole but ESP is absent. AT and AI are measured from the start of early systole to the point of slope change. Figure 12.9c shows waveform corresponding to critical 80 per cent or more RAS or occlusion of the renal artery. No point of abrupt change in slope exists between early and late systole.

Accurate assessment of AT and AI and for absence of ESP requires large crisp spectral waveforms. Proper chance of patient position, sonographic window. Doppler probe carrier frequency PRF or velocity scale setting scope speed and Doppler power settings are

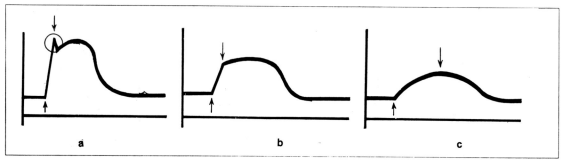

Figures 12.9a to c
The renal artery waveform morphology is RAS (a) 0 to 59 per cent RAS, (b) 60 to 79 per cent RAS, and (c) 80 or more per cent RAS
Note: Top arrow: early stystolic peak (ESP) and Bottom arrow: begining of early systolic

all necessary to achieve this goal.[31] In addition variations in the size of the normal ESP relative to the second part of systolic wave must be recognised.[31] Small and ill-defined spectral waveforms obtained without proper attention to detail will cause false positive tardus parvus appearance. Few terminal criteria have been set to ensure that the apparent tardus and parvus waveform are real and not artifacts of poor technique and suboptimal Doppler sensitivity.[31] These include:

1. No liver or spleen visible between skin window and kidney. This ensures that the approach has been sufficiently posterior or lateral to minimise the depth of the segmental arteries and the angle of incidence.
2. Highest frequency probe possible (3.5 MHz or high). The signal from segmental arteries is stronger and the waveforms larger and more well-defined in higher Doppler carrier frequency.
3. Lowest spectral display velocity scale or PRF setting possible. Improper use of higher velocity scales than necessary is the most common cause of waveforms that are too small and ill-defined to interpret or are falsely interpreted as normal.
4. Standard or full pulsed Doppler power settings segmental arterial waveforms obtained with low pulsed Doppler power settings are frequently too ill-defined to measure accurately or to evaluate for absence of ESP.

Limitation

Because tardus and parvus waveforms may be seen distal to slight stenosis or occlusion with collateral arteries, indirect Doppler studies cannot enable distinction between these two conditions.

Stenosis of only one of multiple renal arteries or of segmental renal arteries may cause false negative finding with this techniques. However obtaining sample from both the upper pole and another from the lower pole improves changes of detecting stenosis in an accessory renal artery or segmental renal artery.[31]

Colour Doppler imaging in even more helpful in the setting of RAS because in the presence of RAS fewer vessels have blood flow that is detectable by means of Duplex sonography alone. Colour Doppler imaging indicates which segmental arteries have the strongest signals and blood flow at optimum angles, thus providing guidance for pulsed Doppler. In the paediatric population. Patriquinn *et al*[36] reported an AI < 4.0 measured in segmental or interlobar arteries had a sensitivity and specificity of 100 per cent detection of severe RAS (> 75% stenosis). However moderate stenosis which may nontheless be of clinical significance. In addition narrowing of aorta upstream to the intrarenal arteries for example in patients with aortic abdominal coarctation produces a similar decrease in AI.

Renal Transplant

Renal transplantation is the most commonly performed abdominal organ transplant worldwide over 10,000 patients receive renal transplants each year.

Most often the indication for transplantation is the presence of irreversible chronic renal failure.

Effective evaluation following transplantation requires familiarity with the surgical technique used for transplantation. These are two main types of arterial anastomosis, the choice of which is guided by the type of allograft available for transplantation. Cadaver kidneys are usually harvested with an intact main renal artery and an attached portion of aorta.

KEY POINTS

Renal cell carcinoma
- Peak systolic frequency shift > 2.5 kHz, or above main renal artery.
- Tumor extension into renal vein—thrombus with neovascularity.

Renal vein thrombosis
- Acute cases—no renal venous signal.
- Ancillary signs-absent or reversed end diastolic flow in intraparenchymal arteries.
- Elevated RI.
- In chronic cases. Venous collaterals present.
- Ancillary signs absent.

RAS
- Pulse Doppler—non-invasive screening method.
- Haemodynamically significant stenosis (50-60%).
- PSV > 100 cm/sec (renal artery at site of stenosis).
- RAR > 3.5.
- Alternatively segmental renal arteries-tardus parvus waveform.
- AT > 0.07 sec, AI < 3.78.

The piece of aorta is trimmed to a circular or oval configuration (Carrel patch) and then sutured end to side to the external iliac artery of the recipient's external iliac artery or sometimes end to end to the recipient's internal iliac artery. Venous anastomosis is one almost always performed end to side to the recipient external iliac vein.[35]

In case of multiple donor renal arteries or veins patch grafts to the recipient external iliac vessel are performed. When paediatric kidneys are transplanted to an adult recipient a segment of donor aorta with both kidneys is patched to the iliac artery. Ureteric drainage is usually established by ureteroneocystomy or occasionally by pyeloureterostomy using the reciepient's native ureter. Following transplantation a variety of immunosuppressive regimen are used to prevent rejection.[36]

Pretransplant work up includes evaluation of the recipient general medical condition and diagnostic studies to exclude conditions that are contraindicates to transplantation including presence of outflow tract obstruction, active infection and severe debilitating systemic disease or disseminated malignancy. Ultrasound is of value in the pretransplant evaluating of recipient's native urinary tract for evidence of obstruction calculi and neoplasm.

The sonographic evaluation of the transplanted kidney combines imaging and Doppler because transplant dysfunction arises from both vascular and non-vascular causes.

Protocol for ultrasound of renal transplant includes:[36]
a. Documentation of renal size and position.
b. Presence or absence of dilatation of collecting system.
c. Presence, location, dimension of any extrarenal fluid collection.

Imaging examination also documents corticomedullary contrast, the appearance of renal parenchyma and the presence of renal in masses or calcification. The size and configuration of urinary bladder and urinary anastomosis are also recorded.

Transplant dysfunction may result from vascular complication such as vessel stenosis or occlusion or parenchymal changes secondary to rejection, tubular necrosis, or drug toxicity.

Vascular Complications

Vascular complications are reported to occur in upto 10 per cent of transplantation patients with the most types being arterial and venous stenosis and thrombosis and intrarenal and extrarenal arteriovenous fistula (AVF) and pseudoaneurysm.[37] If detected early, many are amenable to graft sparing surgical or radiologic intervention. However, clinical presentation of these lesion is often ambiguous and imaging is required to differentiate them from the more common nonvascular causes of dysfunction.

For most transplant vascular application, both colour and Duplex Doppler imaging should be performed with the lowest filter setting maximal gain without background noise and smallest scale that will accommodate the highest normal peak velocities without aliasing. Gate size should be between 3 and 5 mm and angle connection which should be adjusted when quantifying peak flow.[35]

Renal Artery Stenosis

Arterial stenosis with a reported prevalence of approximately 10 per cent are the most common vascular complication of renal transplants.[38] They usually occur within the first 3 years after transplantation and are more common in grafts from cadavers especially those of young donors than in grafts from living donors.[38] The hallmark of significant stenosis is hypertension. However upto 80 per cent of transplant recipients may exhibit hypertension unrelated to arterial stenosis. Therefore suspicion of stenosis is reversed for patients with specific hypertensive profiles such as newly developed or progressive hypertension, marked hypertension resistant to medical therapy hypertension with graft dysfunction in the absence of rejecting or hypertension in the presence of a systolic bruit over the graft.[35] Three main types of stenosis have been described: anastomoses distal donor and recipient artery anastomotic stenosis occur more frequently in end to end anastomosis distal stenosis occur more frequently in end to side anastomosis and recipient artery stenosis occur equally in both types anastomotic lesions are primarily short segment stenosis composed of variable amounts of intimal fibrosis and calcium that have been ascribed to surgical difficulties such as tight sutures, incomplete intimal approximation, excessive vessel length, twisting of vascular pedicle and large discrepancies in donor and recipient arterial size. Distal donor stenosis are single or multiple long segment stenosis composed primarily of diffuse intimal hyperplasia that are caused by haemodynamic turbulance distal to anastomosis initmal injury caused by graft perfusion catheter or excessive dissection around the main renal artery that results in destruction of vasa vasorum. Both anastomotic and distal donor stenosis may also be caused by rejection. Recipient stenosis are uncommon and usually due to either native atherosclerotic disease or intraoperative clamp injury.[38,39]

The combination of colour and Duplex Doppler sonography provides a very sensitive method for the detection of arterial stenosis.

The vessels of interest are insolated throughout their extent looking for abnormally elevated peak systolic velocities and turbulent flow indicative of stenosis.

The most reproducible criteria for renal transplants were published by Taylor *et al.*[40] Using a 3 MHz transducer they found that significant stenosis (those requiring intervention) were associated with peak Doppler shifts greater than 7.5 MHz (2 m/sec) at the stenosis and turbulence in the immediate post-stenotic segment. As stenosis occurs in different locations in both the main and segmental renal arteries, these vessels must be insolated throughout their entirety. Unfortunately visualisation of these vessels is often quite difficult. Thus the Duplex Doppler examination is commonly a prolonged and tidious procedures in which the arteries are located by a trial and error method.

Colour Doppler sonography with its larger field of view and ability to detect vessels invisible to gray scale sonography is both faster and less likely to miss a stenosis than is Duplex Doppler with properly adjusted colour controls the abnormally increased velocities associated with stenosis appear as regions of focal aliasing. Once located these region can be examined with Duplex Doppler sonography to determine the nature and severity of flow disturbance. If a Doppler study is of reasonable quality and no significant flow abnormalities have been identified then significant stenosis can be excluded with a relatively high degree of confidence. If a strong clincial suggestion of stenosis persists, then angiography should be performed to exclude an undetected stenosis of a segmental or accessory renal artery.

Gottilibe *et al*[41] have suggested that the use of intrarenal waveform parameter substantially improves the accuracy of detecting a haemodynamically significant proximal arterial stenosis compared with the use of the peak systolic velocity measured from the main renal artery as the sole criterion.

An acceleration index > 0.1 sec or a subjective assessment of dampening of the waveforms results in greater accuracy of detecting proximal arterial stenosis.

Renal Artery Thrombosis

Thrombosis of the main renal artery occurs in less than 1 per cent of renal transplantation patients.[35] It is usually an acute event in the early postoperative period (< 1 month) and invariably results in graft loss. Hyperacute and acute rejection are by far its most common causes. However intraoperative intimal trauma, faulty intimal approximation, wide disparity in vessel size, and it end anastomosis, vascular kidney hypotension, hypercoagulable states, cyclosporine and atherosclerotic emboli have all been cited as precipitators of thrombosis.[42] Segmental renal artery thrombosis is clinically less obvious than is main renal artery thrombosis symptoms may be absent or consists of graft tenderness, decreased function or haematuria. Most limited infarcts result in a focal scar rather than complete graft loss.[35] In the presence of an occlusive arterial thrombus, neither Duplex nor colour Doppler sonography will detect flow in the arterial branches distal to the occlusion.[40] Venous flow likewise will be absent. As long as Doppler equipment is functioning properly these findings are highly specific for renal artery thrombosis.

However, false positive reading may occur if the Doppler equipment is poorly calibrated, or in rare cases with high grade stenosis and minimal flow. Colour Doppler sonography because of its larger field of insolation is more likely to detect segmental infarcts than is Duplex Doppler sonography.[35]

Intrarenal Arteriovenous Fistulas and Pseudoaneurysms

Intrarenal AVF's and pseudoaneurymas are almost exclusively the result of trauma induced during percutaneous needle biopsy. AVF's occur with simultaneous laceration of adjacent arteries and vein whereas pseudoaneurysm result from isolated laceration. Most AVF's are small and resolve simultaneously AVF's that produce symptoms do so when they become large enough to cause decreased renal perfusion via marked arteriovenous shunting or when they communicate with caliceal system and produce haematuria.

Pseudoaneurysm cause symptoms when they rupture into the perinephric space or renal collecting system.[43] Majority of these lesion can be treated effectively by percutaneous transcatheter embolisation.[43]

The Duplex Doppler findings of both AVF's and pseudoaneurysms are fairly specific AVF's exhibit high velocity low impedance arterial waveforms with associated arterialised venous tracings. Pseudoaneurysms show highly turbulent pulsatile flow in their central lumen with classic to and fro flow at their neck.[40]

The spectral aberration of both AVF's and pseudoaneurysm are always localised to a portion of the kidney with normal haemodynamics in the remaining parenchymal vessels.

Colour Doppler owing to its wide field full of view greatly increases the detection for AVF.[44]

The colour appearance of AVF's depends on their size. Small lesions appear as focal areas of colour abasing that reflect increased arterial velocities. Larger produce considerable perifistula tissue vibration that causes a focal flurry of disorganised colour at normal Doppler setting.[44] Regardless of size AVF's detected by Colour Doppler sonography should be verified with Duplex Doppler sonography to exclude con-

fusion with similar colour aberrations that may be caused by segmental stenosis or focally prominent vessels.[44]

The colour appearance of pseudoaneurysm consists of disorganised colour flow within an apparent cyst with the same surrounding parenchymal vibration colour as in seen with AVF's.[44] Close interrogation may reveal the communicating neck which appears as alternating jets of forward and reverse flow.[44]

Extrarenal Arteriovenous Fistulas and Pseudoaneurysms

Extrarenal AVF's and pseudoaneurysms are less common and usually have a different cause and work prognosis than their intrarenal counterparts do. They are commonly asymptomatic. Occasionally they cause renal dysfunction by excessive arteriovenous shunting or direct compression of the main renal artery. The most serious complication of these lesion is exsanguination due to spontaneous rupture of the pseudoaneurysm. The severity of this complication makes extrarenal pseudoaneurysms a relative clinical emergency requiring timely intervention.[45]

Extrarenal pseudoaneuryms appear as predominantly anechoic spherical paranephric fluid collections that exhibit Doppler characteristics identical to those of intrarenal pseudoaneuryms. However, recognition of the external lesions is more difficult because of involvement of larger common vessels. In the main renal arteries the increased velocity and turbulence that occur in AVF feeding arteries may be mistaken for abnormal haemodynamics of the more common arterial stenosis.

Recognition of associated increased diastolic flow will suggest the correct diagnosis. Presence of arterialised vein will help in confirmation. However, the arterialisation will be diffuse rather than focal as occur with intrarenal AVF's. This diffuse venous pulsation can be confusing because it also occurs in normal transplanted kidney. Thus diagnosis of extrarenal AVF requires careful evaluation of both arterial and venous Doppler spectra.[35]

Renal Vein Thrombosis and Stenosis

Renal vein thrombosis is a rare complication of transplantation that occurs mostly in the early postoperative period. Symptoms are usually abrupt in onset and consist of graft tenderness swelling oliguria, proteinuria and decreased renal function.

Predisposing factors include hypovolaemia, faulty surgical technique, propogation of ipsilateral common femoral or iliac deep venous thrombosis and renal vein compression by postoperative fluid collections (haematoma, lymphocele, urinoma, abscess).[35]

Renal vein thrombosis are rarely visualized by gray scale sonography. Instead the allograft can appear normal or enlarged with decreased parenchymal echogenicity and non-visualised renal veins. The duplex Doppler findings of renal vein thrombosis consist of absent renal venous flow and reversed plateauing diastolic arterial flow.[46] Venous stenosis are readily detected by colour Doppler sonography as region of focal aliasing that reflect the increased velocities associated with stenosis.[40]

ATN, Rejection and Drug Toxicity

Important causes of altered renal blood flow resulting in transplant dysfunction are ATN, acute and chronic rejection and drug toxicity.

In the normal transplant flow in the segmental interlobar and diastole and RI values range from 0.50 to 0.70 in the segmental and interlobar arteries.[36] In patients with rejection, ATN and drug toxicity elevation of RI values may be observed. High RI values have also been associated with renal vein thrombosis, renal compression, pyelonephritis and obstruction. Conversely it is possible to have acute transplant rejection without RI elevation. The value of using RI measurements to predict rejections has been extensively studied, however most workers now acknowledge the non-specific nature of mild to moderate RI elevation.[47] This limits the use of this measurement in differentiation of causes of renal transplant dysfunction and when the clinical setting does not permit differentiation, renal biopsy is required. ATN is a result of ischaemia and is common following transplantation, particularly of cadaveric kidneys where the incidence may be as high as 50 per cent.[48] Doppler abnormalities including significant elevation of RI (0.9) or greater may accompany ATN but differentiation of ATN from acute rejection is not possible.[47,49]

Transplant rejection a major complication of renal transplantation results in impaired renal function. Two forms of rejection are recognised. Acute vascular rejection and cellular or interstitial rejection.[36]

In acute vascular rejection a proliferative endovasculitis narrows the vessel lumen leading to vascular occlusion and ischaemia. In cellular or interstitial rejection perivascular oedema and infiltrate cause impaired

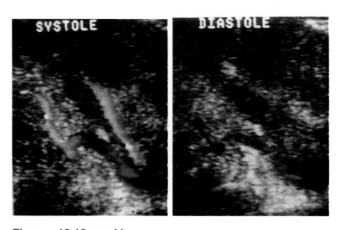

Figures 12.10a and b
Renal transplant rejection: Colour Doppler showing a forward flow during systole (a) while no flow in diastole (b)

circulation. Pure vascular rejection is uncommon and in most cases interstitial changes predominate. In either case an increase in peripheral renal arterial resistance frequently results in elevation of RI. This may be detected by spectral waveform analysis and can also be seen with Doppler colour imaging (DCI). DCI shows reduced duration of systolic arterial flow and reduction or loss of antegrade diastolic flow as the RI in the renal artery increases (Figs 12.10a and b).

Nishioka *et al*[50] have correlated visualisation of segmental and parenchymal branches of the renal artery using DCI with transplant function, nothing more pronounced changes in parenchymal vessels.

A comparison of DCI and Duplex Doppler in evaluation of 50 renal allografts performed by Mostbeek *et al*[51] has revealed a good correlation of measurement of RI and DCI findings. Allografts with pathologic RI measurements greater than or equal to 0.9 showed abnormal colour flow characterised by absence of flow in arcuate and/or interlobar arteries. In children RI has also been shown to be of little value in the identification of rejection with Doppler induce less than 0.7 reported in acute and chronic rejection as well as in cases of ATN and cyclosporine toxicity.[52] The function of renal transplant requires a balance between the beneficial effects of immunosuppressive agents in prevention of rejection and the toxic side-effects of these agents. Cyclosporine is routinely used as an immunosuppressive agent following renal transplantation. Impaired renal function and transplant loss may result from the nephrotoxic effects of cyclosporine. Although changes in vascular impedance in patients with cyclosporine toxicity may be normal, elevation of RI with cyclosporine toxicity may occur, making differentiation from rejection difficult or impossible.

Perella *et al*[54] have summarised that RI measurements do not appear capable of differentiating between these major causes of renal transplant dysfunction, i.e. acute rejection, acute tubular necrosis and cyclosporine. A nephrotoxicity specifically the RI, at any threshold cannot distinguish between acute rejection and acute tubular necrosis. Because of the very different therapy regimens for acute rejection versus acute tubular necrosis and the significant number of cases of acute rejection that can occur in the low RI ranges a biopsy must be performed in all cases.

Differentiation between vascular rejection and cellular rejection as it relates to the RI is of questionable value. However, Duplex and colour Doppler ultrasound remain valuable tools for assessing response to therapy and for evaluating the allograft for other vascular abnormalities such as acute venous and arterial thrombosis, arterial stenosis or arteriovenous fistulas.

Renal Transplant Pyelocaliectasis

Urinary obstruction is an infrequent but serious complications of renal transplantation. Obstruction is a common cause of an elevated RI > 0.75 in a transplanted kidney with pyelocaliectasis.[53] In the setting of renal transplant dysfunction and a collecting system seen at US to be dilated an abnormal RI is not conclusive for obstruction but reinforces that obstruction should be strongly considered and its presence excluded. An abnormal Doppler waveforms (increased RI) may also be helpful in the setting of a high clinical suspicion of obstruction but only mild dilatation on the realtime US examination.

In conclusion, the importance of correlation of Doppler spectral analysis, imaging and clinical observation in determining the most likely cause of transplant dysfunction deserves emphasis. Abnormal Doppler indices although not specific usually signal pathologic changes in an allograft. Biopsy remains the only definitive procedure for establishing the cause of dysfunction in many cases.

COLOUR DOPPLER SONOGRAPHY IN DETECTION OF VESICOURETERIC REFLUX

Vesicoureteric reflux is an important condition leading to renal scarring and deterioration of renal failure and hypertension. To date the most accurate and sensitive investigation has been voiding cystourethrography.[58] Radionuclide cystography is considered to be a sensitive alternative investigation of reflux.[59] Colour flow Doppler sonography is an attractive alternative to these imaging modalities as it eliminates the danger of ionising radiation and the need for urethral catheterisation and contrast agent.

Doppler study is conjunction with conventional sonography can evaluate the kidneys for echotexture, parenchymal thickness and scars while dilatation of the pelvicalyceal system helps is grading VUR.

Colour Doppler examination is carried out using 3 and 5 MHz phase array convex sector probes. Colour gain settings and filters should be optimised for slow flow sensitivity, colour map selected is red towards the probe and blue away from probe.

The patients are asked to drink water and hold their urine until they have a strong sensation of bladder fullness or to the point of reflex voiding in infants. Doppler examination is carried out in supine position. Both ureterovesical junctions (UVJ) are identified on a transverse scan and the ureteric jets are easily detected and depicted in red. Bilateral UVJ's and distal ureters are scanned in sagittal and oblique sections.

Dilated distal ureter is seen as an anechoic tubular structure posterior to the urinary bladder and entering it at the vesicoureteric junction. The presence of reflux of urine into the ureter is seen as a colour jet in blue (Figs 12.11 and 12.12).

In cases of doubt these colour jets were differentiated from nearly vascular structures by combining pulsed Doppler and colour Doppler. Colour Doppler examination is also carried out during straining and later while voiding.

VUR is graded on colour flow Doppler sonography as:[60]

Grade I	=	Low grade reflux present
Grade II	=	Reflux present and lower ureteral filling. US does not show pelvicalyceal system dilatation
Grade III	=	Reflux $\pm$ mild dilatation of ureter and pelvis on ultrasound
Grade IV	=	Reflux with moderate dilatation of pelvis on USG
Grade V	=	Reflux with massive dilatation of pelvis and ureter on USG.

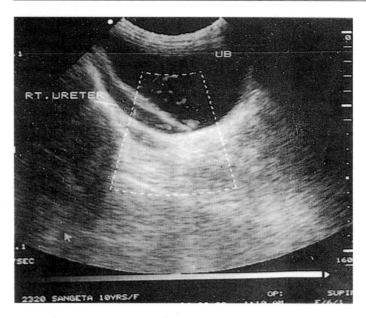

Figure 12.11
Sagittal scan CDFI showing dilated right lower ureter with VUR seen as blue colour

Since it is not possible to differentiate Grade I from Grade II VUR on combined and conventional colour flow Doppler sonography both are appropriately grouped under low grade reflux.

Studies have demonstrated low sensitivity of CFDS in detecting grade I and II reflux.[61]

However, asymptomatic grade I and II reflux may be a physiological condition in children and CFDS can be used as a possible alternative to standard cystoure-thrography for the screening and follow-up of low grade reflux.

Patient found to have higher grades (Grade III to V) can be accurately graded by performing colour Doppler sonography study.[61]

The major limitation of CFDS is suboptimal imaging of the posterior urethra, an important point to be evaluated is a male child with VUR. However, a trabe-culated bladder with bilateral hydronephrosis and hydroureters and a partially seen dilated posterior urethra can suggest distal obstruction.

The results of CFDS depends upon patient compliance and therefore is unsuitable in very young patients below 2 years of age.

DOPPLER EVALUATION OF THE PROSTATE

Anatomy

The prostate is histologically composed of glandular cancer and non-glandular elements. The non-glandular elements are the prostatic urethra and the anterior fibromuscular stroma.

The glandular prostate consists of outer and inner components.[62] Both the outer and inner prostate are subdivided, the inner prostate consists of periurethral glandular tissue and transition zone and outer prostate consists of central and peripheral zones.

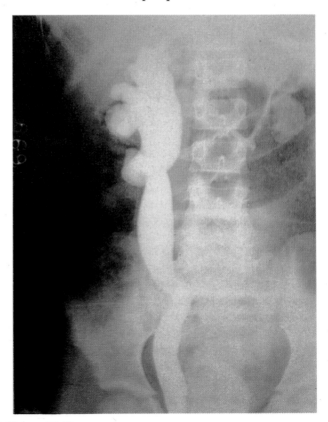

Figure 12.12
VCUG of the same patient showing GR V reflux

In total, zonal anatomy recognises five components to the prostate (1) anterior fibromuscular stroma, (2) periurethral glandular tissue, (3) transition zone, (4) central zone, and (5) peripheral zone.

From a radiologic view point, there are two important subdivisions of the glandular prostate—the peripheral zone and central gland.[63] Central gland collectively refers to periurethral, transitional and central zone.

The transitional and central zone are in variable proportion depending on the degree of benign prostate hyperplasia. In young men central gland is composed mainly of central zone whereas in older men with benign prostatic hyperplasia the central gland in composed mainly of transition zone.

Imaging

The prostate can be visualised from a suprapubic position with trans-abdominal transducers but detailed assessment of the zonal anatomy is performed using a transrectal approach. In normal young men, the zones of prostate are not sonographically evident.[62,63] With the development of benign prostate hypertrophy the central gland becomes distinguishable as a well demarcated area of heterogeneity which may contain visible nodules cysts or calcification.[63, 64]

The surgical or pseudocapsule may be evident as discrete change in echogenicity or a hypoechoicrim. The peripheral zone forms an area of uniform echogenicity surrounding the central gland. The anterior fibromuscular stroma forms a less echogenic band at the anterior aspect of the prostate.

The seminal vesicles can be seen superolaterally encased in hyperechoic fat that is continuous with fat surrounding the prostate.

Doppler Imaging

Doppler evaluation of the prostate has undergone rapid and continuous development over the last few years. The sensitivity of power Doppler is acknowledged to be superior for detection of blood flow because it relates primarily to the amplitude of Doppler signal and not direction of flow.

Standard colour Doppler however may provide some additional information in flow velocity.

Regardless of which technique is used some important scanning techniques should be emphasized following initial gray scale evaluation.

Any focal hypoechoic area or region of mass effect should be interrogated by Doppler. The initial axial scan is performed with the Doppler sample window covering the entire prostate to allow easy bilateral comparison. Any region of increased flow should be assessed further by placing that region within the centre of the image. This is particularly important for the bases of the prostate which can have normal increased capsular vessels from adjacent neuro-vascular bundles. The superior neurovascular bundles provide more prominent capsular flow than the inferior neurovascular bundles at the apex. Therefore, documenting intraparenchymal components to the flow at the bases helps decrease false positives from normal increased capsular flow.[65] Because the mid-gland is less prone to these capsular flow artefacts from the adjacent neurovascular bundles, even subtle increased intra-parenchymal flow in the mid-peripheral zone should be considered more suspicious.

Regions of increased flow need to be taken in context with gray-scale findings and other risks assessment.

Littrup and Bailey[65] have attempted to categorise increased flow patterns to normal, mildly increased or distinctly increased foci.

Normal vascularity is categorised as minimal intraparenchymal flow with symmetric capsular vessels. Subtle vascularity constitutes regions with mild increased intraparenchymal flow or asymmetric capsular vessels that show minimal penetration into adjacent parenchyma. Distinct vascularity includes areas of focal intraparenchymal flow or prominent asymmetric capsular vessels which penetrate well into adjacent parenchyma.

Distinct increased intraparenchymal flow can relate to normal vessels which are clustered together frequently in areas of atrophy where the intervening parenchyma has receded. Intraparenchymal flow is more suspicious when it has a speckled appearance perhaps suggesting much smaller vessels associated with angiogenesis.

It remains well established that prostatic carcinomas have a much higher number of microvessels per high power field than benign parenchyma.

Prostatic Cancer

Small prostatic cancers are generally hypoechoic because of the nodular cellular appearance of the carcinoma against the background of normal peripheral zone glandular tissue. Hypoechoic lesions in addition tended to be better differentiated with lower Gleason glands.[66]

However, other reports have found that hypoechoic tumors were poorly differentiated and better seen with ultrasound.[67] Hyperechoic cancer although seen infrequently has been identified. This appearance may be caused by a desmoplastic response of the surrounding glandular tissue to the presence of tumor or to infiltration of neoplasm into a background of benign prostatic hyperplasia.[66]

A significant number of prostate cancers are difficult or impossible to detect because they are isoechoic with surrounding prostate. Secondary signs such as glandular asymmetry and capsular bulging may then be helpful in diagnosis.

Colour Doppler in conjunction with transrectal ultrasound has increased the sensitivity and specificity of prostate ultrasound and ultrasound guided biopsy.

Initial reports on colour Doppler were disappointing, showing only a minimum advantage for adding colour Doppler to gray scale but suggesting that in isoechoic areas colour Doppler may give additional information.[68]

In a recent study[65, 69] Doppler findings were correlated with biopsy findings with the conclusion that colour Doppler is a useful adjunct to define areas of neovascularity that correlate with high grade cancers (Fig. 12.13). Colour Doppler also helps guide biopsies to potentially more clinically significant neoplasm.

More recent studies evaluating role of colour Doppler in the isoechoic cancer also confirm the ability of colour Doppler to identify higher grade cancers in the isoechoic gland.[70]

Importantly investigators are now studying the cause of hypervascular colour Doppler images as a function of neovascularity that has been identified in prostate and other cancers. These studies[71,72] indicate that increased microvessel density is higher in cancer than is benign tissue. In addition angiogenesis associated growth factors have been implicated is angiogenesis seen in malignant tumors. It is further suggested that angiogenesis and its associated hypervascularity seen by colour Doppler may have stage and grade implications for prostatic cancer.[72]

About 70 per cent of prostate cancers arise in the peripheral zone, 20 per cent in the transition zone and 10 per cent is the central zone. With ultrasound peripheral zone cancers are the most commonly detected and the clinician must strongly suspect cancer to identify and biopsy lesions outside the peripheral zone with gray scale imaging. With colour Doppler any area seen with small irregular vessels should be biopsied.

The contours of both the prostate and the surgical capsule are important morphologic landmarks in the evaluation of neoplastic disease. Any contour bulge of more than 1.5 cm with an associated gray scale or colour Doppler finding is suspicious for early extracapsular extension. Contour bulges along the anterior capsule need to be interrogated with colour Doppler to confirm increased blood flow differentiating cancer from BPH asymmetry.

Other abnormalities of the prostate can produce focal hypoechoic area and have to confusion regarding the significance of this finding. These include ductal ectasia, infarct atrophy, prostatitis and prostatic epithelial neoplasia.[65]

Ductal ectasia is easy to exclude because gray scale images generally demonstrate a parallel pattern of reflective interfaces when viewed is both axial and sagittal projections. Ductal ectasia is also compressible when the probe is pushed anteriorly.

Atrophy generally produce a more vague hypoechoic appearance without any mass effect and has no distinct vascularity. Granulomatous prostatitis is generally very hypoechoic focal and can produce a palpable nodule. Frequently there is history of prior infection. Granulomatous prostatitis may show increased vascularity if it is in a more active phase, which also corresponds with a recent PSA elevation. Prior or chronic granulomatous prostatitis generally does not have increased Doppler flow.

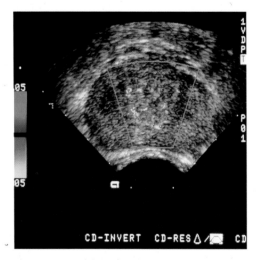

Figure 12.13
Focal hypoechoic lesion in the prostate showing increased vascularity with haphazard vessels which on pulsed Doppler

KEY POINTS

Renal transplant
- US for renal size, PCS dilatation, extrarenal collection.
- Doppler for vascular complications
  - Renal artery stenosis (m/c-10%)/ thrombosis (1%).
  - Intrarenal and extrarenal AV fistulas and pseudoaneurysm.
  - Renal vein thrombosis and stenosis.
- Transplant rejection
  - RI ≥ 0.9.
  - Reduced duration of systolic arterial flow.
  - Reduction or loss of antegrade diastolic flow.
- VUR
  - CDFI accurately grades III to V grade VUR.
  - Colour jet from bladder into distal ureters.
- Prostatic malignancy
  - Usually hypoechoic with hyper vascularity on CDFI.

Prostatic epithelial neoplasia remains difficult to differentiate from focal early neoplasms and requires biopsy confirmation.

REFERENCES

1. Desbergt AL, Paushter DM, Lammert GK, *et al*: Renal artery stenosis evaluation will colour Doppler flow imaging. *Radiology* **177**: 749-53, 1990.
2. Platt JF, Rubin JM, Ellis JH: Distinction between obstructive and non obstructive pyelocaliectasis with Duplex Doppler sonography. *AIR* **153**: 997-1006, 1989.
3. Platt JF, Rubin JM, ELlis JH, *et al*: Duplex Doppler US of the kidney differentiation of obstructive from non obstructive dilatation. *Radiology* **171**: 515-17, 1989.
4. Buds RO, Dipitro MA, Platt JF: Age dependence of the renal resistive index in healthy children. *Radiology* **184**: 469- , 1992.
5. Killer MS: Renal Doppler sonography in infants and children. *Radiology* **172**: 603-04, 1989.
6. Craonan JJ: Contemporary concepts in imaging urinary from obstruction. *Radiol Clin North Am* **29**: 527-42, 1991.
7. Klahr S, Buerkert J, Morrison A: Urinary tract obstruction. In Brenner BM, Rector FC (Eds): The Kidney (3rd edn) Philadelphia, Saunders 1449-82, 1986.
8. Yarger WE, Schocken DD, Harris RH: Obstructive uropathy in the rat. *J Clin Invest* **65**: 400-12.
9. Dodd GD, Kaufman PN, Svachen KB: Duplex Doppler evaluation of urinary obstruction in dogs. *J Urol* **145**: 644-46, 1991.
10. Wilson DR: Pathophysiology of obstructive nephropathy kidney. *Int* **18**: 281-92, 1980.
11. Leahy AL, Ryan PC, Mcentec GM: Renal injury and recovery in partial ureteric obstruction. *J Oral* **142**: 199-203, 1989.
12. Platt JF, Rubin JM, Ellis JH: Acute renal failure: Possible role of duplex Doppler ultrasound in distinction between acute prerenal failure and acute tubular necrosis. *Radiology* **179**: 419-23, 1991.
13. Patriquin HB, O'Regan S, Rabitaille P: Hemolytic uremia syndrome: Intrarenal arterial Doppler Pattern as a useful guide to therapy. *Radiology* **172**: 625-25, 1989.
14. Kier R, Taylor KJW Fejock AL: Renal masses: Characterisation with Doppler US. *Radiology* **176**: 703-07, 1990.
15. Kuijperi D, Jaspers R: Renal masses: Differential diagnosis with pulsed Doppler US. *Radiology* **170**: 59-60, 1989.
16. Dubin PA, Wills I: Renal carcinoma: Duplex Doppler evaluation. *J Radiol* **59**: 231-16, 1986.
17. Gonwa TA, Poplawski S, Paulsen W: Pathogenesis and outcome of hepatorenal syndrome in patients undergoing orthoptic liver transplant. *Transplantation* **47**: 395-97, 1989.
18. Gentiline P, Laffe G, Buzzelli G: Functional renal alteration in Chronic liver disease. *Digetion* **20**: 73-78, 1980.
19. Platt JF, Ellis JH, Rubin JM: Renal Duplex Doppler ultrasonography: Non invasive indicator of kidney dysfunction and hepatorenal failure. Liver Disease. *Hepatology* **20(2)**: 362-69, 1994.
20. Pozniak MA, Dodd GD, Kelcz F: Ultrasonographic evaluation of renal transplantation *Radiol Clin N Am* **30**: 1053-66, 1992.
21. Platt JF, Ellis JH, Rubin JMA: Intrarenal arterial Doppler sonography in the Detection of Renal vein thrombosis of native kidney. *AJR* **162**: 1367-70, 1994.
22. Keating MA, ALthausen AF: The clinical spectrum of renal vein thrombosis. *J Uroe* **133**: 938-1045, 1985.
23. Parvey HR, Eisenberg RL: Image directed Doppler sonography of intrarenal arteries in acute renal vein thrombosis *J Clin Ultrasound* **8**: 512-16, 1990.
24. Laplante S, Patriguin HB, Robitaille P: Renal vein thrombosis in children: Evidence of early flow recovery with Doppler US. *Radiology* **189**: 37-42, 1993.
25. Haber E, Slater EE: High blood pressure. *Sci Am* **i(VII)**: 1-30, 1992.
26. Mann SJ, Pickiring: Detection of renovascular hypertension. *Ann Intern Med*, 117.
27. Chen CC, Hoffe PB, Vahjen G: Patients at high risk for renal artery stenosis: A simple method of renal scintigraphic analysis with Tc99m DTPA and captopril. *Radiology* **176**: 365-70, 1990.

28. Kohler TR, Zierler RE, Martin RL: Non invasive diagnosis of renal artery stenosis by Ultrasonic duplex scanning. *J Vaso Surg* **4**: 450-56, 1986.

29. Taylor DC, Killer MD, Moneta GI: Duplex ultrasound scanning in the diagnosis of renal artery stenosis: A prospective evaluation. *J Vase Surg* **7**: 363-69, 1988.

30. Berland LL: Koslin Db, Routh WD: Renal artery steonsis: Prospective valuation of diagnosis with colour duplex US compared with angiography. Work in progress. *Radiology* **174**: 421-23, 1990.

31. Stavros ATA, Parker SH, Yakes WF: Segmental stenosis of Renal artery: Patt recognition of the Tardus and Parvus abnormalities with Duplex sonography. *Radiology* **184(2)**: 487-02, 1992.

32. Handa N, Fukunaga R, Etani H *et al*: Efficacy of echo Doppler examination for the evaluation of renovascular disease. *Ultrasound Med Biol* **14**: 145, 1988.

33. Kotval PS: Doppler waveform parvus and tardus: A sign of proximal flow obstruction: *J Ultrasound Med* **8**: 435-40, 1989.

34. Patriguin HB, Lafortune M, Jequic JC: Stenosis of renal artery: Assessment showed systole in the downstream circulation with Doppler sonography. *Radiology* **184**: 479-85, 1992.

35. Dodd GD, Tublin ME, Shah A *et al*: Imaging of vascular complication associated with renal transplants. *AJR* **157**: 449-59, 1991.

36. Meerut CRB: Organ Transplants. In Taylor KJW, Burns PN, WIlls PNJ (Eds): *Clinical Application of Doppler Ultrasound* (2nd edn). Raven Press 203-330, 1995.

37. Hohnke C, Abendroth D, Schleibnee S *et al*: Vascular complication in 1,200 kidney transplantations. *Transplant Proc* **19**: 3691-92, 1987.

38. Roberts JP, Ascher NL, Fryel DS *et al*: Transplant renal artery stenosis. *Transplantation* **4**: 580-83, 1989.

39. Honto D, Simmons R: Renal transplantation: Clinical considerations in organ transplantation. *Radiol Clin North Am* **25**: 239-48, 1987.

40. Taylor KJW, Morse SS, Rigsby CM *et al*: Vascular complication in renal allografts: Detection with Duplex Doppler ultrasound. *Radiology* **162**: 31-38, 1987.

41. Gottlish RH, Lirberman JC, Pahico RC *et al*: Diagnosis of renal artery stenosis in transplanted kidneys value of Doppler waveform analysis of the intrarenal arteries **165**: 1441-46, 1995.

42. Ahula ND, Greenberg A, Banner BF *et al*: Atheroembolic involvement of renal allografts. *Am J Med Dis* **12**: 329-32, 1989.

43. Beneit G, Charepntier B, Roche A: Arterio calyceal fistula after grafted kidney biopsy: Successful management by selective catheter embolisation. *Urology* **24**: 487-90, 1984.

44. Middleton WD, Kellran GM, Melson GL: Post biopsy renal transplant arteriovenous fistula: Colour Doppler versus US characteristics. *Radiology* **171**: 253-57, 1989.

45. Pigott JP, Sharp WV: Arteriovenous fistula involving tansplant kidney: Brief communications. *Transplantation* **44**: 1, 1987.

46. Kaveggia LP, Parella RR, Grant EG: Duplex Doppler sonography in renal allografts the significance of reversed flow in diastole. *AIR* **155**: 295-98, 1990.

47. Taylor KT, marks WH: Use of Doppler imaging for evaluation of dysfunction in renal allografts Comment. *AJR* **155**: 536-37, 1990.

48. Tiggeler RG, Berdin JH, Hoitsma AI *et al*: Prevention of acute tubular necrosis in cadavesic kidney transplantation by the combined use of manitol and moderate hydration. *Ann Surg* **201**: 246-51, 201.

49. Kelez F, Pozniak MA, Pirsch JD: Pyramidal appearances and resistive and nonspecific sonographic indicators of renal transplant rejection (See Comments). *AJR* **155**: 531-35, 1990.

50. Nishioka N, Ikegami M: Imanishim: Renal transplant blood flow evaluation of colour Doppler echography. *Transplant Proc* **21**: 1919, 1989.

51. Mostbeeh GH, Rachlatter C, Stockenluber F: Comparison of Duplex sonography and colour Doppler imaging in renal allograft evaluation: A prospective study: *Eur J Radiol* **10**: 201-07, 1990.

52. Drake DG, Day DL, Letourneau JG: Doppler evaluation of renal transplant in children: A prospective analysis with tests pathologic correlation: *AJR* **154**: 785-87, 154.

53. Platt JF, Ellis JH, Rubin JM: Renal transplant pyelocaliectasis: Role of Duplex Doppler US in evaluation *Radiology* **179**: 425-25, 1991.

54. Perrella RR, Duerincky A, Tessler FN: Evaluation of renal transplant dysfunction by duplex Doppler sonography: A prospective study and review of literature. *Am J Med Dis* **15(6)**: 544-50, 1990.

55. Laing FC, Jeffrey RB, Wing VW: Ultrasound versus excretory urography in evaluating acute flash plain. *Radiology* **154**: 613-16, 1985.

56. Plat JF, Rubin JM, Ellis JH: Acute renal obstruction: Evaluation with intrarenal duplex Doppler and conventional US. *Radiology* **186**: 685-88, 1993.

57. Killer MS, Korsvih HE, Weiss RM: Diuretic Doppler sonography with correlative scintigraphy in children with hydronephrosis. *Sco Pediatr Radiol* **35**: 4972, 1992.

58. Tremewan RN, Bailey KR, Little PJ: Diagnosis of gross vesicoureteric reflux using ultrasonography. *Br J Urol* **48**: 431-35, 1976.

59. Nasrallah PF, Conway JJ, King LR: Quantitative nuclear cystogram and in determining spontaneous resolution of vesicoureteric reflux. *Urology* **12**: 654-58, 1978.

60. Haffman AD, Le Roy AJ: Uroradiology: Procedures and anatomy. In Kelalils PP, King LR, Belman AB (Eds): *Clinical Pediatric Urology* (3rd edn). Philadelphia WB Saunders: **97**: 1992.

61. Hanburg D, Coulden R, Farman P: Ultrasound cytography in the diagnosis of vesicourteric reflux. *Br J Urol* **65**: 65-68, 1990.

62. Stamey TA, McNeal JE: Adenocarcinoma of the prostate. In Walsh PC, Retik AB, Stamey TA, Vaughan ED (Eds): *Campbells Urology* (6th edn) Philadelphia, WB Saunders: **1**: 643-58, 1992.

63. Older RA, Watson LR: Ultrasound anatomy of the normal male reproductive tract. *J Clin Ultrasound* **24**: 389-409, 1996.

64. Rifkin MD, Dahnert W, Kurtz AB: State of the art: Endorectal sonography of the prostate gland. *AJR* **154**: 691-700, 1990.

65. Littrup PJ, Bailey SE: Prostate cancer: The role of transrectal ultrasound and its impact on cancer detection and management. *Radiol Clinics North Am* **38 (1)**: 87-113, 2000.

66. Rifkin MD, McGlynn ET, Choi H: Echogenicity of prostatic cancer correlated with histologic grade and stromal fibrosis: endorectal ultrasound studies. *J Urol* **170**: 549-52, 1989.

67. Shinohara K, Wheeler TM, Scardino PT: The appearance of prostatic cancer on transrectal ultrasonography: corrrlation of imaging and pathological examination. *J Urol* **142**: 76-82, 1989.

68. Patel V, Rickards D: The diagnostic value of colour Doppler flow in the peripheral zone of prostate with histological correlation. *Br J Urol* **74**: 590-95, 1994.

69. Brce RC: The prostate. In Rumach CM, Wilson SR, Charbonean JW (Eds): *Diagnostic Ultrasound* (2nd edn) *Mosby Year Book* **1**: 399-429, 1988.

70. Decarvalho V, Kuligowska E: The role of colour Doppler for improving the detection of cancer in the isoechoic prastate gland. Presented at the annual meeting of the American Institute of Ultrasound in Medicine, New York, 1996.

71. Bigler SA, Deering RE, Brawer MK: A quantitative morphometric analysis of the microcirculation in prostate carcinoma. *Human Pathol* **24**: 220-26, 1993.

72. MeNeal JE, Redwine EA, Frciha FA: Zonal distribution of prostatic adenocarcinoma. *Am J Surg Pathol* **12**: 897-906, 1988.

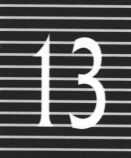

The Retroperitoneum and Great Vessels

Shefali Gupta
GP Vashist
Suchi Bhatt
Shashank Jain
Rohini Gupta

Pulsed Doppler equipment is becoming widely available as an additional facility on many realtime scanners whether mechanical, electronic or linear array. The principle on which these instruments rely for the ultrasonic detection of blood flow is described by the Doppler equation. An ultrasonic beam of frequency of scattered by red blood cells moving with a velocity suffers an change in frequency Δf.

$$\frac{\Delta F = 2f\upsilon \, \text{Cos} \, \theta}{c}$$

where θ is the angle between the axis of beam and direction of flow and c is velocity of ultrasound.

Thus for a given ultrasonic frequency the Doppler shift is proportional to the blood flow velocity and the cosine of the beam vessel angle. A range of velocities within the vessel lumen will give risk to a range of Doppler shift frequencies. Most instruments provide a realtime display of this range of frequencies with time on horizontal axis, Doppler shift frequency on the vertical axis.

A Doppler examination can be made simply to confirm the presence or absence of flow or determine direction. Such a qualitative use of Doppler imaging can be clinically valuable. In patients with cirrhosis, reversed flow in the portal vein may accompany severe portal hypertension. The presence of flow in portal vein or renal vessels can be most helpful in excluding occlusion, while flow signals from solid mass can indicate neovascularisation associated with malignancy.

In addition to such qualitative uses of Doppler technique spectral analysis of the signals allows more detailed quantitation. The outline of the maximum Doppler shift frequency corresponds to the time variation of the maximum flow velocity within the vessel. The pulsatility of this waveform is related to the vascular impedance downstream to the point of measurement.[1] In addition the range of frequencies present in the Doppler spectrum yields information about distribution of velocities across the vessel lumen. This provides evidence of the flow conditions, whether there is a plug or parabolic flow profile, whether there is flow disturbances or turbulence related to vessel wall abnormality.

Figure 13.1 for example shows how different velocity profiles in a vessel with laminar flow give rise to different spectral distributions and how this is reflected in the distribution of the gray scale in Doppler display.[1] When all the flow laminae are moving at the same velocity one Doppler shift frequency predominates: this is the plug flow profile typical of the aorta (Fig. 13.1a).

A parabolic velocity profile from a smaller vessel such as hepatic artery results in a more even distribution of power in the Doppler spectrum (Fig. 13.1b).

Intermediate profiles are present in such arteries as the caeliac trunk (Fig. 13.1c). These Doppler characteristic which can be quantified using a variety of parameters, enable a discription of a signal that is fairly specific to a particular vessel or even vessel site.

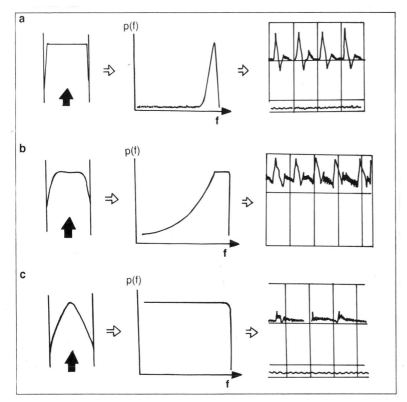

Figures 13.1a to c
Showing the relationship between differing velocity profiles in a vessel with laminar flow (left column), the Doppler power spectrum (middle), and the resulting spectral display (right)

Aorta

The abdominal aorta is a compliant tube that supplies blood to the digestive organs, the kidneys, the adrenals, the gonads, the abdominal and paraspinal musculature and the pelvis and lower limbs. It contributes significantly to the continuous forward flow of blood during diastole by acting as a reservoir of fluid during systole when it has a very pulsatile, inflow. It decreases in size during diastole by discharging blood into rest of the circulation in a much less pulsatile manner.[2] The abdominal aorta tapers from its cranial to caudal extent in 95 per cent of people and usually measures less than 2.3 cm in diameter for men and 1.9 cm for women.[3] The upper limit of normal for aortic diameter varies with age as the diameter normally increases by upto 25 per cent in the seventh and eight decades.

The abdominal aorta enters the abdomen through the aortic hiatus of the diaphragm, immediately anterior to the twelfth dorsal vertebra. The upper abdominal aorta lies posterior and slightly to the left of the gastroesophageal junction. The median arcuate ligament of the diaphragm about its anterior surface and it is flanked on either side by the diaphragmatic crura. To the right lies the azygous vein and thoracic duct on its left lies the hemiazygous vein. Below the level of the crura it lies to the left of IVC and posterior to the coeliac artery, superior mesenteric artery, inferior mesentric, left renal vein, gonadal vessels and root of mesentery. At the L_4 level, it bifurcates into paired common iliac arteries which are about 5 cm long and generally run slightly anterior to the corresponding veins. The common iliac arteries bifurcates into external and internal iliac arteries. The external iliac artery lies just on the medial aspect of psoas muscle.

The main aortic branches that are frequently seen on ultrasound are the iliac artery the paired renal arteries, the superior mesenteric artery and the common iliac arteries.

The coeliac artery is typically bifurcates into hepatic and splenic arteries within 3 cm of its origin. The left gastric artery is given off superiorly is sometimes seen. The internal iliac arteries have numerous branches immediately after the common iliac artery bifurcation but are rarely seen on routine sonograms. The external iliac artery gives off the inferior epigastric artery and deep circumflex iliac artery before continuing below the inguinal ligament as the common femoral artery.

Other aortic branches not usually identified include paired inferior phrenic, paired middle suprarenal, gondal arteries, the inferior mesenteric artery and

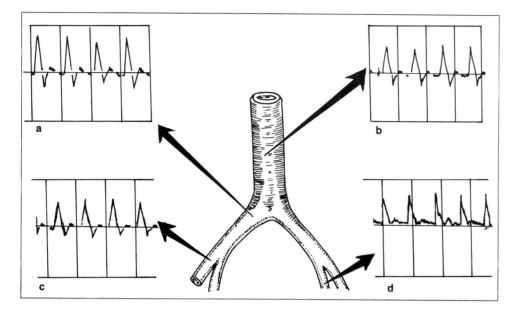

Figure 13.2
Time velocity spectra in common iliac artery (a), distal aorta (b) external iliac artery (c) and internal iliac artery (d)

paired first to fourth lumbar artery. At the aortic termination, the middle sacral artery is given off postero-inferiorly.

At sonography aorta is shown as a hypoechoic tubular structure with echogenic walls. It is usually located just to the left of the midline, although it becomes variable in position when it becomes ectatic. The mid-abdominal aorta at the level of renal arteries is frequently difficult to visualise well because of overlying bowel gas.

The normal flow pattern in the aorta is classified as plug flow, a situation in which most of the blood is moving at the same velocity. In the aorta and iliac arteries, flow is typically of the high resistance type with a sharp increase in antegrade velocity during systole followed by a rapid decrease in velocity and culminating in a brief period of reversed flow (Fig. 13.2). The aortic signals show a clear window below the systolic time velocity pulse implying that most cells are moving at same velocity. During the remainder of diastole there is some low velocity antegrade flow. Of note is the decrease in flow at the end of diastole which begins to reverse in direction at the level of bifurcation.[1] This is due to blood actually rebounding up the aorta as the velocity wave is reflected from high impedance of the peripheral vascular bed of legs. The fact that this flow is found below the renal vessels results in the renal arterial flow being maintained during diastole. Relatively continuous flow in the renal artery may be of importance in renal function.

The main aortic branches supply numerous low resistance areas and as such, these have a lower resistive index and a lower pulsatility index. These smaller vessel show a more variable velocity pattern across the blood vessel and so the thickness of the spectral line is broadened. Good acoustic window for scanning the abdominal aorta include:

- The midline in the upper abdomen.
- The left flank with patient. Supine or right lateral decubitus.
- Along the lateral aspect of the lower rectus abdominis muscle for evaluating iliac vessels.

The entire aorta should be visualised in transverse and longitudinal planes and its maximum antero-posterior and transverse diameter measured accurately.

Aortic Pathology

The abdominal aorta and its main branches are affected by atheroma, aneurysm formation, connective tissue disorders, rupture, thrombosis, infectious and displacement by and invasion from disease in adjacent structures.

Atheromatous Disease

Atheroma or arteriosclerosis is a vascular wall disorders characterised by the presence of lipid deposits in the intima atherosclerotic changes in the aorta are virtually universal beyond the age of 20 years and it affects more men than women. It affects both the aorta, the iliac arteries and the other aortic branch arteries and is most common on the posterior wall in the aorta iliac area.[4] It is associated with cigarette

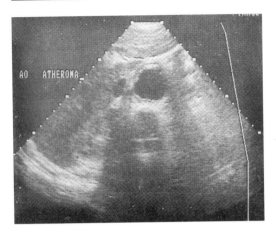 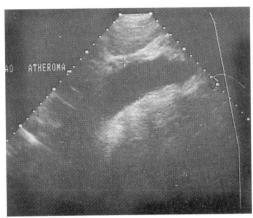

Figures 13.3a and b
Dilated abdominal aorta in (a) transverse, and (b) longitudinal scan with atherosclerotic plaques

smoking, diabetes mellitus, hypertension and increased levels of low density lipoprotein (LDL) fraction of serum cholesterol.

If significant lower limb pain is present, it is prudent to assess the entire lower limb arterial tree to rule out emboli and to look for further stenosis. Similarly in down limb analysis the presence of a dampened waveform in the common femoral artery should provoke a search for a stenotic lesion more proximal in arterial tree.[5]

Ultrasound can demonstrate thickening and calcification within the aortic wall (Figs 13.3a and b). If calcification is extensive, acoustic shadowing may result. In these cases, visualisation of the aortic lumen may be limited. Atheromatous plaque is a soft porridge like material which may discharge into the vessel lumen causing a distal embolus or a thrombus or both at the donor site. Thrombus within the vessel usually has a low level echogenicity but may be anechoic (Figs 13.4a and b). An occluded vessel can appear patent because of echo free lumen but will not pulsate.[6] Plaque cause mural irregularity[6] and frequently narrow the vessel lumen with resulting distal

ischaemia. Stenotic or occlusive disease most often occurs in the infrarenal portion of the aorta. Atheroma may also be associated with mural weakening and aneurysm formation.

Patency of the aorta and its branch vessels can be confirmed with colour Doppler analysis and where aliasing occurs, a Doppler spectral tracing helps to determine whether a true stenosis is present or not.

Angle corrected spectral Doppler analysis at stenosis typically shows increased pulsatility (increased pulsatility index and resistive index) proximal to stenosis, increased peak systolic and peak diastolic velocity immediately at the stenosis, turbulence immediately post- stenosis and dampening of waveform further distal to stenosis.[7]

Several workers[8,9] have classified arterial stenosis. Each arterial segment is graded into five categories of stenosis (i) Normal (ii) 1 to 19 per cent diameter reduction (iii) 20 to 49 per cent diameter reduction (iv) 50 to 99 per cent diameter reduction (v) Total occlusion.

Normal arteries have a triphasic signal and minimal spectral broadening. The spectral band is narrow with a clear area below the systolic peak (systolic

Figures 13.4a and b
(a) Longitudinal and (b) transverse scans of aorta showing a thrombus in the lumen just at the point of origin of superior mesenteric artery

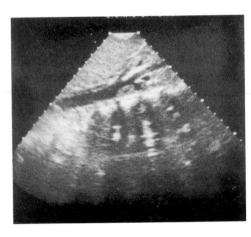 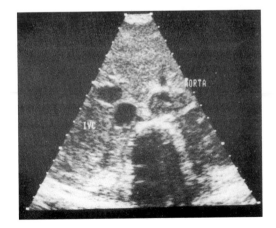

window). A diameter reduction of 1 to 19 per cent causes only spectral broadening and loss of systolic window waveform contour and peak systolic velocity remain normal. In moderate stenosis (20-49% diameter reduction) the peak systolic velocity increases 30 to 100 per cent with respect to the normal segment immediately proximal to the stenosis and spectral broadening is marked. Stenosis of 50 to 99 per cent diameter reduction are consider haemodynamically significant. Reverse velocity is absent in these stenosis, the systolic peak is increased by 100 per cent or more and spectral broadening is usually prominent. Occluded arteries have no detectable flow and velocity is markedly decreased in the segments proximal to occlusion.

Angiography has long been the definitive test for symptomatic aortic iliac disease. However, this approach provides anatomic rather than functional data and has many limitation. Because atherosclerotic lesion are often concenteric, the angiographic appearance may be misleading, especially if only unipolar views are obtained. The best way to determine the haemodynamic significance of arterial lesion is to measure the pressure gradient at angiography but this is not always practical or anatomically possible. Finally the invasive nature and relatively high cost of angiography make it unsuitable for screening purpose or routine follow-up.

Duplex scanning can localise and classify peripheral arterial stenosis nearly as well as angiography.[8] A normal Duplex study virtually excludes significant occlusive disease. When the Duplex study localises the suspected area of disease, it can be helpful to the angiographer who may be able to tailor the angiography technique to fit the needs of patient.

In addition Duplex scanning provides a baseline for assessing the early and long-term results of PTA. Duplex scanning can detect restenosis of segments dilated by angioplasty or bypass graft stenosis before pressure drops occurs.[8]

Flow velocities less than 40 cm/sec in femoropopliteal bypass[8] grafts are associated with a high rate of graft failure.[18] Thus, the ability of Duplex scanning to distinguish high grade stenosis from occlusion to detect haemodynamically in-significant disease and to localise disease accurately is unique among non-invasive tests and represents the first practical means of documenting arterial disease progression.[18]

Aortic Aneurysms

Abdominal aortic aneurysm is a common disease with potentially catastrophic complications. Untreated, these aneurysms enlarge and eventually rupture with a high mortality of 50-90 per cent. Conversely elective surgical resection has an excellent prognosis and low mortality (2-4%) and currently is the treatment of choice.[10] Because most patients are asymptomatic the diagnosis of abdominal aortic aneurysm is frequently unsuspected. Evaluation of these patients is heavily dependent on imaging and the radiologist is in a unique position to direct the work-up.[11]

A true aneurysm of abdominal aorta is a localised dilatation of wall greater than 3 cm in diameter. All these layers of the vessel (intima, media and adventitia) are involved. A false aneurysm (pseudo-aneurysm) is essentially a perforation of the aorta with subsequent haematoma formation limited by adventitial or surrounding vascular tissues (Fig. 13.5).

Most abdominal aortic aneurysms are secondary to atherosclerosis. Other causes include trauma,

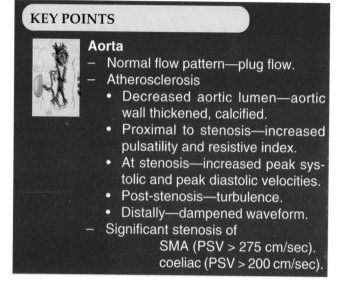

KEY POINTS

Aorta
- Normal flow pattern—plug flow.
- Atherosclerosis
  • Decreased aortic lumen—aortic wall thickened, calcified.
  • Proximal to stenosis—increased pulsatility and resistive index.
  • At stenosis—increased peak systolic and peak diastolic velocities.
  • Post-stenosis—turbulence.
  • Distally—dampened waveform.
- Significant stenosis of
  SMA (PSV > 275 cm/sec).
  coeliac (PSV > 200 cm/sec).

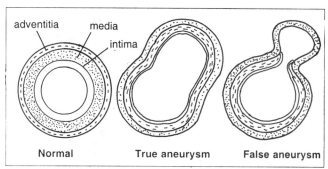

Figure 13.5
Types of aortic aneurysm

infection, syphilis, cystic medial necrosis, inflammation and Marfan's syndrome.

Atherosclerotic plaques cause fibrosis and atrophy of the underlying media of aortic wall. Loss of medial elastic fibres seen with advancing age compounds this insult. The weakened media can no longer adequately support the vessel wall, resulting in aortic dilatation. The weakened media can no longer adequately support the vessel wall resulting in aortic dilatation. Increasing dilatation and decreasing wall thickness result in a rapid increase in wall tension (Laplace's law). This leads to progressive dilatation and eventual rupture.[11]

Inflammatory aortic aneurysm is a distinct clinical entity distinguished from uncomplicated atherosclerotic aneurysms by dense perianeurysmal fibrosis and thickened aortic walls of abdominal aortic aneurysms 4 to 23 per cent are estimated to be inflammatory in origin. They are very difficult to diagnose as they often present with pain and mimic retroperitoneal bleed.[15] While less than 25 per cent of idiopathic abdominal aneurysm present with pain, pain was present in 84 per cent of patients with inflammatory aneurysms.

Surgical repair of these aneurysms is difficult with increased morbidity and mortality compared with simple aneurysm. Abdominal aortic aneurysms 3-6 cm in diameter grow approximately at 4/mm year. The risk of rupture relates primarily to the size of aneurysm with a clear increase in risk over 5 cm. Even small aneurysms are more likely to rupture of significant enlargement is demonstrated on sequential studies. Consequently it has been proposed than even small asymptomatic aneurysms be re-examined 3-6 months after diagnosis and then at 12 months intervals. Regardless of size symptomatic aneurysm imply rapid growth or rupture. The most common surgical treatment is endo-aneurysmorrhaphy which consists of placement of a prosthetic graft within the aneurysm. The aneurysm wall is then wrapped around the graft, providing protection against aortoenteric fistulas. Complete resection of the aneurysm with graft-placement can be performed also.

Currently imaging methods for the diagnosis of abdominal aortic aneurysms include US, CT conventional angiography or digital subtraction angiography and MRI.[12]

Ultrasound and colour Doppler US[13] are the standard methods in the screening and follow-up of abdominal aortic aneurysm although in many cases they are not able to visualise the renal arteries and can be limited by the extremely variable body weight and bowel gas of the patient.

The CT technique is excellent in both pre and postoperation evaluation of abdominal aortic aneurysms but some controversies exist about the efficiency of CT in evaluating the involvement of renal arteries.[14] Moreover, CT is not always able to discriminate between a thrombus filled aneurysm and a lot within the false lumen of a dissection.[11]

Digital subtraction angiography is the gold standard in the detection of the involvement of increased branches and/or variants of vascular anatomy[11] but it can underestimate both the size and extension of a thrombus filled aneurysm, due to opacification of the lumen alone.

The first MRI reports in the study of abdominal aortic aneurysms, obtained by using spin echo or gradient echo sequences have been encouraging, but more recently by magnetic resonance angiography seems to be the most promising non-invasive method in the assessment of abdominal aortic aneurysms.[12]

Sonography is the standard method for screening and follow-up of aortic aneurysms. It approaches 100 per cent accuracy in detection and measurements correlate within 3 mm of surgical specimen. Sonograms may show thrombus, periaortic abnormalities, dissection cephalic and caudal extent as well as complication such as hydronephrosis.

Sonography is limited in obese patients or those with abundant overlying bowel gas. In addition the renal arteries are rarely visualised directly and suprarenal extension frequently can only be inferred by the relationship of the aneurysm to the superior mesenteric artery. Availability, cost, non-invasiveness combined with accuracy in detection and measurement make sonography ideal for screening and follow-up of uncomplicated aneurysms.

Diagnosis of an aneurysm is made sonographically by finding a focal dilatation of the aorta or a generalised dilatation bigger than 3 cm. Aneurysms elongate as they grow and as the lower end of aorta rarely moves significantly caudally, most abdominal aortic aneurysms defect to the left side or kink anteriorly or both as they enlarge.[5]

The anterior or posterior borders of the aneurysms are usually better seen than its lateral borders which are indistinct. The adventitia is usually continuous with adjacent fibrofatty tissue and in echogenic. Mural thrombus, which frequently makes up most of the wall is usually of low to medium echogenicity and it may or may not have a lamellated appearance. The intimal lining may be smooth or irregular and calcification may also be present.

Sonography measurement of these aneurysms may be challenging and it is important to get an accurate outer layer to outer layer measurement in a plane perpendicular to the long axis of the vessel.

Analysis of an aneurysms would include its maximum true length width and transverse dimension, documentation of its shape and documentation of its location including suprarenal extension or involvement of common iliac vessels. This analysis is of great practical importance, as different surgical approaches are used with the different types of aneurysms. The aetiology, complications rate and post- procedure morbidity are also quite distinct. The nature and type of wall thickening should be found and flow pattern characterised. Effort should be made to detect any dissection and to evaluate hypoechoic channels for flow with Doppler. Both kidneys should always be examined, their size measured and pelvic caliectasis excluded.[5]

Following descriptive terms and sonographic criterion as used for abdominal aortic aneurysm:
- *Bulbous* Sharp junction between normal and abnormal
- *Fusiform* Gradual transition between normal and abnormal
- *Saccular* Sharp sudden transition between normal and abnormal
- *Dumbbell* Figure eight appearance to the aneurysm

The decision to operate on an aneurysm is based on[5]:
- Absolute size especially when diameter > 6 cm
- Documented enlargement over-time
- Associated pain or tenderness
- Associated distal emboli
- Renal obstruction or vascular compromise
- Gastrointestinal bleeding
- Suspected rupture.

In a study by Carriero *et al*[12] results suggested that MRA together with colour Doppler US represented a valid alternative to invasive imaging in the assessment of abdominal aortic aneurysm. In their study colour Doppler US proved to be effective in the determination of aneurysm diameter, cranio-caudal extension and thrombotic and calcific components. It showed better results than MRA in the evaluation of the relation between aneurysm and main arterial branches (renal and iliac) due to the possibility to detect colour encoded flow signals which make it easier to identify the vessel. In particular it always detected the iliac arteries and correctly documented their involvement in 50 per cent of cases. The detection rate of renal arteries proved less satisfactory than MRA due to technical problems.

The recognised complications of abdominal aortic aneurysm includes rupture, thrombosis, dissection, distal embolism, infection and obstruction and invasion of adjacent structures. Most common complications are branch artery occlusions or stenosis which have more to do with atheromas than with aneurysm. They can occur anywhere but are most commonly seen in the inferior mesenteric artery and renal artery.[15]

Aortic Rupture

The most catastrophic of aortic aneurysm complication is aortic rupture which has a mortality rate of at least 50 per cent.[15] Because of the critical nature of problem few of these patients have ultrasound preoperatively. Computed tomography is the test of choice.[16] It is better at detecting acute bleeds is not tampered by bowel gas and provides a greater overall perspective. Some aortic rupture may be contained in the retroperitoneum; they are referred to as chronic ruptures. Ultrasonic appearances those of a pulsating haematoma, a hypoechoic collection in the periaortic region extending to the flanks.[17]

Aortic Dissection

A dissecting aortic aneurysm is not a free aneurysm of the aorta but rather a propagating haematoma extending initially within the media of the aorta to eventually rupture into intimately lined aortic lumen[17] (Fig. 13.6).

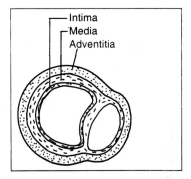

Figure 13.6
Line diagram showing aortic dissection

It is easily recognised on sonography with the classical appearance being a thin membrane fluttering in the lumen at different phases of cardiac cycle.[15] Colour Doppler shows blood flow in both channel, although flow rates frequently differ between the channels.

Effort should be made to distinguish a true dissection from a pseudo-dissection which is caused by liquefaction of aneurysm thrombus.[18] The distinguishing features include no fluttering of the intravascular membrane, no flow in one lumen and a thick membrane in pseudo-lesion.[15]

Abdominal Aortic Pseudoaneurysm

Abdominal aortic pseudoaneurysms may occur as a complication of abdominal aortic aneurysm, abdominal interventional procedure or abdominal surgery. They may also result from vasculitis, mycotic aneurysms or abdominal surgery and may be associated with post-procedural haematomas particularly in patients receiving anticoagulant or antiplatelet medication.[19]

A pseudoaneurysm is an organised paravascular haematoma that has a lumen is continuity with the vascular lumen. Formation of a pseudoaneurysm generally involves an arterial injury, local haemorrhage and tamponade by surrounding tissues.[20] Pseudoaneurysm of the abdominal aorta is a rare finding accounting for only 1 per cent of all abdominal aneurysms.[21]

On gray scale sonography pseudoaneurysms appear as anechoic saccular collections in proximity to arteries (Figs 13.7a and b). These collections are more easily perceived by colour flow mapping. Pulsed Doppler studies show turbulent or arterial-like flow (swirling or whirl wind flow) within the pseudoaneurysm lumen and systolic and diastolic continuous flow, the classic 'to and fro' spectral wave pattern, in the communicating channel. This pattern consists of high speed flow directed outward from the artery into the pseudoaneurysm during systole and slower flow out of the pseudoaneurysm during diastole.[22]

The 'to and fro' sign is helpful in identifying the exact point of communication between the pseudoaneurysms and aorta when planning a surgical approach.[3]

Haematomas or other fluid collections adjacent but not communicating with the aorta may move vigorously as the aorta pulsates. Such movement should not be mistaken for the concentric pulsations of a pseudoaneurysm.

The final diagnosis with Duplex Doppler sonography requires identification of the typical flow pattern within the neck of the pseudoaneurysm. This finding usually demonstrated in postcatheterisation pseudoaneurysms' can be absent or less obvious in those that are due to a dehiscence of the anastomotic connection of synthetic bypass grafts, those due to involvement of peripancreatic arteries by chronic pancreatitis, or those complicating organ transplants.[22] The reason for this can be due to either the absence of or difficulty in locating a communicating channel or it can be due to the presence of a broad channel that shows a highly turbulent and disorganised atypical

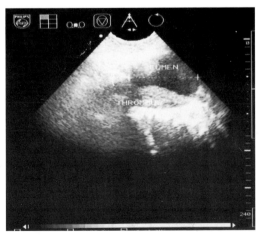

Figure 13.7a
Gray scale image in transverse plane at mid-aortic level showing well defined, anechoic saccular collection in continuity with the aorta. An echogenic thrombus is seen in the posterior wall of the pseudoaneurysm

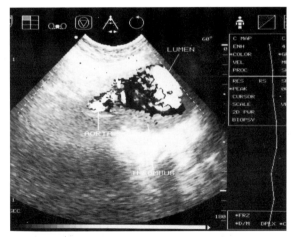

Figure 13.7b
Colour flow Doppler image of same patient showing luminal blood flow in the pseudoaneurysm

flow throughout the cardiac cycle. Combined Duplex and colour flow sonography is the screening modality of choice to evaluate a pulsatile mass in the abdomen.

Aortic Grafts

Distal Aortic Graft

The operative procedure for a patient with an isolated infrarenal abdominal aortic aneurysms who has no evidence of peripheral vascular disease is a simple tube graft. This is appreciated sonographically by a rather sharp definition of parallel echogenic walls in the distal aorta.

Aortic aneurysms are repaired by incising the aneurysms, implanting the graft, then wrapping the aneurysmal sac around the implanted graft as a stabilizing force.

The relatively high incidence of complications following endovascular aneurysms surgery mandates rigorous postoperative surveillance programme. Endo leaks have been described in all initial series of endovascular aneurysm repairs with an incidence ranging from 10 to 43 per cent. Endoleaks may be early or late and may arise from the proximal anastomosis, the distal anastomosis or as a result of retrograde filling from the lumbar, inferior mesenteric or common iliac vessels. Irrespective of the origin of the leak the consequences are potentially serious. Establishment of flow within the aneurysm sac may facilitate continued aneurysm expansion and rupture. Conventionally CT has been used to follow patients after endovascular aneurysm repair. Recent study has suggested than Duplex imaging may be useful in the setting.[23]

It bleeding occurs postoperatively haematoma tends to dissect between the graft and the encircling aneurysmal wall producing a characteristic ultrasonic appearance of a lumen within a lumen.

Duplex imaging demonstrates the presence of flow within the aneurysm as at the site of leak.[23]

Majority of patients with a proven endoleak have continued expansion of aneurysm sac.[23]

Studies have shown that successful exclusion of the aneurysm sac results in a reduction in aneurysm size.[23,24]

One theoretical problem associated with endovascular aneurysm repair concerns the fate of the proximal aortic neck. The proximal aortic neck may continue to dilate, which could cause migration and displacement of the proximal aortic stent.[23]

Duplex Doppler imaging may be used as the first line investigation to monitor patients following endovascular aneurysm repair. Cross-sectional imaging may then be reserved for patients with a demonstrable endoleak or increase in aneurysm diameter.[23]

Aortoiliac Graft

Often patients with extension of abdominal aortic aneurysm into iliac arteries have an aortoiliac prosthesis placed with an end to end proximal and distal anastomosis.

These grafts can be appreciated sonographically because of their very parallel echogenic walls.

Aortofemoral Graft

Aortofemoral grafts are placed in patients who have some vascular compromise below the distal aorta. These aortofemoral grafts have either end to end or end to side anastomosis. Sonographically the end to end grafts produce slight dilatation at the proximal anastomosis.

Complications of Graft Implantation

Pseudoaneurysms

Pseudoaneurysms are by far the most common complication of vascular prosthetic surgery. Aortic anastomotic pseudoaneurysm is defined as a type of pseudoaneurysm due to extravasation of blood caused by a defect in the suture line at the junction of the prosthetic graft and the native aorta.[25]

A pseudoaneurysm is not surrounded by any layer of the wall of the native aorta. Usually partial thrombosis of the pseudoaneurysms occurs with blood flowing into non-thrombosed part.

False aneurysms can result from a number of causes, late failure of suture material, endarterectomy at the site of anastomosis, graft dilatation, hypertension and atherosclerotic degeneration of native vessel.[25]

Graft infection is another dreaded complication and leads to false aneurysm formation at the suture line as does the communicating haematoma from a leak of the suture line at the time of a fresh anastomosis.[17] With Duplex Doppler imaging pulsatile or turbulent flow within the pseudoaneurysm may be seen.[25]

Proximal anastomotic false aneurysm of the aorta have a serious prognosis and are associated with a high mortality.

Aneurysms when they occur in patients with vascular prosthetics are almost always anastomotic in location either proximally or distally, the only exception being those related to trauma or those secondary to an intrinsic defect is the prosthetic wall, a distinct rarely.[17]

Perigraft Fluid

Fluid around the graft-either proximally, distally or along its length is a serious and important finding best seen with ultrasound or CT. Perigraft fluid produces a similar appearance sonographically whether it is secondary to haematoma, serum, lymph node or abscess.

If the collection is large or echogenic or increasing in size or far away from the graft then infection must be considered[16] and fine needle aspiration is indicated. Lymphocele around the graft may be very hypoechoic and may simulate a dissection.[5]

Ordinarily ultrasound distinguishes between false aneurysm and perigraft fluid collections.

False aneurysms have definite discrete pulsations throughout other fluid collections may have some transmitted pulsation where the fluid abuts upon the pulsatile vessel but are never intrinsically pulsatile. Colour spectral Doppler are very useful in there instances.

KEY POINTS

- Aneurysm
  - True aneurysm—localized dilatation > 3 cm diameter.
  - Pseudoaneurysm—organized paravascular haematoma, lumen contiguous will aortic lumen.
  - Doppler reveals swirling within pseudoaneurysm, continuous systolic and diastolic flow.
  - To and fro move pattern at neck.

Aortic dissectionv

- Thin membrane fluttering in lumen—blood flow in both channels with different flow rates.
- Aortic grafts—complications
  - Duplex Doppler distinguishes pseudoaneurysms, (Pulsatile/turbulent flow) from perigraft fluid (transmitted pulsation).

Coeliac Trunk

Classically the coeliac artery has a high resistive pattern at its origin with a small amount of reversed early diastolic flow.[5] As one goes distally it losses its early reversed diastolic flow. Distally the artery has continuous forward flow throughout the cardiac cycle of low resistance type.

With the cursor appropriately positioned waveforms can be sampled in the hepatic artery, splenic artery and the left gastric artery.

The gastric artery demonstrated surprisingly high shifts and is easily seen ascending from the coeliac trunk. The splenic artery shows low resistance flow and has a turbulent flow presumbambly associated with its common tortuosity.[1]

The hepatic artery rises solely from the coeliac axis 72 per cent of the time. The superior mesenteric artery given off the common hepatic artery in 4 per cent of the cases the right hepatic artery in 11 per cent of cases and the left hepatic artery in 10 per cent of cases.[5]

The common hepatic artery can easily be sampled as well as its branch, the pancreatoduodenal artery lying on the superficial surface of the pancreas. Real-time imaging allows the proper hepatic artery to be traced up to the portahepatitis and the right hepatic artery can be sampled as it crosses anterior to the portal vein. The hepatic artery usually has a low resistance pattern (Fig. 13.8).

Superior Mesenteric Artery

The normal SMA spectral pattern demonstrates organised flow throughout the cardiac cycle and in the fasting states. Characteristically has flow reversal in early diastole. This is similar to the higher resistance outflow vessels in the periphery. Normal coeliac artery velocity wave form demonstrates organised flow in systolic and somewhat disorganised diastolic flow with continuous forward flow throughout diastole and no diastolic flow reversal. These waveforms are reminiscent of the low outflow resistance system seen in the internal carotid artery.[33]

Fasting peak systolic velocities of SMA and coeliac artery have ranged from 103 to 196 cm/sec and 118 to 163 cm/sec respectively[33] (Fig. 13.8).

Flow Responses to Physiology Stimulus

Jager *et al*[34] have measured postprandial velocities in the SMA after 1000 calories test meal: within 15

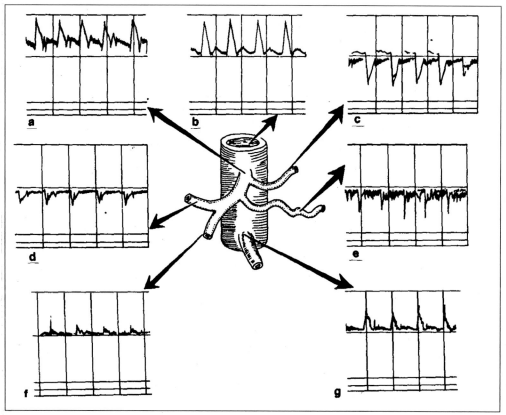

Figure 13.8
(a) Time velocity spectra in celiac trunk (b) proximal aorta, (c) left gastric artery, (d) common hepatic artery, (e) splenic artery, (f) gastroduodenal artery, and (g) superior mesenteric artery

minutes after eating a significant increase in peak systolic velocity was observed. This reached a maximum of almost double the baseline flow velocity 45 minutes after eating and returned to normal by 90 minutes. During this time diastolic velocity increased to almost three times fasting levels. This dramatic postprandial increase in diastolic velocity appeared to be the most predictable spectral change in SMA velocity waveforms. There is also a complete disappearance of diastolic flow reversal in SMA after eating.

Moneta and coworkers[35] measured coeliac and SMA flow velocities post- prandially. There was 20 to 24 per cent increase in iliac systolic and diastolic flow velocities after meals but the difference was not statistically significant. In contrast SMA flow velocities increased significantly after test meals.

Mesenteric Doppler

The arteries primarily responsible for mesenteric circulation include the SMA, IMA and branches of coeliac artery which provide anastomotic links in case of occlusive disease. The branches which provide collateral flow include common hepatic artery and gastroduodenal artery. Chronic mesenteric ischaemia results due to atherosclerotic involvement of a least two of the three major vessel supplying the bowel. Abundant collateral exist in the mesenteric circulation hence it is possible at times that all three mesenteric vessels are occluded without bowel infarction or symptoms due to the rich collateral network. Mesenteric Duplex scanning represents a noninvasive technique for anatomic and physiologic assessment of visceral vessels. It provides a rapid accurate method for the evaluation of patency of major splanchnic vessel. This aids in the selection of patients for arteriography and allow rational selection of alternative diagnostic studies.

Moneta and colleagues[35] found that a peak systolic velocity more than 275 cm/sec indicates a significant obstruction of SMA. A peak systolic velocity more than 200 cm/sec for the coeliac also correlated with a significant stenosis of the vessel.

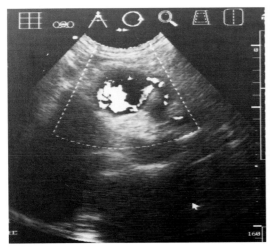 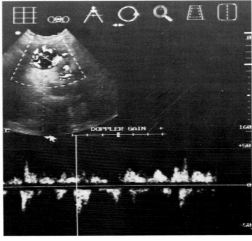

Figures 13.9a and b
(a) Colour and
(b) Duplex Doppler
images in a case of
splenic artery aneurysm

When mesenteric ischaemia requires surgical intervention bypass grafting from the aorta to the mesenteric arteries is frequently employed. Mesenteric Duplex scanning may provide an improved, noninvasive technique for objective assessment of postoperative graft patency as well as a method for long-term follow-up of these arterial reconstruction procedures.[36]

Splanchnic Aneurysms

Splanchnic aneurysms may be congenital, athero-sclerotic, post-traumatic, myotic or inflammatory. About 10 per cent of patients with chronic pancrea-titis develop there pseudoaneurysms which occur in the hepatic artery, splenic artery, (Figs 13.9a and b) SMA, gastroduodenal and IMA. They may be saccular or fusiform and usually have no reverse within them. They may have layers of thrombus on the walls. They present a significant risk to the interventional radio-logist as they may be mistaken for simple abscesses. It is prudent to evaluate with Doppler all collections prior to drainage.[15]

Realtime identification of pulsation in the aneu-rysm is helpful in characterising the vascular nature of mass. Pulsation may be absent or be diminished as a result of perianeurysmal fibrosis. Doppler ultra-sound can make a precise diagnosis.[37]

Renal Arteries

The renal arteries originate at or slightly below the origin of the superior mesenteric artery.

The normal right renal artery arises laterally or anterolaterally from the aorta and passes anterior to the right diaphragmatic crus and posterior to the inferior vena cava. The left renal artery arises lateral or posterolateral from aorta. Transverse scanning can usually visualise the renal arteries but coronal scan with the patient in the left lateral decubitus position may help identify the arteries in difficult case. The proximal renal artery waveform has a low pulsatility and a high continuous flow component (indicated by mean height from the zero line) and is dramatically different from that of the adjacent aortic signal. Similar wave-forms are seen in the renal sinus the midregion of the kidney and the arcuate vessels at the corticomedullary junction (Fig. 13.10).

Aneurysms

Renal artery aneurysms are rare. True aneurysms are usually secondary to arteriosclerosis, polyarteritis nodosa or fibromuscular dysplasia and false aneurysm are often the result of trauma. Pulsations in the aneu-rysms may be seen with realtime imaging or arterial flow identified in them using Doppler ultrasound.[32]

Arteriovenous Malformations

Renal arteriovenous malformations may be congenital or acquired. Latter occur as a result of trauma, surgery, renal biopsy or neoplasms. Arteriovenous malfor-mations may appear as a cluster of tortuous arteries and veins or more commonly a cystic structure repre-senting either the aneurysmal artery or vein. A dilated renal vein or inferior vena cava above the renal vein suggest the presence of this lesion. Rim calcifications or mural thrombus may also be present and if a major component of the malformation is arterial pulsation may be identified. Doppler analysis may also be utilised.[32]

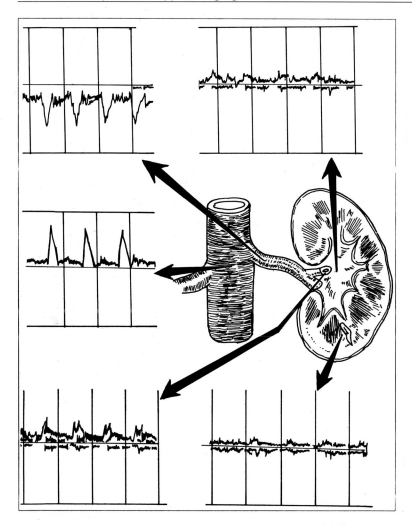

Figure 13.10 Time velocity spectra in: main renal artery at origin (a); mid zone of kidney (b); midaorta (c); renal sinus (d); arcuate artery (e)

Stenosis and Occlusion

Doppler techniques have been applied to the renal artery with 83 per cent sensitivity and 97 per cent specificity in diagnosing stenosis greater than 60 per cent.

A threshold velocity of 180 cm/sec of renal arteries is taken as normal with velocities greater than this suggestive of stenosis.

A ratio of peak systolic velocities in the aorta and stenotic renal artery segment of 3.5 of greater indicates 60 per cent chance of RAS.[38]

Another technique evaluates spectral Doppler waveform intrarenally. The shape of systolic upstroke is evaluated and the acceleration time and index are calculation. An acceleration index of $3\,m/sec^2$ or greater is abnormal.[39] Lack of the normal early systolic peak in the renal artery tracing is also highly specific for diagnosing renal artery stenosis.[39]

Inferior Vena Cava

Anatomy

The inferior vana cava is a large vein that returns blood from the lower limbs, pelvis and abdomen to the right atrium. It is formed by the paired common iliac veins on the anterior surface of the L_5 vertebral body and lies anteriorly and slightly to the right of the spine.[26] It traverses the diaphragm and enters the right atrium at the level of eight thoracic vertebra.

Its main branches are the hepatic veins, the renal veins and the common iliac veins. The walls of IVC are much thinner than those of aorta and the pressure of blood it deals with is also much lower.

Sonography

The intrahepatic portion of the IVC is routinely viewed by using the liver as an acoustic window. The remainder of the vessel is inconsistently seen because

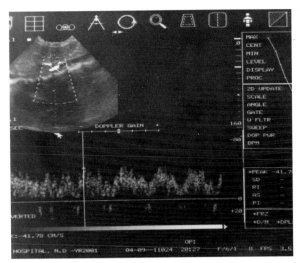

Figure 13.11
Duplex Doppler of normal IVC showing wide variation in flow velocity and direction owing to effects of cardiac and respiratory cycles

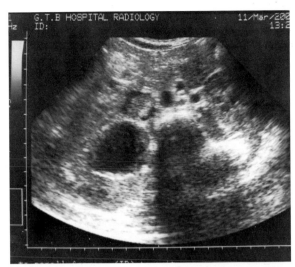

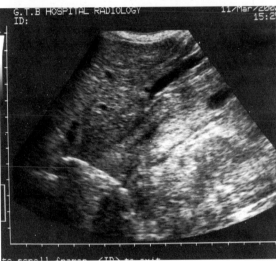

Figures 13.12a and b
Gray scale image in transverse and longitudinal sections showing an echogenic thrombus obliterating the lumen of inferior vena cava and extending along its entire length

it is intermittently flat and oval shaped and may be obscured by overlying bowel gas. Common iliac vein and external iliac veins are seen inconsistently with their arteries on the lateral aspect of the pelvic brim. The IVC lumen is anechoic although with slow flowing blood it becomes more echogenic and may show swirling. This is seen with right heart failure, fluid overload and caudal to an IVC obstruction. The appearance varies with respiration. With deep inspiration, venous return decreases and IVC dilates. With deep expiration, venous return improves and IVC diameter decreases. By doing a valsalva, venous return is blocked and flow temporarily reversed in the IVC: causing it to bulge. The IVC transmits both cardiac and respiratory pulsations, the transmission are more noticeably sonographically the closer one comes to heart. The classical tracing has a saw tooth pattern (Fig. 13.11). Most distally and in the common iliac veins there is a more phasic pattern similar to the pattern in proximal limbs.[5]

Pathology

The most commonly encountered intraluminal pathology of the IVC is thrombosis which usually spreads from another vein in the pelvis, lower limbs, liver or kidney. IVC thrombosis is sonographically diagnosed as an intraluminal filling defect that usually expands the diameter of the vessel (Figs 13.12a and b). The echogenicity of a thrombus depends on its age, chronic thrombi may calcify. If a thrombus is hypoechoic or

isoechoic with the liver, colour Doppler is very helpful in making the diagnosis as colour frequently surrounds the thrombus.[5] Spectral Doppler analysis produces no signal from uncomplicated thrombus. Arterial type tracing may be seen within tumor thrombi. The presence of IVC tumor thrombus is usually diagnosed readily. The kidney is the most likely site of origin.

A variety of vena cava filters are now being used in the IVC to prevent distal venous thrombi from going onto pulmonary embolism. Ultrasound can sometimes see these as echogenic structures within the IVC and can monitor complications such as thrombosis that may occur at their site of insertion.[27] The Kimray Greenfield filter is one of the more common devices and consists of stainless steel wire cage that has a narrow apex with six diverging limb. Its optimal position is above iliac bifurcation but below the level of the renal veins (so as not interfere with blood flow from kidneys). Duplex Doppler demonstrates the patency of the inferior vena cava above and below the filter. Thrombus affecting the filter can be detected by Doppler ultrasound even when it is undetected by realtime scanning.[32]

Mural Lesions

Mural based lesions include adherent thrombus and tumors. Primary tumors are rare but of them the leiomyosarcoma is the most common. It most frequently affects females in the fifth and sixth decade of life.[28] Typically this is a low grade malignancy with an early, relatively quiescent growth period of at least several months, during which collateral vessels may develop.[28] However, it is nearly always lethal because of its late stage at presentation. Frequent sites of metastases include liver and lung. Moreover extension into right atrium usually precludes surgical resection.[29]

The typical gray scale ultrasound appearance of this tumor in a soft tissue mass which distends the IVC and may contain scattered foci of cystic necrosis. IVC thrombus may be bland due to extensive deep venous thrombosis or may represent malignant tissue. The diagnosis of a malignant thrombus is greatly aided by the detection of tumor neovascularity with Doppler ultrasound. Such vessels demonstrate opacity of smooth muscle in the intima and media, which causes arteriovenous shunting and low impedance high diastolic flow. Colour Doppler demonstrates continually fluctuating colour indicating pulsatile arterial flow. The detection of such arterial vascularity distinguishes this from the chief entity in the differential diagnosis, bland thrombus which is avascular.[29]

Although imaging studies may strongly suggest an IVC leiomyosarcoma biopsy is needed for definitive diagnosis.[29]

Metastatic lesions include direct spread from lymphoma, hepatocellular carcinoma, breast and renal cell carcinoma mural IVC lesions can exert mass effect and affect structures like the ureter (retrocaval ureter) or the lesions can spread into IVC branches such as renal hepatic veins.[5]

IVC rupture Usually follows severe abdominal trauma or surgical or interventional therapy. It frequently results in large retroperitoneal bleed and it is associated with damage to other structures.

IVC Branches and Tributaries

Renal Veins

The right renal vein is very short while the left renal vein has a much longer course as it travels between the aorta and the SMA to reach the IVC. Both renal veins (especially the left) frequently collect blood from varies in portal hypertension patients. Circumarotic veins are rare. The left renal vein retroaortic variant which occurs in about 2 per cent of patients is of great importance when contemplating surgery.

Renal vein thrombosis is associated with acute glomerulonephritis, lupus, amyloidosis, sepsis, trauma and dehydration.[5] Of those who have undergone renal transplants 1 per cent develop this problem. On sonography one may see dilatation of vein proximal to the occlusion. The kidney enlarges and there is decreased echogenicity secondary to oedema in the kidney. Doppler study shows no renal vein flow and a high resistive arterial flow pattern.[5]

Hepatic Veins

Hepatic vein Doppler spectral tracings are usually triphasic and pulsatile reflecting transmitted cardiac pulsations. This pattern is abolished in about 20 per cent of cases of cirrhosis and hypertension, and it is exaggerated in right heart failure.[30]

Iliac and Ovarian Veins

The common and external iliac veins with the adjacent arteries. They are predominantly medial and anterior at the inguinal ligament and they become posterior and lateral to the accompanying vessels close to the IVC. They have a respiratory phasicity and can be compressed by adjacent structures and pathology including lymphoceles, haematoma transplant kidney, abscess and aneurysm.

They collapse with a Valsalva manoeuvre because of their intra-abdominal position but increase in diameter following augmentation by a squeezing of iliac or by elevation.

Ovarian vein thrombosis usually occurs postpartum and is associated with endometritis and surgery. Sonography frequently shows massive enlargement of all part of the ovarian vein often with an echogenic thrombus within it.[31] It usually occurs on the right side. Sonography detection should include evaluation of the expected entry of the vein directly into IVC.

Intraoperative Applications of Doppler

Doppler ultrasound can be used in abdominal surgery to help assess intestinal viability.

Colonic ischaemia may follow aortic reconstruction in 1.5 to 10 per cent of patients. The ischaemia is related to inadequate collateral flow following division of inferior mesenteric artery. After temporarily occluding the inferior mesenteric artery, a Doppler probe is applied to the colon. Marked diminution or loss of the arterial signal identifies those patients who need reimplantation of the inferior mesenteric artery. Doppler ultrasound can also assess colonic viability in colon oesophageal bypasses and can delineate the borders of resection in surgery for small bowel ischaemia.[40]

Intraoperative detection of abdominal and renal arteriovenous malformations is possible with Doppler.[41] It has also been employed in order to avoid damage to the major arteries of kidney during nephrotomy.

REFERENCES

1. Taylor KJW, Burns PN, Woodeock JP: Blood flow in Deep Abdominal and pelvic vessels: Ultrasonic pulsed Doppler analysis. *Radiology* 15: 487-93, 1985.

2. Burns PN: Hemodynamics: In Taylor KJW, Burns PN, Wills PNT (Eds): *Clinical Applications of Doppler Ultrasound* (2nd edn) New York Raven Press: 35-53, 1995.

3. Abu Yousef MM, Wirse JA, Shamma AR: Case report. The to and fro sign: Duplex Doppler evidence of femoral artery pseudoaneurysms. *AJR* **150**: 632-34, 1988.

4. Allison DJ: Arteriography. In Grainger RG, Allison DJ (Eds): Diagnostic Radiology: *An Anglo American Textbook of Imaging*. Edinburgh: Churchill Livingstone **1**: 2014-15, 1986.

5. Downey DB: The Retroperitoneum and great vessels. In Rumack CM, WIlson SR, Charboneau JW (Eds): *Diagnostic Ultrasound*. Mosby Year Book **12**: 455-86, 1998.

6. Gooding EAW, Effeney DJ: Static and real time B mode sonography of arterial occlusion. *AJR* **139**: 4949-52, 1982.

7. Zwiebel WJ, Fracto D: Basics of abdominal and pelvis Doppler intrumentaion, anatomy and vascular Doppler signatures. *Semin Ultrasound CT MR* **13**: 3-21, 1992.

8. Koher TR, Nance DR, Crames MM *et al*: Duplex scanning for diagnosis of aorto iliac and femoropopliteal disease: A prospective study. *Circulation* **76(5)**: 1074-80, 1987.

9. Jager KA, Ricketls HJ, Strandness DE: Duplex scanning for the evaluation of lower limb arterial disease: In Bernstein EF (Eds): Non invasive diagnostic techniques in vascular disease. St Louis: The CV Mosby 10p-619, 1985.

10. Pasch AR, Ricotta JJ, May AG: Abdominal aortic aneurysm: The case for elective resection. *Circulation* **70 (Suppl 1)**: 1-4, 1984.

11. Laroy LL, Cormier PJ, Matalon TAS *et al*: Imaging of abdominal Aortic Aneurysms. *AJR* **152**: 785-92, 1989.

12. Carriero A, Jezzi NM, Filippone A *et al*: Magnetic resonance angiography and colour Doppler sonography in the evaluation of abdominal aortic aneurysm. *Eur Radiol*, 1997.

13. Schroeder WB, Holeg SW: The definition assessment of aneurysm by colour flow Doppler. *J Diagn Med Sonogr* **7**: 201-09, 1991.

14. Giron J, Senae JP, Francois F *et al*: Place de la TDM Dans pevaluation pre-operative dis aneurisms de l' aorta abdominals *J Radiol* **71**: 49-55, 1990.

15. Pennel RC, Hollier LH, Lui JT *et al*: Clinical and therapeutics evaluation of inflammatory aortic aneurysms: A thirty year review: *J Vase Surg* **2**: 839, 1995.

16. Zwiebel WJ: Aortic and iliac aneurysm. *Semin Ultrasound CT MRI* **13**: 53-68, 1992.

17. Gooding GAW: Aneuryms of abdominal aorta, iliac and femoral arteries. *Sem in Ultrasound* **2**: 170-79, 1982.

18. King PS, Cooperberg PL, Madigan SM: The anechoic cresent in abdominal arotic aneurysms: Not a sign of dissection. *AJR* **146**: 345, 1986.

19. Erturk H, Erden A, Yusdakul M: Pseudoaneurysm of Abdominal Aorta diagnosed by colour Duplex Doppler. *Sonography J Clin Ultrasound* **27(4)**: 202-05, 1999.

20. Bennet DE, Cherry JK: The natural history of traumatic aneurysm of the aorta. *Surgery* **61**: 516, 1967.

21. Richard GP, Patrich CA: Pseudoaneurysm of the abdominal aorta. A case report and review of literature. *Am J Med Sci* **301**: 25, 1991.

22. Llornte JG, Gallego MG, Arnaize AM: Chronic post traumatic pseudoaneurysm of the abdominal aorta diagnosed by duplex Doppler ultrasonography. *Acta Radiol* **38**: 121, 1997.

23. Thompson MM, Boyle JR, Hai-I-shorn T: Comparison of computed tomography and duplex imaging in assessing aorta morphology following endovascular aneurysm pair. *Br J Surg* **85**: 346-50, 1998.

24. May J, White GH, Yu W: A prospective study of changes in morphology and dimension of abdominal aorta aneurysm following endoluminal repair: a preliminary report. *J Endovasc Surg* **2**: 343-47, 1995.

25. Guinet C, Buy JN, Ghossain MA: Aorta anastomotic pseudoaneurysm: US, CT MR and angiography. *J Comp Asst Tomography* **26(2)**: 182-88, 1992.

26. Gray G: Gray's Anatomy (3rd edn.) London: Longamans Green and Lo, 859-62, 1954.

27. McWissen MW, Erichson SJ, Foley WD: Thrombosis at venous insertion sites after inferior vena caval filter placement. *Radiology* **12**: 415-19, 1989.

28. Coughlen JH, Andrews S: Growth of a leiomyosarcoma is the inferior vena cava. *Can Associ Radiol J* **43**: 221-224, 1992.

29. Paanghaal SS, Karenek TJ, Waehsberg RH: Inferior vena caval leiomyosarcoma: Diagnosis and biopsy with colour Doppler sonography. *J Clin Ultrasound* 25: 275-78, 1997.

30. Bolondi L, Gaiani S, Semincelli S: Changes in hepatic venous flow in liver disease assessed by Doppler US: Relationship with histology. *J Hepatol* **13 (Suppl)**: 98, 1991.

31. Adkin J, Wilson SR: Unusual course of the gonadal vein a case report of postpartum ovarian vein thrombosis mimicring acute appendicites clinically and sonographically. *JUM* **15**: 409-12, 1996.

32. Needleman L, Rifken MD: Vascular ultrasonography: Abdominal applications. *Radiol Clin North Am* **24(3)**: 461-84, 1986.

33. Flinn WR, Rizzo RJ, Park JS: Duplex scanning for assessment of mesenteric ischaemia. *Surg Clin North Am* **70(1)**: 99-107, 1990.

34. Moneta EL, Taylor DC, Helton WS: Duplex ultrasound measurement of postprandial intestinal blood: Effect of meal composition. *Gastroenterology* **95**: 1294-1301, 1988.

35. Moneta EL, Yeagu RA, Lea RW: Non invasive localisation of arterial occlusive disease: A comparison of segmental pressures and arterial duplex mapping. *J Vasc Surg* **17**: 578-82, 1993.

36. Sandager E, Flinnn WR, McCarthy WJ *et al*: Assessment of visceral arterial reconstruction using duplex scan. *J Vasc Technol* **11**: 13-16, 1987.

37. Derchi LE, Biggi E, Cici GR: Aneurysms of the splenic artery non invasive diagnosis by pulsed Doppler sonography. *J Ultrasound Med* **3**: 41-44, 1984.

38. Olin JW, Piemonte MR, Young JR: The utility of duplex ultrasound scanning of diagnosing significant renal artery stenosis. *Ann Intern Med* **122**: 833-38, 1995.

39. Starros AT, Parker SH, Yakes WF: Segmental stenosis of the renal artery. Pattern recognition of tardus and parvus abnormality with duplex sonography. *Radiology* **184**: 487-92, 1992.

40. Hobson RW, Wright GB, O'Donnell JA: Determination of intestinal viability. *Arch Surg* **114**: 165-68, 1979.

41. Boyce WH: Ultrasonic velocimetry in resection of renal arteriovenous fistula and other intrarenal surgical procedures. *J Urol* **125**: 610-11, 1981.

Current Role of High-resolution Ultrasonography and Colour Doppler in the Diagnosis of Scrotal Diseases

Bharat Parekh

Advent of high-resolution Ultrasonography and high sensitivity of colour Doppler imaging of scrotum has widened the diagnostic spectrum. Ultrasound probes using frequencies ranging from 7.5 to 10 MHz coupled with colour Doppler equipment capable of picking up slow flows are essential modalities currently used for adequate diagnostic imaging of scrotal pathologies. Scrotal Ultrasonography augments clinical examination and when interpreted with appropriate clinical background provides definitive diagnosis and prompt management often limiting the need for surgical intervention. The indications are:

- Palpable scrotal mass
  Hydrocele, epididymal cyst, inguinal hernia, varicocele
- Pain
  Infection, torsion, trauma
- Infertility
  Hypogonadism, varicocele
- Cryptorchism
  Undescended testis
- Follow-up
  Patients with previous disease, retroperitoneal mass, undescended testis
- Search for unknown primary.

NORMAL ULTRASOUND ANATOMY

Scrotal wall Its thickness ranges from 2-7 mm and is formed by various tissue layers, which cannot be separately imaged with present resolution of equipment.

Testes They have ovoid shape, smooth contour and medium echogenicity. It measures 3-5 cm in length and 2-3 cm in transverse diameter. It consists of numerous convoluted tubules, split into various lobules by fibrous septa that radiate from mediastinum to the periphery.

Mediastinum testis This seen as linear echogenic density in the posterior aspect of the testis and the site of attachment to the epididymis. Arteries and veins enter through this site.

Tunica vaginalis It is a fibrous capsule of testis not imagable separate from the testis. It invaginates into the testis in the mediastinal area. It has the visceral and parietal layers with potential space that is filled with minimal fluid.

Epididymis It is located postero-laterally to the testis. The triangular upper portion-head is larger than the rest and measures 8-12 mm and isoechoic with the testis. Body and tail are usually not well differentiated on ultrasound.

Vascular anatomy It can be easily studied with colour Doppler mode. The arterial supply consists of peripheral capsular arteries, centripetal arteries and transmediastinal arteries.

Spectral waveforms of testicular flow typically show prominent diastolic component. Normal low flow in the testis are readily demonstrated on colour Doppler study and it is also possible to diagnose hypo or hypervascular states in various disease processes.

Technique

It is generally helpful to explain the procedure to the patient and reassure them about the safety and simplicity of the procedure. Examination in a quiet dark room with minimal disturbance and in children, warm room temperature to avoid cremasteric reflex is extremely useful to derive utmost co-operation and diagnostic information. Patient is placed in supine position with thighs slightly separated and a towel placed under the scrotum to lift and support the contents. Examination in the erect position of the patient is preferred for diagnosis of varicocele and reducible hernia. Sedation is seldom necessary in infants and young children if they are starved for an hour or two and feed is given during the examination while they rest in their mother's lap. High-resolution linear probes in the range 7.5 to 10 MHz frequency should be used. It is recommended that colour Duplex Doppler equipment be set to lowest possible PRF and wall filters to pick-up low flows. Simultaneous visualisation of both testicles for comparing the vascularity is extremely useful when one of the testis is normal.

TESTICULAR TORSION

Testicular torsion is a result of excessive mobility of testis. Most torsion is seen at puberty (intravaginal) with a peak during neonatal period (extravaginal at the cord) and is usually bilateral requiring bilateral orchiopexy.

Ultrasonography findings vary depending on the time elapsed between the onset of episode and the time of examination.

Acute phase (within 6 hours)
- Normal findings
- Scrotal wall thickening
- Small haematocele
- Enlarged hypoechoic testis and epididymis.

Early subacute phase (1-4 days)
- Acute findings are more obvious
- Echofree area of liquefactive necrosis
- Hypoechoic mass of haemorrhage.

Late subacute phase (5-10 days)
- Progressive decrease of early subacute phase findings

Chronic phase (over 10 days)
- Normalisation of findings
- Testis small and echopoor
- Persistent epididymal enlargement and increased echogenicity.

COLOUR DOPPLER FINDINGS

Acute phase (Fig. 14.1)
- Diminished or absent flow to the testis
- Normal peritesticular flow.

Late phase (3-8 days) (Figs 14.2 and 14.3)
- Persistence of decreased flow to testis
- Increased peritesticular flow.

Although much has been written about the usefulness of colour Doppler to detect torsion of testis, recent studies indicate that surgery need not be delayed by an ultrasound study if high degree of clinical suspicion persists. colour Doppler imaging is rendered less useful in following conditions:

1. Prepubertal testis which normally have low flows
2. Ectopic testis

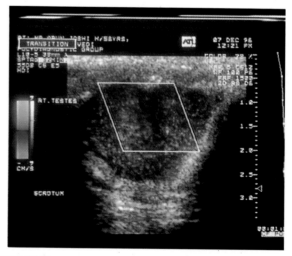

Figure 14.1
Torsion of testis—Complete absence of colour flow in the testis (lowest velocity settings used for Doppler study

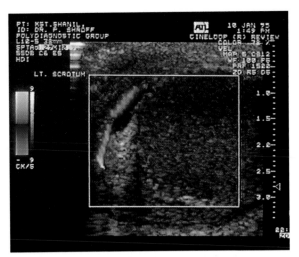

Figure 14.2
Late phase of testicular torsion—No flow is seen in the testis. Peri-testicular flow is present

3. Torsion-detorsion state-previously torsed testis is now reperfused and colour flow may be normal or hypervascular
4. Severe epididymo-orchitis causing secondary ischaemia.

The recently reported most reliable sign is a "snail shell curl" of the epididymis and not the colour flow abnormalities.

INFLAMMATORY DISEASES

Acute inflammation Most frequent cause of acute scrotum in adults is inflammation, particularly epididymitis in about 75 per cent of cases. It is detected in

KEY POINTS

– Testicular vessels show low flow with prominent diastolic component.
– In testicular torsion, there is decreased or absent flow to testis with normal or increased peritesticular flow.
– Most reliable sign for testicular torsion is 'snail shell curl' of epididymis.
– Enlargement of epididymis and testis with increased vascularity is seen in acute inflammation.
– Epididymo-orchitis may mask underlying tumor.

about 44 per cent cases by colour Doppler. Isolated orchitis is commonly seen in viral disease like mumps. This condition exhibits clinical manifestations closely resembling those in acute testicular torsion and need to be differentiated clearly to select the correct management options.

Ultrasound findings (Figs 14.4 to 14.6)
• Enlargement of epididymis and testis
• Focal or diffuse hypoechogenicity
• Scrotal wall thickening
• Fluid in tunica vaginalis
• Increased vascularity on Colour Doppler.

An excellent general rule is that in acute painful enlargement of the scrotum, greater enlargement of epididymis and fewer changes in the testis, usually

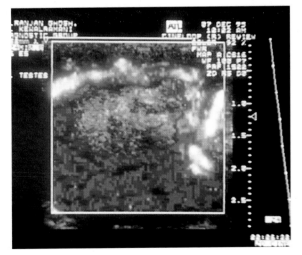

Figure 14.3
Power Doppler highlights exuberant peri-testicular flow and absence of flow in the testis

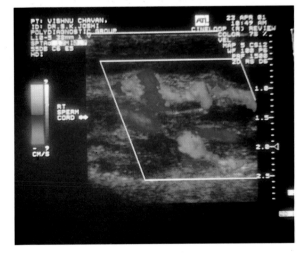

Figure 14.4
Funiculitis-hypervascularity along the spermatic cord (postoperative infection)

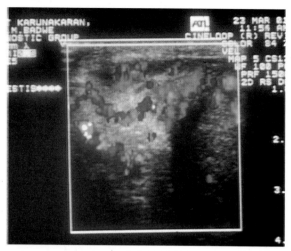

Figure 14.5a
Acute epididymitis-increased colour flow in epididymis

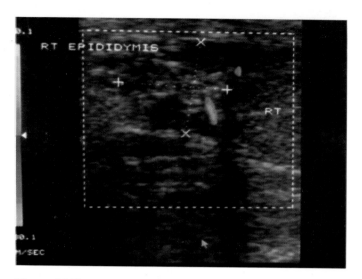

Figure 14.5b
Colour Doppler scan in another patient shows enlarged hypoechoic right epididymis with hypoedic

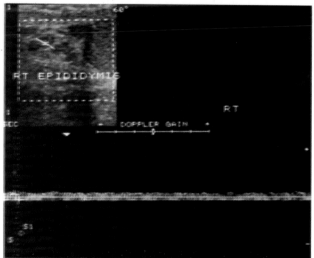

Figure 14.5c
Velocity waveform from vein confirms venous flow in epididymis in this patient

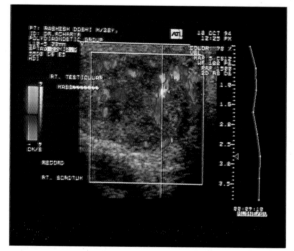

Figure 14.6
Acute orchitis-increased colour flow in the testis

with increased free fluid, points to infective process viz. epididymitis or epididymo-orchitis.

Testicular tumors may be masked by a presenting epididymo-orchitis and hence, it is important to rescan patient after the therapy to detect the tumor.

Chronic inflammation More frequently seen in under-developed countries and evolve with mild symptoms. This might result from inadequate treatment of an acute inflammation or from specific infection caused by *Mycobacterium tuberculosis* or *Treponema pallidum*, etc. Genitourinary tuberculosis is one of the most commonly encountered extrapulmonary sites of infections in our country. Ultrasound features are not specific and the gamut of findings may overlap with those found in acute inflammation. The ultrasound features are (Figs 14.7 to 14.8b):

- Thickening and increased echogenicity of epididymis
- Confluent anechoic areas representing necrosis in testis
- Complex mass of epididymis-testicular complex
- Organised hydrocele
- Testicular calcification
- Scrotal wall calcification
- Color Doppler may reveal hypervascularity in the scrotal wall.

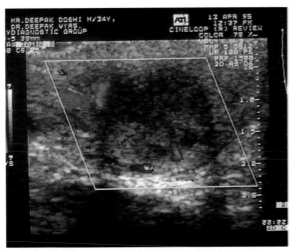

Figure 14.7
Chronic epididymo-orchitis (Tuberculous)

SCROTAL TRAUMA

Ultrasonography plays a profound role in defining the extent of injury in cases of blunt trauma. Early diagnosis and surgical intervention within 72 hours after the injury significantly increases the salvage rate and prevents ischaemic atrophy of the testis. Diagnosis of rupture, torsion and dislocation of testis are indicative of surgical exploration. About 50 per cent of traumatic haematoceles are associated with rupture.

Ultrasonography findings are:

- Haematocele-echogenic or echopoor
- Testicular rupture presents as discontinuity in the normal smooth contour of the testis indicating break in the tunica albuginia
- Intratesticular hematoma may be echogenic or echopoor and may mimic tumors hence followup is recommended to avoid missing an undiagnosed tumor with superimposed hemorrhage secondary to trauma.

HYDROCELE

Hydrocele is the most common cause of scrotal swelling and is caused by collection of fluid in tunica vaginalis. It may be idiopathic or associated with trauma, infection, torsion, tumor and infarction or due to obstructed lymphatic Ultrasound reveals fluid surrounding the testis located posteriorly. Ultrasonography findings are (Figs 14.9a and b):

- Echo-free area representing clear fluid
- Echogenic debris in the fluid suggests presence of blood, pus, protein or cholesterol
- Septation
- Scrotal calculii.

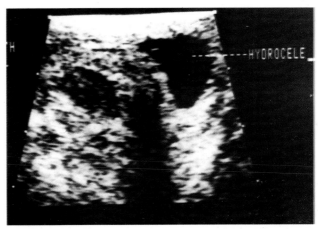

Figure 14.8a
Epididymo-orchitis with testicular abscess: Gray scale image in transverse plane shows enlarged testis within homogenous texture and a hypoechoic mass at the inferior pole (abscess) associated with hydrocele

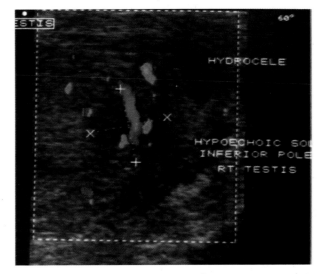

Figure 14.8b
Epididymo-orchitis with testicular abscess: Colour Doppler image in same patient shows generalized increased vascularity in testis

UNDESCENDED TESTIS

Undescended testis is the most common congenital abnormality found in about 1 per cent of boys and men and it occurs due to pathological impairment of hypothalamo-pituitary-gonadal axis. The incidence of malignancies encountered in this testis is upto 45-48 times higher than the general population and are also more prone to rupture, torsion and infertility. If repaired before 5 years of age, the risk for malignancy drops significantly. Fortunately most of the undescended testis are located in superficial soft tissue or

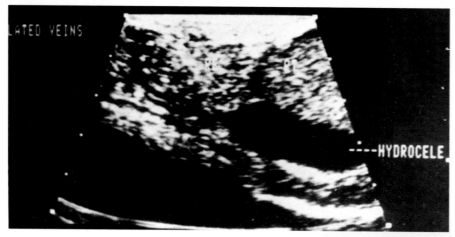

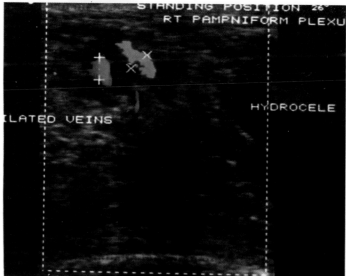

Figures 14.9a and b
(a) Gray scale image in longitudinal plane shows echo free area adjacent to right testis in a case of hydrocele. Dilated veins are also seen superior to the epididymis, suggestive of associated varicocele, (b) color Doppler flow image shows evidence of color flow in dilated veins

inguinal canal and are readily detected in about 97 per cent of cases. The search usually begins from the scrotum upwards. The undescended testis is a small oval structures, may be slightly hypoechoic or isoechoic to the parenchyma of normal testis. The undescended testis can not be imaged if located in the abdominal cavity. Confusion with an enlarged lymphnode in the inguinal region may be avoided by noting following points:

- Enlarged inguinal nodes are uncommon in the age group
- Hilum of the lymphnode is prominently echogenic as compared to faintly echoic mediastinum testis
- Enlarged node is hypervascular as compared to virtual vascular undescended testis
- Lymph-nodes are fairly fixed in position as compared to mobile undescended testis

SCROTAL CALCIFICATIONS

Isolated testicular calcifications are of no clinical significance and usually presents as spermatic granulomas, phleboliths or 'burned-out' tumors. It is seen in atrophic testis as evenly distributed, diffuse small calcifications. Irregular calcifications are seen in teratomas and embryonal cell carcinoma, chronic tuberculosis and as sequel to old trauma. Microlithiasis is seen in cryptorchism, infertility, post-orchiopexy, Klinefelter's syndrome and male pseudohermaphroditism and is considered benign but possible premalignant condition. Extratesticular calcifications are mainly benign in nature.

VARICOCELE

Varicocele is the most common correctable cause of male infertility. Ultrasonography and colour Doppler

KEY POINTS

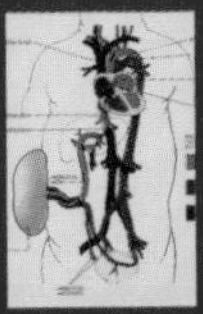

- Intratesticular hematoma may mimic a tumor.
- Undescended testis is usually located in superficial soft tissue or inguinal canal.
- In varicocele, veins are > 2 mm in diameter with retrograde flow in internal spermatic veins.
- Majority of testicular tumors arise from germ cells.
- Testicular tumors have variable echogenecity and may show flow in the periphery of the lesion.

play an important role in the diagnosis, particularly in sub-clinical cases (10%). The veins of the Pampiniform plexus are dilated to exceed 2 mm in diameter. The veins are characterised by retrograde flow in the internal spermatic vein. The examination performed in standing posture and during valsalvas the veins often dilate to 3 mm and more (Figs 14.10 to 14.11b).

SCROTAL HERNIAS

Scrotal hernias are common para-testicular masses. Clinical history and physical examination are primary basis of diagnosis, however, sonography helps in

atypical cases. The contents of the hernia sac may be small bowel, colon, and omentum. Presence of peristalsis and bowel mucosal pattern help in distinguishing the nature of the contents. Highly echoic content within scrotal sac may be due to presence of omentum or fatty tissue. Sonography of the inguinal canal can establish the extension of the bowel/omentum from the scrotal sac. In the absence of peristalsis and signature bowel mucosal pattern, differentiation from other extra testicular masses may be difficult. Often a strangulated

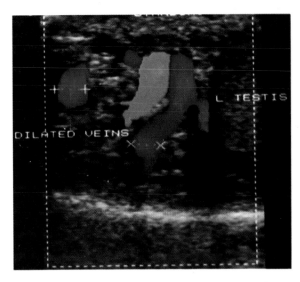

Figure 14.11a
Colour Doppler in another patient shows dilated veins in standing position

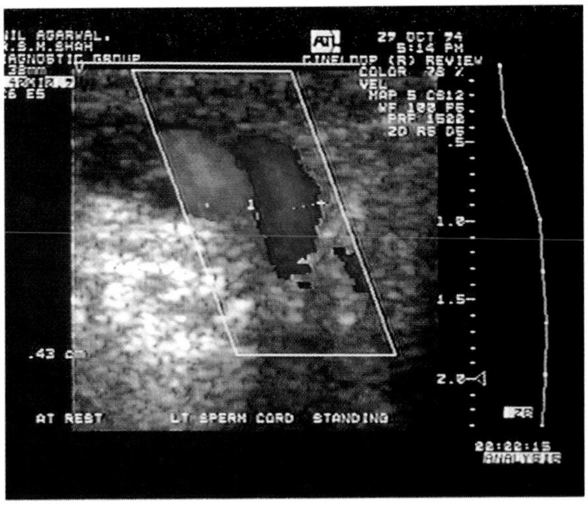

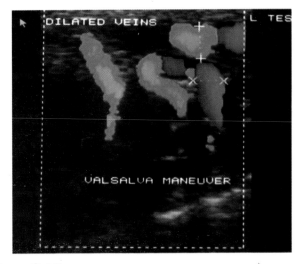

Figure 14.11b
Colour Doppler in another patient shows dilated veins during Valsalva manoeuvre

Figure 14.10
Longitudinal colour Doppler image of the left spermatic cord demonstrating dilated vascular channels suggestive of varicocele

inguino-scrotal hernia may present as an "acute scrotum".

TESTICULAR TUMORS

Most neoplasms of testis are malignant and commonly present as a mass. The peak incidence occurs between the age group 25-35 years and majority of them arises from germ cells. There is a wide spectrum of ultrasonographic features ranging from hypoechoic, isoechoic, hyperechoic and even complex echoic. Colour Doppler sonography may reveal flow in the periphery of the mass lesion. Focal orchitis may mimic neoplasm and hence the importance of follow-up studies.

Seminoma is the most common occurring germ cell tumor (40-50%) which is radiosensitive with excellent prognosis. The only exception being an anaplastic seminoma which carries poorer prognosis. It shows hypoechoic uniform echotexture with poor margins (Figs 14.12a and b).

Embryonal cell carcinoma It is the next common tumor (20-25%). It is aggressive causing early invasion of surrounding tissues, haemorrhage and cystic degeneration. The ultrasound shows a large tumor with distortion of testicular configuration and cystic-echoic areas. It carries poor prognosis.

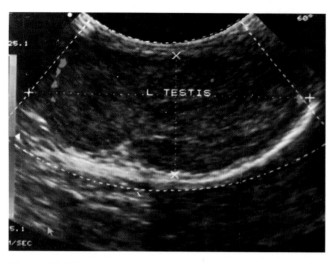

Figure 14.12b
Seminoma: color Doppler image shows increased vascularity at the periphery of the lesion

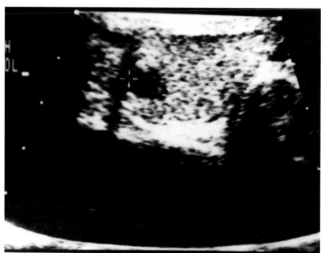

Figure 14.13a
Gray scale image in a patient with teratoma shows: hypoechoic mass with ill-defined margins at superior pole of left testis

Teratomas They are less common (5-10%). In adults they are usually benign but in children they are also found to be malignant. Usually small, 2 mm size tumors composed of germ cell layers and may show calcifications, cyst, mixed echogenicity and whirled appearance (Figs 14.13a and b).

Early preoperative diagnosis can often salvage the unaffected part of the testis (partial orchiectomy).

Teratocarcinoma It is a combination of teratoma and embryonal cell carcinoma, which is the most frequent tumor after seminoma.

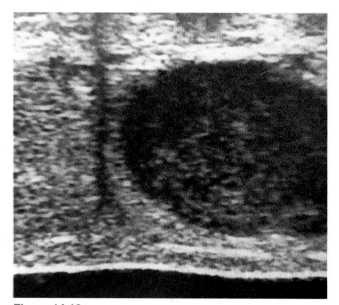

Figure 14.12a
Seminoma: gray scale images show enlarged testis with uniform hypoechoic echotexture

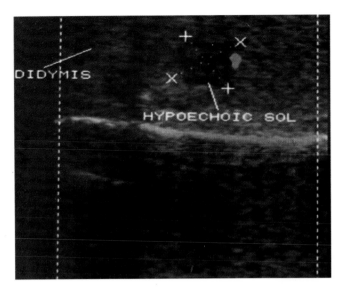

Figure 14.13b
Gray scale image in a patient with teratoma shows: peripheral vascularity is evident on color Doppler image

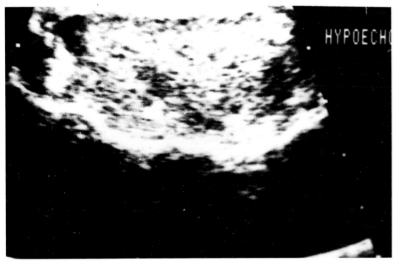

Figure 14.14a
Findings in a 62-year-old man with senile testicular atrophy: gray scale image reveals multiple hypoechoic areas within the testis

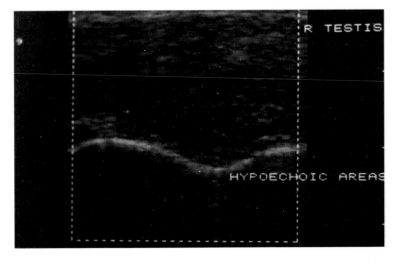

Figure 14.14b
Findings in a 62-year-old man with senile testicular atrophy: colour Doppler flow image shows avascular nature of hypoechoic areas

The other tumors occurring are yolk sac carcinoma, choriocarcinoma and 'burned-out' tumor. The non-germ cell tumors are Leydig cell and Sertoli cell type tumors.

Secondary tumors comprising of 5 per cent of tumors are lymphoproliferative diseases, acute and chronic leukaemia and non-Hodgkin's lymphoma. The ultrasound pattern is of diffusely hypoechoic, ill-defined lesion with normal or larger testis.

Secondary non-lymphoproliferative diseases are metastasis arising from primary tumors in kidney, prostate, stomach, melanoma, Wilm's tumor, neuro-blastoma, histiocytosis, retinoblastoma and rhabdo-myosarcoma. Ultrasound may show multiple lesions of variable echogenicity, usually hypoechoic.

The majority of extra testicular tumors are benign and originates from the spermatic cord. Lipomas are the most frequent benign while sarcomas are the most frequent malignant tumors seen.

Senile Atrophy of Testis

Age related atrophy is evident ultrasonographically by multiple hypoechoic areas within the testis. On color Doppler imaging, hypoechoic areas appear avascular (Figs 14.14a and b).

Duplex Ultrasonography of Erectile Dysfunction

Sanjay Thulkar
Deep N Srivastava

Erectile dysfunction (ED) or impotence is defined as an inability to achieve rigidity of the penis, which is sufficient for penetration. It is broadly classified into two categories—organic and psychogenic. Vasculogenic impotence is the most common cause of organic impotence. Many patients with erectile dysfunction have combination of both organic and psychogenic components. Therefore, the term vasculogenic ED does not rule out the presence of underlying psychological factors. It merely means that vascular factors are predominant cause of ED. Vascular ED has two different possible mechanisms—obstruction in penile inflow tract, termed as arterial ED and the inability to trap the incoming blood at sufficient pressure in the cavernosa, termed as veno-occlusive ED.

Anatomy and Physiology of Penile Erection

Paired internal pudendal arteries give rise to common penile arteries on both sides. These divide into four arteries, one each to spongiosa, cavernosa, proximal urethra and dorsum of the penis (deep dorsal artery). The cavernosal artery provides blood to cavernosa via multiple helicine arteries that open directly into the cavernosal sinusoids. Venules located within the subintimal space between the periphery of erectile tissue and the tunica albuginea provides venous outflow channel from corpora cavernosa via peripheral lacunae.

Penile erection is a neuro-vascular phenomena in which the neurological stimulus via parasympathetic nerves from sacral 2,3,4 leads to smooth muscle relaxation in helicine arteries leading to vasodilatation. There is also relaxation of trabecular smooth muscle relaxation in cavernosa, which coupled with increased blood flow leads to increase in size and length of the penis causing tumescence. In the next phase, subtunical venules are compressed against tunica albuginea due to dilatation of sinusoids and increase in intracavernosal pressure, leading to erectile response. If this veno-occlusive mechanism is competent, the arterial inflow leads to increase in intracavernosal pressure to the level of mean arterial pressure. Perineal muscles contractions generate to further increase in pressure and erectile response leads to the rigidity.

Evaluation of Erectile Dysfunction

Various tests available for evaluation of vascular ED includes papaverine induced penile erection (PIPE) test, pharmacopenile Duplex ultrasonography (PPDU), cavernosometry with cavernosography, penile angiography and radionuclide imaging. PPDU is sufficient for majority of patients, other more invasive tests are reserved for patients actually considered for surgical treatment.

Traditionally, evaluation of ED begins with PIPE test in which the erectile response of the penis is studied after intracavernosal injection of papaverine or some other vasoactive agent. Normal erectile response is suggestive of normal vascular status and hence neurological or psychological factors are considered as a predominant cause. If only partial or short-lived erection is resulted, then the vascular ED is presumed.

Pharmacopenile Duplex Ultrasonography (PPDU)

PPDU is fast becoming the firstline investigation to define vascular ED and to differentiate between arterial insufficiency and incompetent veno-occlusive mechanism.

The different vasoactive agents used for PPDU are papaverine, prostaglandine (PGE_1) and combination of papaverine and phentolamine. Papaverine may lead to false negative erectile response in some patients or may lead to persistent painful erection (priapism) in others. Prostaglandine (PGE_1) has better erection rate and lesser incidence of priapism.[1] Genital self-stimulation, visual erotic stimulation or application of light tourniquet at penoscrotal junction may augment the erectile response to these agents.

Technique

The examination must be carried out in an atmosphere of privacy. Anxiety and resultant sympathetic stimulation may interfere with the response to pharmacological stimulus, hence every effort should be made to relax the patient during the procedure. A rubber band is preferably placed at the root of the penis. The sonographic evaluation begins with scanning of the flaccid penis in transverse plane to measure the diameter of the cavernosal arteries. Then, under aseptic precautions, intracavernosal injection of 60 mg of papaverine is made with 26/27 G needle in either of the cavernosa. Injection on the contralateral side is not required as cross communications exist between both sides. Care must be taken not to inject in subcutaneous tissue, vessels or urethra. Erectile response is graded visually from E0 to E5 as described by Broderick.[2] E0 refers to no response, E1 to partial elongation of the shaft only, E2 to moderate tumescence without any rigidity. E3 erection achieves full tumescence but there is no rigidity and the penis is easily bendable. E4 and E5 grades show full erection with partial rigidity or full rigidity for at least 20 minutes respectively. After evaluating the erectile response, scanning is started from root of the penis to the distal part; both in transverse and longitudinal plane. Dorsal scanning in longitudinal plane is necessary to identify penile deformities and cavernosal collaterals. Post-injection diameters of both cavernosal arteries are measured in transverse plane. Angle corrected flow velocities are measured in cavernosal arteries as proximal as possible (Fig.15.1). Initial flow velocities are taken five minutes after the injection. The measurements are repeated after short intervals till peak rigidity. Most accurate flowmetry values coincide with peak rigidity of the penis. If no rigidity is achieved initially, the flowmetry may be obtained at least till 15 minutes before termination of the examination, as some individuals may reach to that stage after some time.

Post-papaverine injection normal spectral waveform cavernosal artery normally has five reproducible phases[3] (Fig. 15.2). In phase 1, there is increase in both systolic and diastolic velocities. In phase 2, there is progressive decrease in end diastolic velocity and

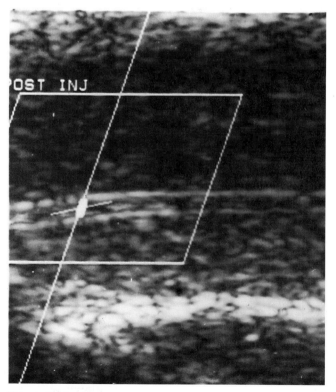

Figure 15.1
PPDU examination shows technique for placement of sample volume in the cavernosal artery with angle correction

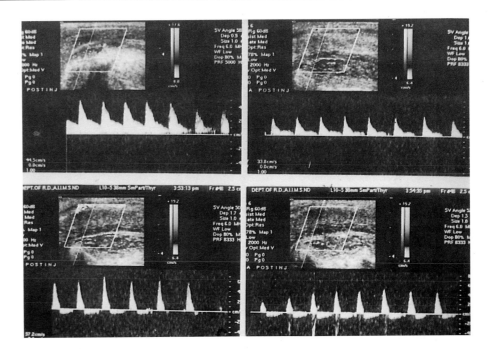

Figure 15.2
Serial spectral tracings during PPDU shows various phases of flow pattern (refer text)

appearance of the diachrotic notch. Patients with severe venous leakage do not progress beyond phase 2. In phase 3 diastolic flow approximates zero and it is reversed in phase 4. Phase 5 is characterized by eventual loss of both systolic and diastolic flow signals. Various parameters and there accepted normal values studied on flowmetry are maximum recorded peak systolic velocity (PSV) of 30 cm/second or more, minimum end diastolic velocity (EDV) of 5 cm/second or less (zero or reversed diastolic flow included as normal), Acceleration time (AT) of 0.11 second or less, and Resistive index (RI) of 0.85 or more. Mild variations are seen in cut off values as described in various reported studies.

The studies that have been published regarding the normal Doppler flowmetry values have been on small number of healthy volunteers.[3,4] There has been no such study on Indian patients. At our institution, we could not conduct our study on normal healthy volunteers because of invasive nature of the procedure and feasibility and ethical considerations. Therefore, it was decided to study patients with psychogenic impotence with a normal erection elicited on pharmacological stimulus test since these patients can be presumed to have a normal vascular status.[5,6]

In our study comprising 30 men, the mean age was 24.8 years. This is significantly less than the mean age of patients in the earlier studies by Valji *et al* and Quam *et al* who reported the mean age of 51 and 56 years respectively in their studies[7, 8.] This lower mean age

of patients in our population is difficult to explain but probably it is related to observation of our clinical psychologist that elderly men are usually hesitant to seek medical advice for their sexual problems (personal communication). They also have a tendency to regard it as part of aging rather than a disease problem. All 30 men in our study were diagnosed to have nonvasculogenic ED. Their younger mean age emphasize the fact that the younger men have less incidence of organic impotence than older men as the later group are likely to suffer from atherosclerosis and a replacement of elastic collagen with non-distensible collagen leading to vasculogenic erectile dysfunction.[9] All the patients had peak systolic velocity above 35 cm/sec, which correlates well with that reported by Benson *et al*.[10] However, mean PSV was 61.3 cm/second which is significantly higher than all previously reported studies.[3,8] Analysis of PSV variation with age has shown that there is a negative correlation and thus a higher mean PSV in the present study can be attributed to younger age of the study population. Similar results have been reported by Chung WS *et al*.[11] The mean acceleration time, which is now considered the best discriminator of arterial impotence, was 0.06 sec and none of the patients had AT of more 0.1 sec which is in conformity with existing literature.

The mean end diastolic velocity was–1.2 cm/seconds (negative sign indicates flow reversal) and it also correlates well with the prevailing consensus in literature.[3] Mean RI was 0.93 in whom diastolic flow reversal was not achieved. Majority of the patients had either absent or reversed diastolic flow (20 patients) or EDV 5 cm/sec or less (six patients). Four patients had end diastolic velocity more than 5 cm/sec, however, these patients had a very high PSVs and normal resistive indices. They also showed normal rigid erection on pharmacological stimulation. Thus, it appears that EDV > 5 cm/sec alone may not be a specific indicator of veno-occlusive insufficiency and it should be correlated with resistive index for diagnosis of veno-occlusive insufficiency. Normal mean PSV is dependant upon the age of the individual and it decreases with advancing age.[12]

In summary, abnormal PSV and AT are suggestive of arterial cause while abnormal EDV and RI indicates venous leakage. RI is considered more accurate than EDV for assessment of venous competence as probe vessel angle, the most important variable associated with the process of sampling and velocity calculation is filtered out in calculation of RI. Any increase in cavernosal artery diameter by less than three-fourth of the baseline is also suggestive of arterial insufficiency. If arterial disease is present, intracavernosal pressure remains below systemic pressure and veno-occlusion cannot occur, even if this mechanism is intact, and diastolic flow will continue to persist. Therefore, veno-occlusive mechanism cannot be assessed in presence of arterial disease.

Treatment of Complications

The most common complications during the diagnostic work-up and especially during the PPDU, is a papaverine induced prolonged, painful erection or priapism. Not all of them require specific treatment as penile detumescence generally occurs within few hours. In case the duration of erection exceeds six hours, the corpora cavernosa are drained to decrease the pressure and 10 microgram of adrenaline is injected intracavernosally to induce cavernosal smooth muscle contraction, effective venous drainage and restriction of arterial flow. The adrenaline of 1 in 1000 strength can be diluted with appropriate amount of normal saline to produce adrenaline injection of the desired strength. Compression bandage is also applied for few minutes. In case the erection has recurred, the procedure can be repeated.

KEY POINTS

– Vasculogenic impotence is most common cause of organic impotence.
– PPDU differentiates arterial insufficiency and incompetent veno-occlusion.
– Abnormal peak systolic velocit and acceleration time suggest arterial cause.
– Abnormal end-diastolic volume and resistive index indicate venous leakage.
– Veno-occlusion cannot be assessed in presence of arterial insufficiency.

Peyronie's Disease

This is a benign condition resulting from inelastic scar of tunica albuginea, which produce curvature deformities of penis and ED. On sonography, the penile plaques are seen as echogenic focal thickening of tunica albuginea which may displace or encase cavernous vasculature. Dense plaques may contain calcification and produce acoustic shadowing (Fig. 15.3) however, calcification can be seen even without evidence of calcification on the plain radiographs. Most plaques are located on the dorsal surface of middle third of the shaft of the penis.

REFERENCES

1. Meuleman, Diemont WL: Investigation of erectile dysfunction. *Urol Clin N Am* **22**: 803-19, 1995.
2. Broderick GA, Arger P: Duplex Doppler ultrasonography: noninvasive assessment of penis anatomy and function. *Semin roentgenology* **28**: 43-56, 1993.
3. Shwartz AM, Lawe M, Berger RE *et al*: Assessment of normal and abnormal erectile function–colour Doppler sonography versus conventional techniques. *Radiology* **180**: 105-09, 1991.
4. Shabsigh R, Fishman IR, Quesda ET *et al*: Evaluation of vasculogenic erectile impotence using penile duplex sonography. *J Urol* **142**: 1469-74, 1990.
5. Lue TF, Tanagho EZ: Physiology of erection and pharmacological management of impotence. *J Urol* **137**: 829-35, 1987.
6. Merckx LA, DeBruyne RMG, Goes E *et al*: The value of dynamic colour Doppler scanning in the diagnosis of venogenic impotence. *J Urol* **148**: 318-20, 1992.
7. Valji K, Bookstein JJ: Diagnosis of arteriogenic impotence: Efficacy of duplex sonography as a screening tool. *AJR Am J Roentgenology* **160**: 65-69, 1993.

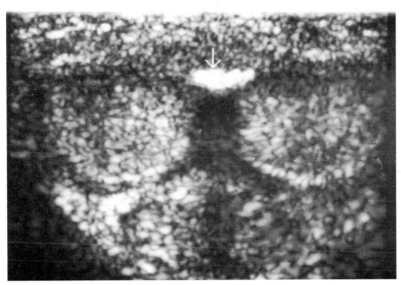

Figure 15.3
Peyronie's disease: dense echogenic plaque of tunica with distal shadowing
is seen on the dorsal surface of the penis

8. Quam JP, King BF, James EM *et al:* Duplex and colour Doppler sonographic evaluation of vasculogenic impotence. *AJR Am J Roentgenology* **153**: 1141, 1989.

9. Padma Nathan H, Boyd SD, Chung D: The biochemical effect of ageing, diabetes and ischemia on corporal and tunical collagen. *J Urol* **145**: 342-518, 1991.

10. Benson CB, Aruny JE, Vickers MA: Correlation of duplex sonography with angiography in-patients with erectile dysfunction. *AJR Am J Roentgenology* **160**: 71-73, 1993.

11. Chung WS, Park YY, Kwon SW: The impact of aging on penile hemodynamics in normal responders to pharmacological injection: Doppler sonographic study. *J Urol* **157**: 2129-31, 1989.

12. Bhargava R, Srivastava DN, Thulkar S *et al:* Colour duplex Doppler ultrasonography evaluation of non-vasculogenic male erectile dysfunction: an Indian perspective. *Australian, Radiology* 2002 (in press).

16

Colour Doppler of Small Parts

Lalendra Upreti
GP Vashisht
Satish K Bhargava
Anju Yadav

Musculoskeletal System

Ultrasound is often the first step in the assessment of musculoskeletal soft tissue masses. It can confirm the presence of a lesion, and provide information regarding its size, location, margin and internal structures. It can easily differentiate solid from fluid masses. Further characterisation of the solid masses is not very specific. Sonography is usually not able to distinguish benign from malignant mass lesions. Newly formed tumor vessels in a malignant neoplasm shows some distinct features like abnormal branching pattern, irregular size, wide sinusoids and arteriovenous shunts. Such features and resulting blood flow abnormalities can be detected by colour Doppler and pulsed Doppler sonography

Instrumentation and Technique

An adequate frequency probe should be chosen depending upon the size and depth of the lesion. Frequency varies from 3.5-7.5 MHz. Colour Doppler parameters should be optimised for low blood flow velocities. For spectral analysis low value of PRF and low wall filters should be used. The values can be adjusted upwards if medium to high velocities are encountered. Sample values should be adjusted to the vessel size. For each lesions, a minimum of three values should be taken. Absolute velocities should be obtained after angle correction. When different peak systolic values are found within a lesion. Highest value should be considered for evaluation.

Colour Doppler evaluation should be preceded by thorough gray scale examination. The lesion should be examined for growth pattern, margins, echogenicity and internal texture. On gray scale imaging, feature which are suggestive of a malignant lesion are: infiltrating or mixed pattern of tumor growth, blurred or irregular margins, hypoechoic pattern and heterogenous texture.

On colour Doppler flow imaging extent and configuration of tumor vascularity should be assessed on the basis of following features:
a. Flow signals: present or absent
b. Number of vessels
c. Vessel arrangement within the lesion—regularly distributed or randomly dispersed
d. Vessel course—linear or tortuous
e. Presence or absence of abrupt variation in calibre.

On pulsed Doppler evaluation, systolic and diastolic velocities and pulsatility index should be measured.

Colour and pulsed wave Doppler data are more helpful in categorizing a lesion as benign or malignant compared to gray scale sonography alone. Absence of flow is now specific in evaluation of these lesions. Colour Doppler sonography increases the specificity of the

KEY POINTS

Doppler in Musculoskeletal mass lesions
- Regular arrangement of vessels with linear course suggests presence of a benign mass.
- Malignant lesions have randomly distributed vessels with abrupt variations in size as well as flow signals.
- Peak systolic velocity more than 50 cm/sec. Is highly suggestive of a malignant lesion

is a characteristic feature of the benign lesion. Presence of flow however, can be found in both benign and malignant lesions. The number of vessels in the lesion is also not of much help in distinction. It co-relate more with the tumor size and not with benign or malignant nature. Arrangement of the vessels within the lesion is more useful. A regular arrangement with a linear course is usually suggestive of a benign mass. Randomly distributed vessels with abrupt variation in size as well as spot flow signals are seen in malignant lesions. On spectral evaluation peak systolic velocity is the single most reliable parameter for discriminating benign and malignant lesions (Figs 16.1a and b). A threshold of 50 cm/sec is the best criterion. Diagnostic accuracy is enhanced by composite analysis of sonographic, colour and pulsed Doppler findings.

Skin and Subcutaneous Tissues

Evaluation of the skin and subcutaneous tissue is one of the most recent achievements of sonography. Availability of very high resolution probe (10-20 MHz) enables acquisition of excellent image with great anatomic details, including an accurate definition of various layers of the skin. Lesions of the skin are a frequent and possibly serious dermatological problems, as some of the most aggressive neoplasms arise from the skin and are clinically indistinguishable from benign ones. High frequency sonography alone

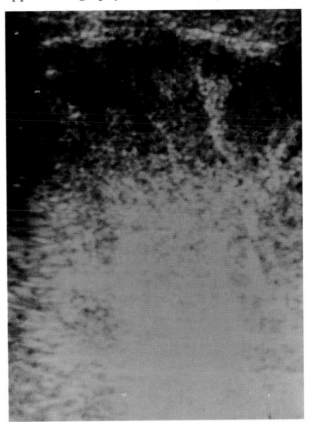

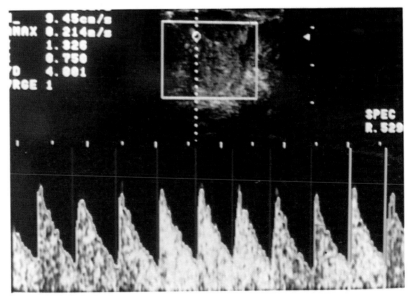

Figures 16.1a and b
Rhabdomyosarcoma—(a) gray scale image reveals a large hetero-genous mass in the neck, (b) colour and pulse Doppler image shows central, high velocity flow signal in the lesion

sonography by providing realtime evaluation of the vascularity, which is an important clue in distinguishing benign from the malignant lesions. Malignant tumours are expected to show increased vascularity compared to their benign counterparts.

The sonographic examination should be carried by a high resolution linear transducer. Doppler parameters should be adjusted to detect low velocity or low volume flow. Power Doppler can be used to increased vessel conspicuity and demonstrate vessel continuity.

The lesion should be scanned slowly with minimum probe pressure, as even slight compression with transducer can obliterate thin vessel pedicles supplying the nodules. Nodules are classified as:

Type I : Avascular

Type II : Hypovascular with a single vascular pole in the hilum

Type III : Hypervascular with multiple peripheral poles, and

Type IV : Hypervascular with internal vessels.

| Type I | Type II | Type III | Type IV |

Majority of the malignant nodules show both peripheral (Type III) and intralesional vascularity (Type IV), where as hypovascularity is seen mainly in the benign lesions. Malignant tumors of the skin

produce angiogenic factors that promote the development of multiple small arterial vessels, which enter the tumor peripherally at right angles and give rise to multiple intralesional vessels which contain stagnant blood. The subsequent central necrosis progressively obstructs and destroys the intralesional vessels and eventually progresses to stop blood flow in the peripheral arteries, because of high resistance of the intralesional blood vessels. Thus, Type IV pattern is more likely to be present in a malignant tumor without necrosis (Fig. 16.2a), whereas Type III pattern would be found in tumor with central necrosis. Type I (avascular nodule) [Figs 16.2b(i, ii)] is the least specific, because it can be found in totally necrotic malignant, as well as benign tumors. Type II pattern is probably a variant of Type I and can be observed when the main artery of a benign tumor is large enough to be detected, possibly because the benign lesion is larger than usual. Pulse Doppler may also

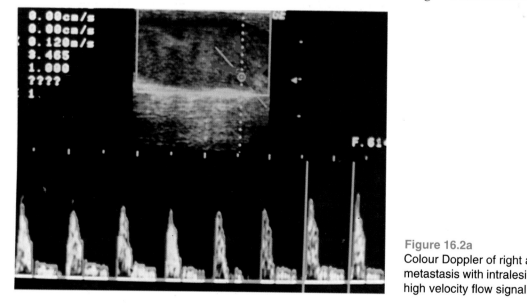

Figure 16.2a
Colour Doppler of right arm shows a subcutaneous metastasis with intralesional vascularity and central high velocity flow signal

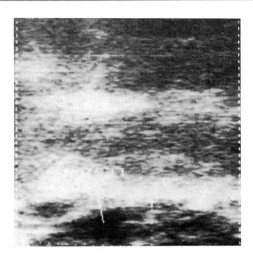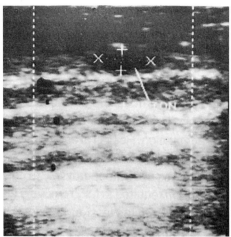

Figures 16.2b(i, ii)
Basal cell carcinoma: A well-defined hypo to anechoic skin lesion showing no color flow in color Doppler analysis

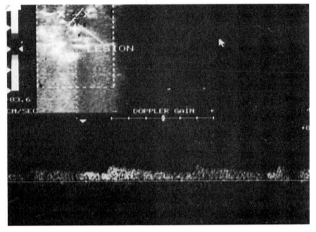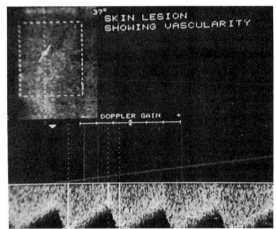

Figure 16.2c(i)
Pyogenic granuloma: a well-defined hypoechoic skin lesion seen with Doppler analysis showing low systolic and end diastolic velocity suggestive of a benign lesion

Figure 16.2c(ii)
Metastasis: A large well-defined hypoechoic skin lesion is seen in the scalp from carcinoma thyroid showing a high systolic and end-diastolic velocity suggestive of a malignant lesion

sometimes help in distinguishing benign and malignant lesions. Benign lesions show low systolic and diastolic velocities while high velocities are seen in malignant lesions [Fig. 16.2c(i, ii) and Table 16.1].

Colour Doppler sonography has still not found acceptance as a primary diagnostic modality, because the superficial nodule can be effectively evaluated by physical examination and biopsy alone. So dermatologist are reluctant to perform further investigations. Differentiation of local relapse of malignant tumors from scar may be potential application of colour Doppler imaging.

	Colour flow doppler findings in skin lesions				
Table	*Lesion*	*Vascularity*	*Max-systolic (cm/sec)*	*End-diastolic (cm/sec)*	*RI*
16.1	Pyogenic granuloma	+	6	3	0.50
	Pyogenic granuloma	+	5	3	0.40
	Pyogenic granuloma	+	6	3	0.50
	Pyogenic granuloma	+	6	3	0.50
	Squamous cell Ca	+	36.20	16.00	0.50
	Squamous cell Ca	+	36.00	14.00	0.60
	Metastasis	+	34.00	17.00	0.50

VASCULAR LESIONS

Haemangioma

Haemangiomas are among one of common soft tissue masses in infants. Clinically they appear as slightly raised bluish red subcutaneous masses. They regress as the child grows older. Some haemangiomas however do not have this typical experience because part of or all of the lesion is deep in the soft tissue and the overlying skin appears normal. These lesions are difficult to distinguish clinically from more suspicious soft tissue masses such as soft tissue tumours and infantile myofibrosis.

Gray scale imaging shows a heterogenous density soft tissue density mass. Some times vessels may also be visualised within the lesion, calcification may also be present (Fig. 16.3a).

On CDFI haemangiomas show presence of large number of intra-lesional vessels. Presence of more than five vessels per square centimeter has been seen. On spectral imaging a high frequency shift measuring more than 2 kHz is seen (Fig. 16.3b).

Arteriovenous malformations may also show similar features on CDFI and pulse Doppler imaging, viz number of vessels more than five per square centimeter and Doppler shift greater than 2 kHz. However, distinction can some times be made on gray scale imaging in these cases, because of multiple sites of arteriovenous shunting large number of prominent vessels may be seen (Figs 16.4a and b). Doppler evaluation may show arterialisation of the waveform.

Breast

Incidence of carcinoma of the breast has been rising steadily, and this along with the carcinoma of cervix is the leading cause of cancer in India. Early detection of this lesion is therefore extremely important as it offers chance of getting cured. X-ray mammography is the most frequent imaging modality used for evaluation of the breast abnormalities. Ultrasound was first used in the diagnostic work up of breast lesions in 1954. Since then many ultrasonic modalities dedicated to the examination of the breast have been developed. Advent of high resolution realtime sonography has enabled excellent visualisation and characterisation of breast nodules. In addition, it provides an accurate guidance for aspiration and biopsy of these lesions. Though sonography is not better than conventional mammography for screening of breast cancer. It is the most beneficial aid to the mammography. Certains features observed on sonography raise a high suspicion of malignancy, but none of them appears to be specific for malignancy. Combination of features are more reliable than presence of a single finding. Various findings which may arouse suspicion of a malignant lesion on B-mode imaging include:

- Irregularity of borders
- Round shape, long axis perpendicular to skin
- Hypoechoic relative to surrounding breast parenchyma
- Presence of heterogeneity and posterior acoustic shadowing
- Echogenic rim of variable thickness.

Other investigative modalities have also been used in the evaluation of suspected breast disease for achieving the hitherto elusive goal of obtaining non-invasive diagnosis of breast carcinoma. These modalities include spectral and colour Doppler flow imaging, MRI, CT, radionuclide studies with ^{99m}Tc

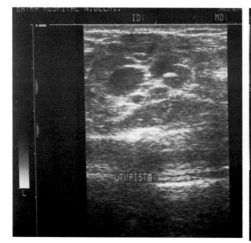
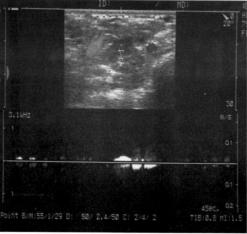

Figures 16.3a and b Haemangioma superficial—(a) on Gray scale sonogram of wrist a mixed echogenic mass lesion is seen with multiple tortuosities suggestive of a vascular lesion, and (b) spectral Doppler shows evidence of flow with frequency shift of 3.1 kHz, suggestive of haemangioma

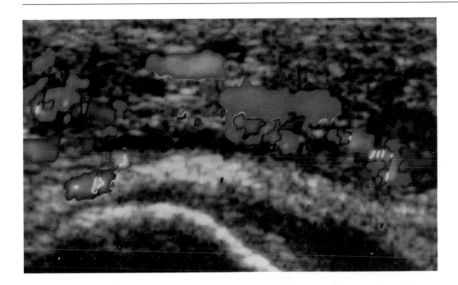

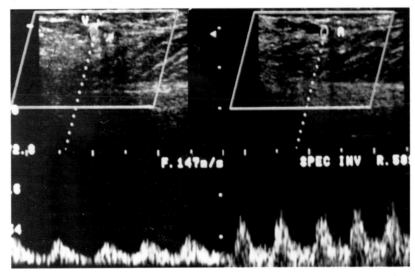

Figures 16.4a and b
Arteriovenous malformation in the leg—
(a) colour Doppler image shows multiple
vascular spaces in a swelling of knee,
(b) spectral tracing shows arterialisation
of venous flow

sestamibi and ^{99}Tc sulphur colloid and digital mammography. Application of Doppler studies in differentiation of benign and malignant lesions is based on premise that the malignant lesions are likely to be more vascular.

For the sonographic and Doppler examination of the breast 7.5 MHz linear transducer is usually required. For the Doppler, gain settings are adjusted so that the clutter noise disappears. Velocity range is adjusted to avoid aliasing. Minimal transducer pressure is applied so that the slow blood flow is not obscured. The tumor vessels are visualised with the help of CDFI and power Doppler imaging and the vessels with the largest diameters are interrogated with pulsed Doppler for spectral analysis.

Blood vessels are more clearly seen with the power Doppler imaging than with colour Doppler. Vascular

continuity is also better demonstrated by power Doppler imaging. Blood flow signals are more numerous in breast cancers than in benign lesions. This is consistent with the fact that malignant lesions are more vascular (Figs 16.5a and b) than their benign counterparts. Due to increased sensitivity of flow detection with PDI, some benign lesion may also appear hypervascular. These include benign phylloid tumours, intraductal papillomatosis, inflammatory lesions, fibroadenoma and fibrocystic disease.

Various Doppler parameters have been evaluated for their use in differentiating between benign and malignant lesions (Tables 16.2 to 16.4).[*] These include

---

* Khanna AK *et al:* From situ duoted Doppler flowmetry and breast lump as a pharametea to Distinguish

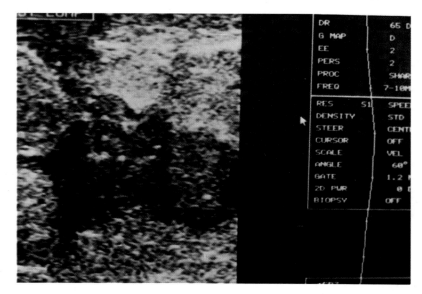

Figure 16.5a(i)

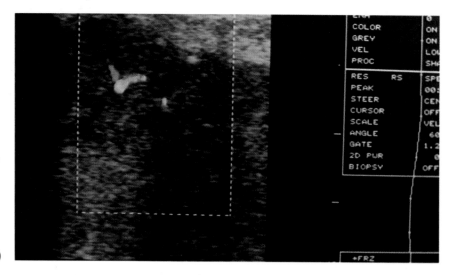

Figure 16.5a(ii)

peak systolic velocity, pulsatility index and resistive index. In malignant neoplasm peak systolic velocity is increased but there is no universal agreement in the cut off velocity beyond which lesion can be classified as malignant. A PI value of > 1.4 and RI value of > 0.8 have been suggested as clinically useful cut off points. With these threshold values CDFI has 80 per cent specificity with higher sensitivity and positive predictive value. Use of intravenous contrast agents such as microphilized albumin in increasing the specificity and sensitivity of colour Doppler flow imaging and power Doppler imaging in tumour detection and differentiation between benign and malignant lesion glands, is being studied at present.

Thyroid and Parathyroid Glands

Ultrasound has been successfully used as an adjunct to nuclear scintigraphy in evaluating the thyroid gland. Development of colour Doppler flow imaging has permitted the assessment of blood supply in addition to morphology. Thyroid gland is one of the most vascular organs in the body. So Doppler may be useful in providing information in some thyroid diseases.

High frequency transducers (7-12 MHz) are used for thyroid and parathyroid imaging. Gray scale longitudinal and transverse images of the thyroid gland are obtained from the level of mandibular angle to the sternal notch. The patient is examined in supine

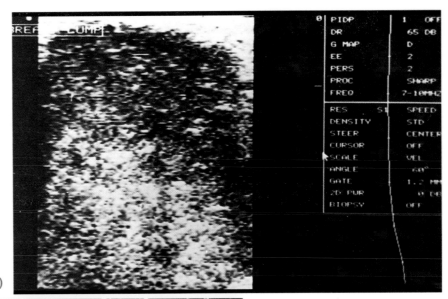

Figure 16.5b(i)

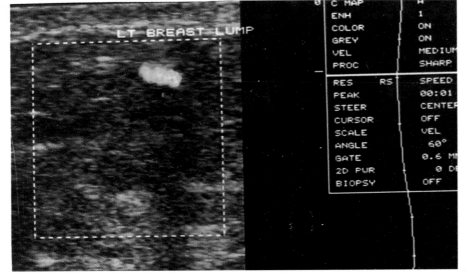

Figure 16.5b(ii)

Figures 16.5a(i) to b(ii)
Carcinoma of breast—(a-i) gray scale sonogram shows a large irregular mass lesion in the right breast, (a-ii) on CDFI Blood vessels are seen in the centre of the lesion, consistent with malignancy, and (b-i) gray scale US shows a large well defined mass with homogenous internal echotexture and no significant change in through transmission, (b-ii) colour Doppler scan shows colour signals located within the mass lesion

	Doppler flow studies in benign vs malignant breast lumps				
Table 16.2	*Malignant lumps*		*Benign breast*		*p value*
	Mean ± SD	*Range*	*Mean ± SD*	*Range*	
1. Doppler signal	+++			±	
2. Peak systolic flow (Hz)	2429.75 ± 521.65	1267-3233	1584.69-726.80	867-2900	< 0.0001
3. Minimum diastolic flow 885 (Hz)	78 ± 862.28	233-1800	574.30 ± 314.97	133-1000	< 0.0001
4. DFT (mm³) Max. frequency envelop	104.07 ± 32.04	42-1520	66.07 ± 28.91	31.133	< 0.0001
5. Pulsality index	0.4810 ± 0.1276	0.239-0.689	0.4868 ± 0.1536	0.233-0.790	NS

Table 16.3	Doppler flow signals vs various clinical parameters in malignant lumps			
	Histopathology	*Maximum systolic freq. (Hz)*	*Minimum diagnostic (Hz)*	*DFT (mm³)*
	Fibroadenoma	1256	492	62
	Fibroadenosis	1067	767	46
	Cystosarcoma phylloides	2744	978	121
	Infiltrating duct carcinoma	2367	686	99
	Lobular carcinoma	2514	707	124
	Squamous cell carcinoma	2867	767	109

Table 16.4	Doppler flow signals vs various clinical parameters in malignant lumps		
	Maximum diastolic Frequency (Mean) Hz	*Minimum diagnostic Frequency (Mean) Hz*	*DFT (mm³)*
Tumour size			
< 2 cm	1643	517	57
2-5 cm	1794	588	72
5-10 cm	2612	1009	118
> 10 cm	3000	1167	121
Tumour area			
0-10 cm²	1948	678	73
11-20 cm²	2006	745	86
21-30 cm²	2095	814	90
31-40 cm²	2192	814	94
41-50 cm²	2192	814	94
> 50 cm²	2793	1280	122
Stage of disease			
Stage II	1294	412	50
Stage III	2013	756	91
Stage IV	2754	1067	86
Grade of tumour			
Well differentiated	1467	707	68
Mod. differentiated	1866	686	83
Poor differentiated	1967	767	75

position with neck extended. A pad may be placed under the shoulder to provide better exposure of the neck. Doppler parameters are optimized for low flow sensitivity in the case of suspected parathyroid adenoma. With presently available Doppler systems, rich vascularisation of thyroid gland can be easily seen, which is most pronounced at the upper and lower pole. Superior thyroid vessels are found at the upper pole of each lobe. Inferior thyroid artery is present posterior to lower third of the lobe. Mean diameter of the arteries is 1-2 mm, the veins may be upto 8 mm in diameter. Peak systolic velocities are 20-40 cm/sec in major thyroid arteries and 15-30 cm/sec in intraparenchymal arteries.

Graves' disease Graves' disease is characterised by generalised enlargement of the thyroid gland with biochemical hyperfunction. Colour Doppler is useful in evaluation of this disease. Markedly increased vascularity is seen on CDFI and power Doppler imaging. This appeerence has been referred to as "Thyroid inferno" (Fig. 16.6). Spectral Doppler shows increased peak systolic velocity, which may exceed 70 cm/sec. None of the other thyroid diseases show such high velocities. Doppler examination can also be used to monitor the response to therapy in these patients. Following treatment significant decrease in vascularity and the velocities of thyroid vessels is seen (Fig. 16.7).

Thyroid nodules Hyperplastic thyroid nodules are less vascular than the normal thyroid parenchyma. Well differentiated carcinomas are relatively hypervascular and show tortuous vessels with arteriovenous shunting. Poorly differentiating and anaplastic carcinomas are rapidly growing tumours with propensity to undergo necrosis and thus are most often hypovascular.

Quantitative analysis of flow velocities is not accurate in differentiating benign from malignant nodules. Doppler finding that may be useful in differentiation, is the distribution of the vessels. With presently avail-

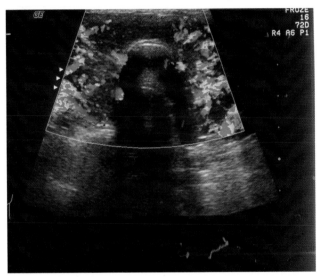

Figure 16.6
Colour Doppler image in a case of thyrotoxicosis. Both lobes of thyroid display marked increase in vascularity, also known as the 'Thyroid inferno' sign

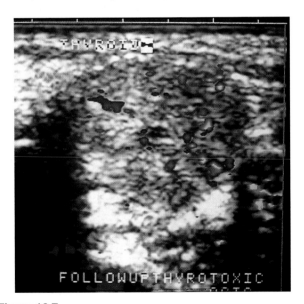

Figure 16.7
Follow-up case of thyrotoxicosis on therapy, colour Doppler image shows decreased flow in the thyroid gland, suggesting response to therapy

KEY POINTS

Doppler in thyroid and parathyroid gland lesions
- "Thyroid inferno" sign on the CDFI with peak systolic velocities greater than 70 cm/sec is virtually pathognomonic of thyrotoxicosis.
- Majority of the benign thyroid nodules show peripheral vascularity.
- Vessels inside the lesion with or without peripheral vessels suggest malignant nodules in the thyroid gland.
- An extra thyroidal feeding artery is a useful guide for localizing a Parathyroid adenoma on the CDFI.

able high definition colour Doppler systems, some degree of vascularity is demonstrated in all nodules. Two types of vascular distribution may be seen:
- Nodule with peripheral vascularity (Figs 16.8a and b)
- Nodule with internal vessels, which may or may not be associated with peripheral vessels (Figs 16.9a and b).

Large majority of hyperplastic, adenomatous and goitrous nodules show peripheral distribution of the blood vessels (Figs 16.8a and b), while majority of the thyroid malignancies show internal vessels with or without peripheral components (Figs 16.9a and b). Role of colour Doppler in evaluation of thyroid nodule is however controversial, and there is no universal agreement regarding its use in evaluation of a suspected thyroid nodule.

Parathyroid Adenoma

Primary hyper-parathyroidism is caused by an adenoma in 80-90 per cent of the cases. Other causes include enlargement of multiple gland (10-20%) and carcinoma (< 1%). Value of preoperative localising studies in patient with primary hyperparathyroidism is controversial. Many surgeon prefer routine bilateral neck exploration as the initial treatment for this condition. Some surgeons advocate unilateral neck exploration, because of following factors:
- Decreased operating room time
- Decreased risk of injury to the recurrent laryngeal nerve and normal parathyroid gland.

When unilateral surgery is being contemplated, accurate preoperative localisation of the adenoma is critical. Sonography has sensitivity of 70-80 per cent for localisation of an abnormal parathyroid gland. Typical sonographic appearence of parathyroid adenoma on gray scale imaging is a hypoechoic ovoid or lobulated mass posterior or lateral to the thyroid gland. Approximately 95 per cent of the adenoma occur in neck and usually obtain their blood supply from the branches of inferior thyroid artery. Parathyroid adenomas are hypervascular (Fig. 16.10). They are suspended by a vascular pedicle consisting of an extra thyroidal artery enveloped in fat. This extra thyroidal feeding artery can be visualised with colour or power Doppler sonography. Identification of this feeding artery can lead to an abnormal parathyroid

gland, which may be inconspicuous on gray scale imaging. Thus, CDFI increases the sensitivity and specificity of sonographic examination, in localising an adenoma.

Salivary Glands

Realtime sonography is a well-established modality for evaluating the head and neck region and its value in diagnosing abnormalities of the salivary gland is well-documented. Sonography helps to clarify clinically equivocal swellings of the salivary glands, and has a high accuracy rate for detection of salivary stone as well as differentiation of inflammation from tumours. In cases of salivary tumors, their location, size, extent in the superficial part of the gland and

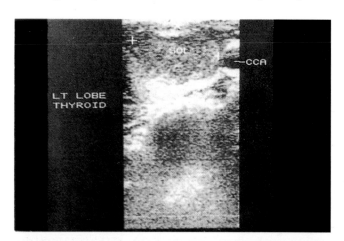

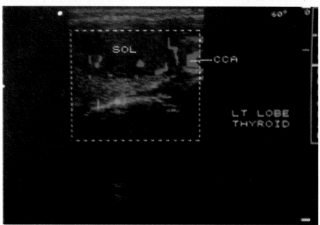

Figures 16.8a and b
Benign lesion of thyroid—(a) grey scale sonogram shows a solitary nodule in thyroid. Hypoechoic halo is visible around the nodule, and (b) Doppler image of same lesion reveals no vascularity in the mass. Colour flow corresponding to the halo is seen

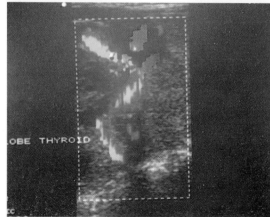

Figures 16.9a and b
(a) Heterogenous parenchymatous pattern seen in thyroid gland. There is obscuration of anatomical planes, and (b) colour Doppler image in a thyroid nodule shows evidence of increased peripheral and central vascularity consistent with malignancy

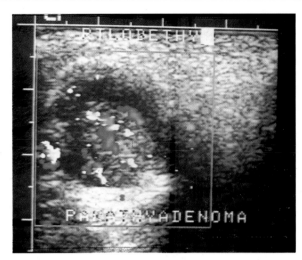

Figure 16.10
Parathyroid adenoma—colour Doppler of neck in a patient with clinical and biochemical evidence of hyper-parathyroidism. A rounded mass lesion is seen posterior to the thyroid gland with increased vascularity. On surgery an adenoma was resected

presence of cystic/necrotic areas can be reliably diagnosed with ultrasound. There are classical ultrasound description of the Pleomorphic Salivary Gland Adenoma (PSGA) and Warthin's tumour and it is possible to demonstrate these pathologies on realtime ultrasound. The ultrasound features of pleomorphic salivary gland adenoma are those of a mass which is round or lobulated, hyperechoic, well-defined and demonstrates through transmission. Warthins' tumors occur in the older age group and appear similar to PSGA, but are more likely to be multiple and show intralesional cystic areas or septations. Differentiation

of benign from malignant salivary gland tumor may be difficult with gray scale sonography alone. Upto 20 per cent of the malignant lesions can have sharp margins, making it difficult to use this criterion alone to differentiate benign from malignant lesions. Incidence of malignant salivary gland lesions is only 5 to 10 per cent of the cases, but it is helpful for the surgeon to be aware of any neoplastic lesion, as the treatment options may vary from local to wide excision, with or without adjuvant therapy.

Increased vascularity in salivary gland tumors can be recognised on colour Doppler flow imaging, a characteristic peripheral pattern for pleomorphic salivary gland adenoma has been described. The lesion may show fine centripetal branches. The RI value ranges from 0.6 to 1.1 and peak systolic velocity is less than 50 cm per sec. Warthin's tumor shows evenly scattered flow throughout the tumor. RI value is 0.55-0.8 and peak systolic velocity is always less than 60 cm/sec. The peak systolic velocity in malignant tumours is more than 60 cm/sec. A study by Bradly *et al* found no correlation between the colour pattern, peak systolic velocity and presence of malignancy. In their study, malignant lesions showed an increased vascular pattern. The Doppler indices (PI, RI) were at the higher end of the spectrum. Most of the malignant lesions had PI > 1.8 and RI > 0.8. PI < 1.8 and RI < 0.8 virtually excludes malignancy (Fig. 16.11). The authors concluded that risk of malignancy rises by a third in those with high PI and RI factors. They suggested that this information should be correlated with ultrasound morphology and clinical history.

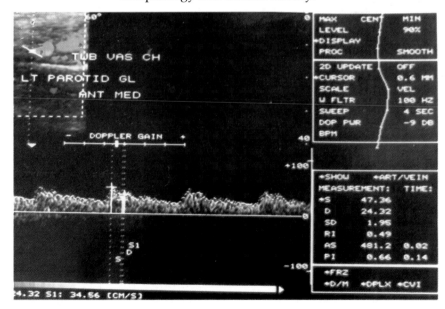

Figure 16.11
Colour Doppler sonography in a benign parotid lesion shows a mass lesion with vascular channels. Few vascular channels show continuous venous flow, arterial waveform shows peak velocity 47.36 and mean RI 0.49

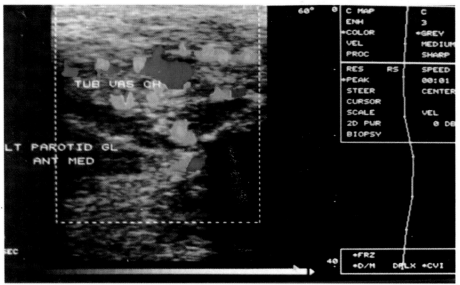

Figure 16.12
Parotid haemangioma—Colour Doppler sonography shows mass lesion with multiple vascular color flow signals

Vascular malformation in the salivary gland have similar feature as in other superficial organ. Multiple tortuous vascular channels with colour flow are seen (Fig. 16.12).

COLOUR DOPPLER IMAGING IN ORBIT

Doppler imaging has been used as an adjunct to routine A and B scanning of orbit since 1960. With the advent of colour Doppler imaging it is now possible to obtain information on the perfusion of the orbital structures in realtime. It is possible to carry out a vessel specific analysis in a fast and easy manner.

The colour Doppler examination can be performed with 7.5 MHz linear transducer. The transducer is applied to the close eyelid using a coupling gel. Patient is scanned in the supine position. Pressure should not be applied, as artifact can occur due to raised intraocular pressure. Horizontal and vertical scan through the eyes and orbit are obtained. The flow is assigned red or blue colour. Flow towards the transducer is coded red and flow away from is coded blue. Spectral analysis can be performed at selected sites. It is possible to distinguish between arteries and veins. Arteries shows evidence of pulsatile flow on colour images and spectral tracing. While the veins show continuous or minimally pulsatile flow. All examinations are performed in a low or medium flow settings. High flow setting may be applied for ophthalmic artery as this vessel has high flow velocity.

The gain settings are adjusted, so as to minimize artifacts by lid and involuntary eye movement.

Normal Orbital Vessels

Central retinal artery (CRA) and central retinal vein (CRV) can be visualized at the level of the optic nerve. These vessels are seen within 2-12 mm of the optic nerve shadow. As the flow in CRA is towards the transducer, it is displayed in red colour. CRV is displayed in blue. Ciliary vessels can be identified on the side of the optic nerves. Ophthalmic artery enters the orbit temporal to the optic nerve. In the middle orbit the ophthalmic artery crosses over the optic nerve to occupy the nasal position relative to the optic nerve. Vortex veins may also be visualised entering into the superior and inferior ophthalmic veins.

Applications

Ocular Tumours

Recruitment of vessels is required for tumour growth. These vessels include the existing and newly proliferating vessels. Most of the tumours can be diagnosed clinically. Imaging techniques are more often used to confirm and document the diagnosis. Diagnostic accuracy of A and B scan for characterisation of the tumours is well-established. Colour Doppler is being increasing used to enhance the efficacy of these techniques. Intraocular mass lesions show evidence

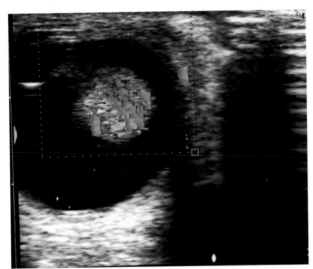

Figure 16.13
Ocular melanoma: colour Doppler flow images reveal evidence of increased vascularity in an intra ocular mass. Melanoma was found at histopathologic examination

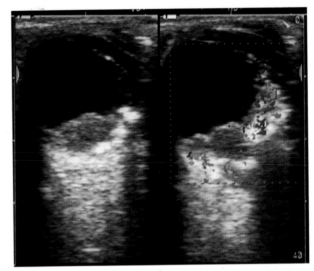

Figures 16.14a and b
(a) Gray scale image of the globe in a child shows a mass lesion in the region of retina. Calcification is also seen within the lesion, (b) CDFI shows a hyper-vascular lesion, suggesting malignant nature. On surgery, retinoblastoma was found

of Doppler signals. **Choroidal melanomas** show abnormal Doppler signals within the lesions (Fig. 16.13). The flow spectrum pattern in these lesions is a medium to high systolic Doppler shift with high diastolic flow velocity. The flow decreases after brachy-therapy in these patients. This is thought to be due to damage and sclerosis of tumour supplying vessels. Post-therapy a decrease is peak systolic and end diastolic velocities is seen. In choroidal haemangiomas, a high maximum systolic Doppler shift is seen along with high diastolic shifts. This is compatible with the pathologic features of this tumor which consist of a network of vascular channels. Evidence of increased flow is also seen in uveal metastases and retinoblastoma (Figs 16.14a and b). Some intra ocular lesions like age related macular degeneration, with subretinal haemorrhage and dense vitreous haemorrhage may simulate the appearance of tumor on B-mode imaging. CDFI can help in differentiating these lesions by demonstrating these lesions by demonstrating lack of abnormal blood flow.

Orbital Tumors and Vascular Lesions

Most orbital neoplasms show presence of intra-tumoral and Doppler signals. In cavernous haemangiomas flow may be seen on decreased gain settings (Fig. 16.15). Significantly increased vascularity is usually seen in malignant tumors. Sometimes benign tumour can cause blindness by pressing upon the optic nerve and its blood suppy and this compression can be easily demonstrated by CDFI. Orbital varices have a characteristic pattern on Doppler imaging. They show dynamic changes throughout inspiration and expiration. During inspiration active filling and distension of the lesion is seen, flow is seen towards the transducer. On expiration the size of the lesion slowly decreases with flow away from the transducer.

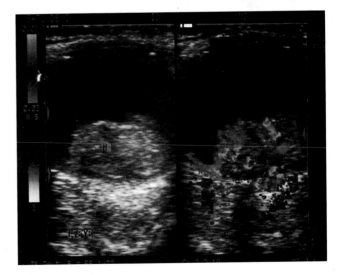

Figure 16.15
Intra ocular haemangioma: colour Doppler image shows a mass lesion in the posterior compartment of globe with increased vascularity

KEY POINTS

Orbital Doppler
– Orbital varices show respiratory variations in caliber with continuous non-pulsatile venous flow on the doppler examination.
– Dilatation of the Superior Ophthalmic Vein with arterialized high velocity flow in the postero-anterior direction is a characteristic feature of the Carotico-cavernous fistula.

On pulsed Doppler evaluation the flow is continuous and non-pulsatile during both phases. This is characteristic of venous flow seen in this lesion.

Carotico Cavernous Sinus Fistulas

A carotid cavernous sinus fistula (CCSF) is an abnormal communication between a branch of the carotid arteries and the cavernous sinus. CDFI clearly demonstrates the dilated arterialised superior ophthalmic vein with high velocity blood flow towards the transducer (posterior to anterior). This finding, well seen on CDFI is highly suggestive of CCSF. High pre septal vascularity and thickening of extra ocular muscles can also be seen. Doppler interrogation of vessels show high systolic and diastolic velocities. CDFI can also be used to document reduced flow after balloon embolisation.

Retinal Vessels Abnormalities

In occlusion of central retinal artery absence or marked reduction in flow can be seen on CDFI. Systolic and diastolic velocities are also reduced. Occlusion of central retinal veins shows a characteristic Doppler pattern. Central retinal artery show reduced flow in systole. Peak systolic waveform is blunted. Markedly decreased or absent flow is seen during diastole indicating high resistance caused by the blockage.

17

Doppler Imaging of Peripheral Arteries

Lalendra Upreti
Satish K Bhargava
Shashank Jain

The diagnosis of diseases involving peripheral arteries can usually be made on the basis of a thorough history and physical examination. Some form of additional testing is usually required for further characterization and/or quantification of the pathologic process. Easy accessibility of the limb arteries to sonography enables it to play a decisive role in the evaluation of disease. With the advent of high resolution ultrasound, it is possible to image the peripheral arteries without the limitations encountered in abdominal and thoracic vessels. Gray scale imaging has a limited role in evaluation. It can detect presence of an atherosclerotic plaque, aneurysm and juxta vascular masses which may appear to be of arterial origin on clinical evaluation. Duplex scanning plays an important role in vascular evaluation. Haimodynamic changes in a vessel can be studied by obtaining spectral waveform. Thus obstructive arterial lesions can be quantified, arterial stenosis can be differentiated from occlusion and the nature of perivascular masses can be determined. The addition of Colour Doppler Flow Imaging (CDFI) has transformed peripheral arterial imaging from a time consuming tedious task to an efficient practical examination. It has also improved the diagnostic accuracy of the examination. A rapid survey by CDFI can identify the zone of abnormal flow in a diseased vessel which can be evaluated by pulsed Doppler. CDFI enables accurate gate placement in the area of maximum flow disturbance. Power mode imaging or Doppler angio displays the peak amplitude of the flowing blood. The colour obtained is uniform, aliasing is not a problem, as with pulsed and CDFI mode and slow flow is better detected, a disadvantage is the lack of information about the flow direction.

INSTRUMENTATION

Peripheral arteries are small in size, so high resolution transducers are required for imaging the vascular wall and the lumen. Frequencies in the range of 5 to 10 MHz are preferred. For larger region like thigh 5 to 7.5 MHz is usually adequate. Examination of small superficial vessels is usually done by 7.5 to 10 MHz transducers. A linear transducer design with electronic steering capability is ideal, as it permits rapid coverage of long arterial segments. For examining iliac arteries and abdominal aorta, a frequency range of 2.5 to 5 MHz is needed depending upon the body habitus of the patient. Doppler frequencies vary between 3-10 MHz, they should be lower than the frequency used for acquiring gray scale image. Colour flow imaging rapidly identifies the area of flow disturbance, which can be evaluated by pulsed Doppler. Lower frequency than gray scale imaging are used, this partially over comes the early aliasing of the colour flow image.

NORMAL ANATOMY AND DOPPLER WAVEFORM

Lower Limb

Common femoral artery is the continuation of the external iliac artery at the level of the inguinal ligament. After a distance of about 4-7 cm, it divides into superficial and deep femoral (profunda) artery. The profunda femoris artery branches just beyond the origin to supply the femoral head and deep muscles of the thigh. Superficial femoral artery continues its downward course along the medial thigh till it reaches the adductor canal. At the lower limit of adductor canal it comes out through the adductor hiatus and continues as popliteal artery in the popliteal fossa. Popliteal artery lies along the posterior aspect of the knee, after giving off geniculate branches it divides into the anterior tibia artery and the tibioperoneal trunk at the lower edge of the popliteal fossa. Anterior tibial artery travels through the interosseous membrane to reach the anterior compartment of the leg. In the leg it is lateral to the anterior border of tibia. It crosses the ankle joint to be known as the dorsalis pedis artery. Tibio peroneal trunk lies posteriorly and divides into the posterior tibial and peroneal artery.

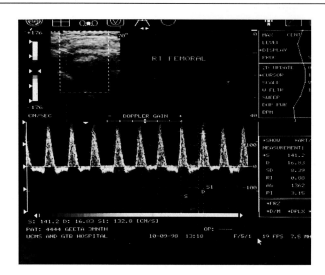

Figure 17.1
Duplex Doppler tracing from right femoral artery shows triphasic waveform characteristic of a peripheral artery

Posterior tibial artery lies in the posterior compartment and in its distal course can be easily localised behind medial malleolus.

Doppler Waveform (Fig. 17.1)

Triphasic flow pattern is seen in all the arteries. There is a phase of early systolic acceleration. This is followed by a period of small flow reversal before antegrade low velocity diastolic flow is seen. This triphasic waveform is characteristic of arteries supplying muscular bed, which has high peripheral resistance. During exercise or transient ischaemia, there is loss of triphasic pattern. A monophasic pattern characterized by persistent antegrade diastolic flow is observed. Peak systolic velocities of arteries vary with location. It is approximately 100 cm/sec at the level of common femoral artery and 40-50 cm/sec in the leg arteries.

Technique

Arterial occlusive disease is the main indication of the lower limb arterial Doppler study. Atherosclerosis is the major cause and as it also involves proximal vessels including aorta and iliac arteries, evaluation of aorto-iliac arteries should be integral part of Doppler study of lower limb arterial occlusive disease.

With the advent of CDFI, the aorta and iliac arteries can be visualised easily. Thus, preparation of the patient to reduce the bowel gas is not usually required. The study begins with the patient supine and transducer placed below the xiphoid process. A 2.5-3.5 MHz

---

KEY POINTS

Lower limb arterial doppler technique
- Complete examination mandates evaluation from the Aortoiliac level to the Dorsalis pedis artery using gray scale, CDFI and pulsed doppler.
- Aortoiliac vessels are examined with 2.5-3.5 MHz transducer with patient in the supine position.
- For Femoral artery evaluation the patient is placed in supine position with abduction at hip and flexion at the knee joint.
- Popliteal segment should be examined with patient in the prone position with slight flexion at the knee joint.
- Anterior tibial artery is localized lateral to the anterior tibial cortex below the knee joint and followed distally till ankle.
- Posterior tibial artery should be looked for behind the medial malleolus and then followed proximally, till it joins the Peroneal artery.

transducer is usually required. 5 MHz probe may be needed in thin individuals. Aorta is imaged in the sagittal section. Celiac axis and the superior mesenteric arteries can be seen arising anteriorly. Renal arteries arise from postero-lateral aspect of the aorta just below the superior mesenteric artery. Aorta is followed to the iliac bifurcation and common and external iliac arteries are examined till the groin. Evaluation of vessels at and below the groin require high frequency transducers. For evaluation of femoral arteries the hip is abducted and leg is flexed at the knees. Common femoral artery is evaluated till its bifurcation. Proximal segment of the profunda femoris is examined. The superficial femoral artery is followed distally. The transducer may have to be placed posteromedially in the lower thigh for examining the adductor canal region. A lower frequency transducer may be used if there is any difficulty in visualisation. Popliteal artery is examined with the patient in prone position with knees slightly flexed. It is followed till its bifurcation. At this point, the anterior tibial artery goes deep to transducer, as it perforates the interosseus membrane to enter the anterior compartment of the leg. Posterior tibial artery is best evaluated by first looking for it behind the medial malleolus with the patient in prone position. Alternatively the patient may be in supine position with leg abducted and flexed at knee. Once localised the artery is followed proximally till it meet the peroneal artery. Peroneal artery is difficult to evaluate as compared to posterior tibial artery. It is seen posterior to fibula with the patient in prone position. Anterior tibial artery is seen below the knee, lateral to the anterior border of the tibia, as it emerges through the interosseus membrane. It can be easily followed along its course till the ankle joint where it becomes the Dorsalis Pedis artery.

Arterial waveforms are obtained from following locations:

- Aorta
- Common and external illiac arteries
- Proximal, middle and distal superficial femoral arteries
- Popliteal artery
- Anterior and posterior tibial arteries

Any sites of increased flow disturbance are noted. Entire length of each vessel must be scanned to avoid missing sites of localised stenosis. Colour mapping provides only a single velocity parameter, which is a mean frequency estimate. Colour imaging is also subject to aliasing, which may be seen as apparent change in direction. Dependance on angle of insolation may result in colour changes caused by change in direction of flow rather than change in velocity. Finally relatively slow frame rate of image acquisition for colour scanning results in spatial and temporal distortion, one portion of the vessel may be imaged in systole and another during diastole, resulting in appearance of a velocity change along the length of the vessel. Thus, it is important to confirm the findings by taking the spectral tracing in the region of abnormality seen on CDFI. Spectral waveforms should be obtained from the centre of the vessel to avoid spectral broadening caused by the steep velocity gradient at the wall.

Upper Limb

Subclavian artery continues as axillary artery lateral to the first rib. It course medially over the proximal humerus to become the brachial artery. Brachial artery divides into radial, ulnar and interosseus artery in the interosseus fossa. Doppler flow pattern of the upper limb arteries is similar to that seen in the lower limb arteries.

Technique

Proximal subclavian arteries can be imaged above the sternoclavicular joint. Caudal angulation of transducer is usually required for optimal visualisation. It can also be seen by placing the transducer in the supraclavicular fossa. Axillary artery can be imaged through the axilla, along the medial aspect of the proximal humerus. Brachial artery can be easily identified in the arm and traced distally. Another alternative approach to image the vessel at the elbow where is superficial and then follow it proximally. Radial artery can similarly be localised at the wrist and followed proximally.

Clinical Aspect of Peripheral Arterial Disease

Most common cause of peripheral arterial occlusive disease is atherosclerosis. Predisposing factors for which include hypertension, diabetes and smoking. Aortoarteritis is a common cause in India, which usually affects proximal vessels in young females. This disease causes marked thickening of the arterial walls with luminal narrowing. Thromboangiitis obliterans or Buerger's disease is seen in males with history of smoking.

Clinical features of the peripheral arterial disease include intermittent claudication, rest pain, non-heal-

Table 17.1	Relation between symptoms and ankle/brachial index	
	Ankle/brachial index	Presentation
	> 1.0	Normal
	0.9-1.0	Asymptomatic or minimal disease
	0.5-0.9	Intermittent claudication
	< 0.5	Rest pain, severe disease

ing ulcer in the leg and gangrene. Extremities may be numb or cold. Patient may have one or more of the features mentioned above. On examination affected limb may be cold on palpation. Skin may show trophic changes. Arterial pulses can be weak or absent. On auscultation a bruit may be heard in the region of stenosis.

Other non-invasive tests are also used for evaluation of peripheral arterial disease. These include pressure studies, segmental pressure measurements, ankle/brachial indices etc. These tests help in establishing the presence of arterial disease, its possible site and severity.

Ankle/brachial index is one of most frequently used test. Blood pressure is taken at the level of ankle joint and in the brachial artery. Normal value of this index is more than one. Value less than 0.9 suggest that an arterial problem is present in lower extremity. Ankle-branchial index co-relates well with clinical symptoms of the disease (Table 17.1).

Once the suspicion of the peripheral arterial disease is aroused on ankle brachial index measurement, segmental pressure measurements are taken in the thigh and the leg for approximate localisation of the diseased segment. A drop of more than 20 mmHg pressure indicates likely presence of disease in that particular segment. However, precise localisation of site of disease is usually difficult and they are of limited value in disease involving multiple segments.

Diagnosis on Doppler Imaging

The waveform of a normal peripheral artery is triphasic (Fig. 17.1). This waveform is altered in presence of arterial stenosis or occlusion. Analysis of the velocity pattern provides the most useful information regarding the haemodynamic significance of atherosclerotic lesion. As already described initial survey carried out by CDFI enables rapid identification of site of flow abnormality, which is then interrogated by pulsed Doppler to obtain the spectral wave forms. Waveforms are also obtained proximal and distal to stenosis. Ratio of peak systolic velocity in the stenosed segment to that in proximal segment is calculated to determine haemodynamically significant stenosis.

Proximal to the stenosis the waveform is usually normal. The findings in the stenotic region depend upon the severity of lesion and help in the determining the degree of stenosis (Table 17.2).

In mild to moderate stenosis, the early diastolic reversal decreases and disppears with increasing severity of the lesion. Along with this increase in the diastolic flow is seen. With increasing severity of the lesion, forward flow through the artery increases and the diastolic velocity may approach near the systolic velocity. This increasing diastolic velocity is probably due to decreased peripheral resistance caused by

Table 17.2	Findings and stenotic region depend on severity of lesion	
	Stenosis	Findings
	1. Normal	• Normal triphasic waveform
	2. 1-19%	• Normal waveform outline • Normal peak systolic velocity • Slight spectral broadening
	3. 20-49%	• At least 30% increase in peak systolic velocity compared to normal proximal segment • Prominent spectral broadening • Normal proximal and distal waveform
	4. 50-99%	• More than 100% increase in peak systolic velocity compared to proximal segment • Loss of reverse flow (monophasic signal) • Extensive spectral broadening • Distal waveform monophasic with reduced systolic velocity
	5. Complete occlusion (Fig. 17.2)	• No colour on CDFI no flow on pulsed Doppler • Echogenic thrombus in artery • Damped waveform proximal to occlusion • Distal waveforms monophasic with decreased velocities (tardus-parvus waveform)

Table 17.3	Efficacy of doppler examination in the evaluation of lower limb arterio-occlusive disease						
	Jager et al (1986)	*Moneta et al (1987)*	*Kohler et al (1987)*	*Cossman et al (1989)*	*Polak et al (1990)*	*Whalen et al (1992)*	*Sharma et al (1996)*
Sensitivity	96	77	82	83	88	92	65.6
Specificity	81	98	92	96	95	97	96.2
Positive predictive value	92	94	80	91	—	90	88.5
Negative predictive value	91	92	93	91	—	98	86.3
Accuracy	76.3	—	—	90	93	96	86.8

dilatation of arterioles in the muscular bed in response to release of metabolites caused by local ischaemia. Opening up of many small collateral pathways also contribute to decrease in peripheral resistance. Peak systolic velocity is less affected by vasodilatation. Therefore, this parameter is used to quantify the degree of stenosis. Artery distal to a high grade stenosis or occlusion show a slow rise, low amplitude (Tardus-Parvus) waveform (Fig. 17.2c).

Accuracy

Many studies have compared sensitivity, specificity and diagnostic accuracy of Doppler with angiography as gold standard. Result of these studies are summarised in Table 17.3. Detection of calcification and thrombus is better with CDFI as compared to angiography. Detection of collateral vessel is poor.

Therapeutic Approaches

Once a haemodynamically significant stenosis or occlusion has been confirmed. Some sort of therapeutic

Table 17.4	Therapeutic options in peripheral arterio-occlusive disease	
	Lesion	*Preferred mode of therapy**
1.	Diffuse aorto-femoral or aorto-illiac disease	Dacron graft
2.	Popliteal artery above the knee joint (occlusion or long segment narrowing)	• Poly tetra fluoroethylene graft (PTFE) • Venous graft • reversed superficial vein • *in situ* superficial vein
3.	Popliteal artery below the knee and other leg vessels (occlusion, long segment of narrowing)	• Venous graft
4.	Short segment narrowing in limb vessels	• Percutaneous interventions • angioplasty • atherectomy • stent

*Extensive lesions may also be recanalised with the help of thrombolytic agents.

intervention is required to stop the progression of disease and to provide symptomatic relief to the patient. The therapeutic approach depends upon site, extent and severity of the lesion. Various options available are listed in Table 17.4.

Evaluation of Bypass Graft by Doppler

CDFI and Duplex Doppler ultrasound are the technique of choice for the post-operative monitoring of the bypass graft patency and to detect focal stenosis or any other cause of graft dysfunction.

In the immediate postoperative period gray scale imaging is useful to evaluate the surgical bed of the graft, to locate perigraft collection which may be due to infection or pseudoaneurysm (discussed later in the chapter).

Synthetic Bypass Grafts

Complications affecting the synthetic graft depend upon the type of graft and time since surgery. In the early period (1-2 year since surgery) graft stenosis and occlusion may be due to technical reasons or development of fibrointimal lesions at the anastomotic site. In the later stage graft failure is usually due to development of stenotic/occluding lesion in the native vessel proximal or distal to the graft. Late anastomotic pseudoaneurysm may occur in femoral anastomosis of aorto-femoral graft.

Development of an anastomotic stenosis will cause significant increase in the velocity signals but increase in velocity, or turbulence of flow may be normal depending upon the nature of connection. This normal increase may be upto 100 per cent without being pathologic. If such finding is noted, serial monitoring is indicated. If there is progressive increase in the velocity at the site of turbulence, it indicates development of stenotic lesion. Absence of signal in a graft is diagnostic of occlusion.

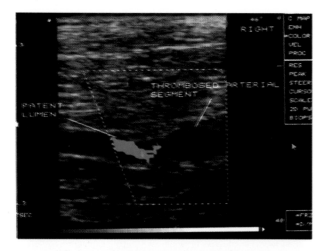

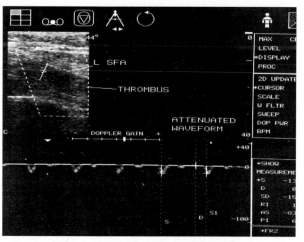

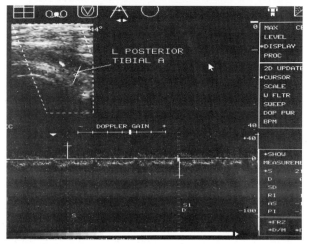

Figures 17.2a to c

Thrombosis of superficial femoral artery—(a) colour Doppler image shows absence of flow in the distal superficial femoral artery, (b) pulse Doppler shows attenuated waveform proximal to the point of occlusion, and (c) spectral tracing from posterior tibial artery in the same patient shows delayed peak with low amplitude (Tardus-Parvus) waveform

Autologus Vein Graft

Two types of venous grafts are used in bypass surgery reverse vein and in situ vein. In the reverse vein type of graft a native superficial vein is harvested and reversed. It is then anastomosed to the native artery, proximal and distal to the diseased segment. In the *in situ* technique the superficial vein is left in its bed (greater or lesser saphenous vein). The valves in the veins are lysed. Perforating branches are ligated. Proximal and distal segments of the veins are mobilised and anastomosed with the arterial segments.

Early cause of graft malfunction differ depending upon the time since the surgery. In *early failure* seen within one month, technical factors are the main causes. These include poor vein selection, poor suture line placement, poor selection of the anastomic site, unsuspected arteriovenous fistula and poorly lysed venous valves. In second period lasting from one month to 2 years following surgery, graft malfunction may occur secondary to fibrointimal hyperplasia at the site of anastomosis or at the site of venous valves. Late failures beyond 2 years period are secondary to progression of atherosclerotic disease in the arteries proximal and distal to anastomosis.

Monitoring of venous bypass grafts has traditionally been performed by serial measurements of the lower extremity pressures, but Doppler sonography is superior to pressure measurements for monitoring and evaluation of suspected graft dysfunction. Measurement of the velocity can be used to identify the graft with high possibility of failure. Previously this approach consisted of measuring the peak systolic velocity in the narrowest segment of graft, with velocity less than 45 cm/sec indicating presence of graft malfunction. But this criterion identifies only the severely diseased graft. Present approach aims at identifying the areas of stenosis in the graft which are likely to progress, causing restriction and finally occlusion of the flow. The graft is surveyed with CDFI. Site of stenosis is identified and spectral analysis is performed. Severity of stenosis can be determined by obtaining ratio of peak systolic velocities in the diseased segment with the velocity obtained in segment 2-4 cm proximal to it. Ratios greater than 2 correspond to 50 per cent diameter stenosis, ratio greater than 3 indicates 75 per cent stenosis. Presence of tandem lesions limits the usefulness of this technique. It has been shown that early lesions can develop within 3 months after surgery and can be detected by Doppler evaluation even before the patient develops symptoms. Intervention in the form of surgical revision of stenosis is indicated. Stenosis with systolic ratios above 3 or 4 usually require this form of intervention.

Aneurysms

Peripheral arterial aneurysms are usually due to arteriosclerosis which causes weakening of the vessel walls. Popliteal artery is the most common site of aneurysm in the lower limb followed by the superficial femoral artery.

Ultrasound is now universally accepted as imaging modality of choice for diagnosis of a suspected aneurysm. A bulge or focal enlargement of 20 per cent of the expected vessel diameter is consistent with diagnosis of aneurysm. Ultrasound can visualise the presence of intraluminal thrombus. With colour Doppler patent lumen can be visualised and complete thrombosis can be diagnosed with more certainty, compared to ultrasound alone (Fig. 17.3a). Ultrasound is the ideal modality for follow-up of these cases. These are no strict criteria to determine the suitability of the patient for surgery. An aneurysm more than 2 cm in size usually requires surgical repair. Presence of distal embolisation is an absolute indication for surgery, irrespective of its size. Since arteriosclerosis is a generalised diffuse process involving all parts of the arterial system, one might expect that aneurysmal degeneration would occur at multiple locations. In fact, the 40 per cent of peripheral arterial aneurysms

KEY POINTS

Peripheral arterial aneurysm
- Arteriosclerosis is the most common cause with involvement of the Popliteal arteries being the commonest.
- Focal enlargement of the artery with diameter more than 20% of the normal is highly specific for the diagnosis.
- CDFI is most helpful in diagnosis of completely thrombosed aneurysm.
- Other peripheral arteries and the aorta must always be examined for presence of associated aneurysm(s), which are present in many of these patients.

are multiple. Thus, detection of any aneurysm in the peripheral artery, mandates a thorough search for detection of aneurysm in the other limbs and aorto-iliac vessels (Fig. 17.3b).

Pseudoaneurysm

Pseudoaneurysm is defined as a contained rupture of the arterial wall. It develops sometimes as a complication of penetrating trauma or arterial catheterisation. Common femoral artery is the most frequent site, because most of these lesions develop following arterial catheterisation. Risk of development depends

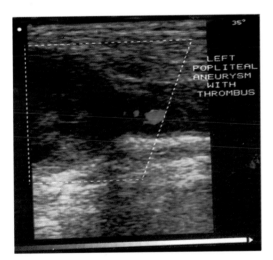

Figure 17.3a
Colour Doppler flow image at the level of popliteal artery. Fusiform enlargement of popliteal artery is seen suggesting presence of an aneurysm. No colour flow is demonstrable

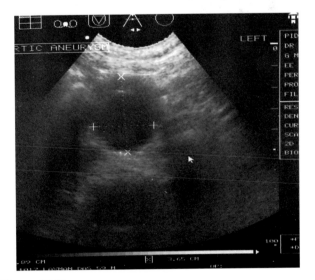

Figure 17.3b
Grey scale image in the same patient shows associated aneurysm, with mural thrombus, in aorta below the level of renal hilum

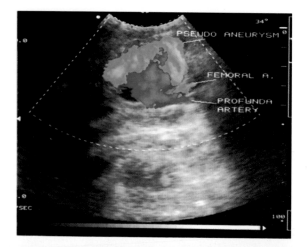

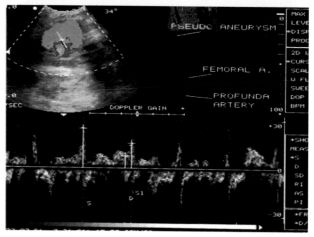

Figures 17.4a and b

upon the size of catheter and anticoagulant therapy. On ultrasound a cystic mass is seen in relation to parent vessel. Communicating channel may be visualised on gray scale sonography. Appearances on CDFI are characteristic. A swirling motion of colour 'ying-yang' sign (Fig. 17.4a) is seen within the cystic mass. The communicating channel or the 'neck' of the pseudo-aneurysm is exceeding well seen with colour Doppler on Duplex sonography, "to and fro" (Fig. 17.4b) sign is typically seen in the neck or the communicating channel. The 'to' component is seen due to blood entering through the communicating channel into the pseudoaneurysm. High velocity settings may be needed for detection. During diastole, the blood present in the cavity returns to main arterial lumen causing the 'fro' component. Pseudoaneurysms can have multiple compartments.

Left to themselves pseudoaneurysms may undergo spontaneous thrombosis and closure on bed-rest. There are two therapeutic approaches to this problem. If the

surgeon decides to do surgery, the site of communication can be marked on skin and preoperative angiogram is not required. Direct "transcutaneous compression therapy" can also be used for obliterating these lesions with CDFI as guide. This intervention is successful if applied to pseudoaneurysm developing within a week of acute event. Later than this, endothelialization of communicating channel occur, which hamper its occlusion. Direct pressure is applied with ultrasound probe over the neck of pseudo-aneurysm. Probe is positioned in the long axis of the artery and flow in pseudoaneurysm cavity is obliterated by firm compression applied till twenty minutes. If initial compression is not successful the procedure can be repeated upto three times. Many reports have documented high success rate of this procedure. Pseudoaneurysm in upper limb arteries can also be treated by this therapy. Arterial or venous thrombosis, may occur rarely. Pseudoaneurysms may also occur following bypass graft. These post-surgical pseudoaneurysms are usually seen with synthetic vascular graft, at the site of distal anastomosis. This is probably due to weakening of the arterial wall at the anastomic site, causing dehiscence. The communicating channel is not seen and the pseudoaneurysm is contiguous with the anastomosis. Thus, the Doppler 'to and fro' sign is not seen. 'Ying yang' appearence is seen on CDFI. A patulous anastomosis should be distinguished from the anastomotic pseudoaneurysm. Surgical anastomosis is made wider to compensate for diameter differences between the graft and artery and subsequent fibrointimal hyperplasia. This causes appearance of vessel dilatation at the site of anastomosis. Patulous anastomosis shows continuation of wall of the artery and the graft, while pseudoaneurysm is seen as an eccentric mass lying in the soft tissues. Thrombus may be seen in the wall of pseudoaneurysm.

KEY POINTS

Pseudoaneurysms
- These are most commonly due to penetrating trauma or arterial catheterization.
- "Color swirl" on CDFI and "to and fro" sign on pulsed doppler examination are diagnostic.
- Transcutaneous compression therapy with the ultrasound probe can obliterate many of these lesion.

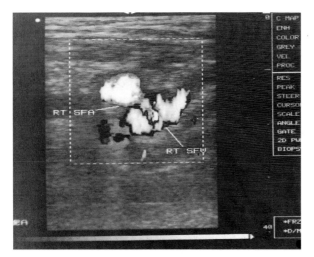

Figure 17.5a
Colour Doppler image at the level of upper thigh shows a communication between superficial femoral vessels

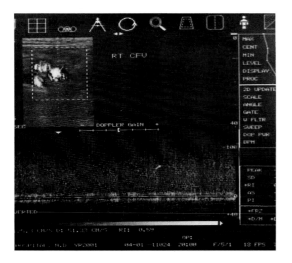

Figure 17.5b
Pulse Doppler in common femoral vein shows turbulent high velocity waveform

Arteriovenous Fistula

Arteriovenous fistula may be:
- Congenital
- Traumatic which may be due to penetrating injury or following angiography
- Created as part of dialysis shunt.

Congenital arteriovenous fistulas are communications between artery and large distended veins. These lesions are clinically obvious, as they cause discolouration of skin and trophic changes. Multiple venous channels with arterial branches feeding them can be seen on the skin. Diagnostic utility of ultra-

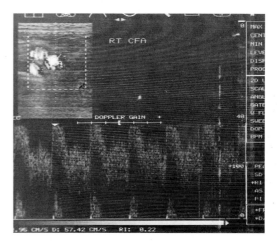

Figure 17.5c
Pulse Doppler in common femoral artery proximal to fistula shows persistent antegrade flow in diastole

sound is limited. It can help in selecting the area for injection of sclerosing compounds and monitor the lesion following sclerotherapy.

Traumatic fistula may develop following penetrating trauma or following catheterisation of the artery or vein. These lesions can be readily diagnosed with CDFI (Fig. 17.5a). The affected vein shows turbulence and is enlarged in size compared to its counterpart in the oppsite limb. the fistulous communication is more easily seen with CDFI than with the Duplex scanning. On Duplex scanning the affected vein shows turbulence and arterialised waveform (Fig. 17.5b). Turbulent waveform in the vein can also been if there is extrinsic compression of the vein due to haematoma, another complication which can occur due to catheterisation. CDFI is extremely helpful in such cases, as it can demonstrate the arteriovenous connection with ease. Arterial waveform proximal to the communication will show increase in the diastolic flow due to reduced resistance in the vein (Fig. 17.5c). Distal artery will

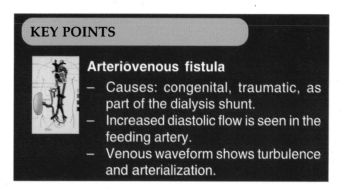

KEY POINTS

Arteriovenous fistula
- Causes: congenital, traumatic, as part of the dialysis shunt.
- Increased diastolic flow is seen in the feeding artery.
- Venous waveform shows turbulence and arterialization.

show a normal waveform. The arteriovenous fistula should also be evaluated for venous flow during *Valsalva's manoeuvre*. In lesion with small communicating channel the venous velocity will decrease. If there is complete cessation of flow, it indicates that the lesion in all probability will undergo spontaneous closure over a period of time. These lesion can be followed with CDFI and active intervention is not needed. Transcutaneous compression therapy under ultrasound guidance has been tried in larger lesions. Success rate for this form of therapy are 30 per cent or lower.

Arteriovenous fistula may be created for haemodialysis. In the present day, clinical practice bypass grafts are most frequently used. They are inserted in the forearm and are made of either synthetic material (polytetrafluoroethylene or PTFE) or autologous vein. Complication which may occur in these access channels include development of small or large aneurysm, pseudoaneurysm or graft stenosis. These complications can be evaluated readily by colour Doppler flow imaging. Pseudoaneurysms can be diagnosed with accuracy greater than 90 per cent. For detection of stenosis accuracy depends upon the type of graft. In straight segment graft the sensitivity and specificity have been reported to be 95 per cent and 97 per cent respectively. In graft having a tortuous path sensitivity and specificity are reportedly less (92% and 84% respectively). Overall accuracy is 86 per cent.

In a normal graft peak systolic velocities range between 100 to 200 cm/sec. Waveform shows turbulence, this is seen as irregular waveform contour and filling of the spectral window. A significant stenosis is diagnosed in presence of a focal area within the graft showing peak systolic velocity ratio greater than two when compared with the velocity of the feeding artery. Presence of velocities less than or equal to 50 cm/sec also indicate presence of high grade stenosis.

Evaluation of dialysis shunts should also include examination of subclavian vein. Stenosis occurs at the site of proximal subclavian vein in 20-50 per cent of the cases. They are seen in individuals, who had temporary haemodialysis access with placement of large diameter catheters.

Lalendra Upreti
Rohini Gupta
Shashank Jain

Venous System

Sonography is the preferred modality for the evaluation of the venous system. Veins are easily visualised on the gray scale sonography. Addition of Duplex and more recently colour Doppler flow imaging has enabled quick visualisation of normal and abnormal venous dynamics. With the advent of CDFI, role of venography has become limited. Additional benefit of CDFI include:

- Short examination time
- Elegant realtime visual demonstration of physiological and pathological states.
- Evaluation of deep seated veins like dubclavian veins.

Lower Limb Veins

These consist of superficial veins, deep veins and perforating veins.

Superficial veins Greater and lesser (small) saphenous veins form the superficial venous system. Greater saphenous vein begins near the medial malleolus and terminates in the common femoral vein below the inguinal ligament. It is the longest vein in the body. It may be duplicated. Lesser saphenous vein begins adjacent to the medical malleolus and terminates in the popliteal vein in the calf.

Perforating veins These are the channels between the superficial and deep venous system, which allow the flow to occur from superficial to the deep venous system. They communicate with the saphenous veins through the arch branches of the saphenous veins.

Deep veins of the limbs comprise of three paired veins in the calf namely posterior tibial veins, anterior tibial veins and peroneal veins. They join to form the popliteal vein in the popliteal fossa. Popliteal vein continues as the superficial femoral vein at the level of the adductor canal. This vein is joined by the profunda femoris vein in the thigh to form the common femoral vein. Above the inguinal ligament, this vein is known as external iliac vein. The external iliac vein joins the internal iliac vein to form the common iliac vein. The common iliac veins from two sides join together to form the inferior vena cava. Deep veins contain numerous valves to prevent backflow of the blood. The veins are accompanied the arteries which bear the same name. The veins are usually larger than the arteries in calibre.

Upper Limb Veins

Superficial venous system of the upper limb consists of cephalic and basilic veins. Cephalic veins run laterally. The Basilic vein runs along the medial aspect of the forearm.

Deep venous system comprises of radial and ulnar veins, which join to form brachial vein in the proximal forearm. This vein continues as the axillary vein at the lower border of the teres major. Axillary vein becomes the subclavian vein at the outer border of the first rib. This vein joins the internal jugular vein to form the brachio-cephalic vein. The brachiocephalic veins from two sides unite to form the superior vena cava.

Instrumentation and Technique

The ultrasound equipment for evaluation for venous system of the extremities should have a high resolution imaging capability with additional facility of Duplex and colour flow imaging capable of picking up slow flow.

In most patients 5-7.5 MHz linear array transducer is adequate for the gray scale evaluation. In obese patients lower frequency transducer may be required. Evaluation of the pelvic veins and the inferior vena cava is done with 3.5 MHz transducer. Doppler evaluation can be performed with same transducer frequency. Additional capability of beam steering is desirable as it allows use of shallower Doppler angles. The Doppler parameters should be adjusted to pick up slow flow. Larger sample volume should be used to cover the entire diameter of the vein.

Lower Limb Veins

Optimum positioning, patient comfort, and co-operation are essential prerequisite for a high quality Doppler examination of the lower extremity venous system. The patient should be in supine position with elevation at the head end. This position increases venous filling and makes them prominent, thus enabling adequate evaluation of small veins. For the evaluation of the femoral veins the leg should be partially flexed at the hip and the hip should be in external rotation. Ultrasound gel is applied from the groin to the knee to facilitate continuous examination. The evaluation, which includes gray scale, Duplex and colour flow imaging, should begin from just above the inguinal ligament in the transverse plane. Longitudinal sections are helpful for pulsed Doppler evaluation. Common femoral vein is identified adjacent to the common femoral artery. Vein can be distinguished from the artery because of following features:

- Medial location
- Larger size
- Lack of pulsations
- Compressibility on applying pressure.

KEY POINTS

Technique for lower extremity venous doppler

- 5-7.5 MHz linear array transducer is required for the limb veins; 3.5-5.0 MHz curvilinear array transducer for pelvic veins and the inferior vena cava.
- Patient position supine with elevation of the head. Hip is kept in flexion and external rotation.
- Identify the Common Femoral vein in the transverse plane, continue examination distally; oblique orientation is needed for adequate visualization of the Saphenofemoral junction.
- CDFI and pulsed doppler is performed intermittently to evaluate phasicity, compressibility, response to Valsalva maneuver and augmentation.
- In adductor canal region CDFI and pulsed doppler examination is a must as compression may not obliterate the vein completely.
- Popliteal vein is evaluated in the prone position.
- Posterior tibial vein is localized posterior to the medial malleolus and followed proximally, Anterior tibial vein is examined from below knee in supine position lateral to the anterior tibial cortex and then followed distally.

The examination continues distally in the transverse plane, with compression of vein at regular intervals. Saphenofemoral junction is identified and examined for competence. Inferiorly bifurcation into the superficial femoral vein and the profunda femoris vein can be seen. Superficial vein is then followed distally till the lower third of the thigh, where it moves away from the transducer to enter the adductor canal. A lower frequency transducer is required for evaluation. The vein is less amenable to compression in this region, thus careful Duplex and colour Doppler evaluation is needed to determine the normal haemodynamics.

Popliteal vein is examined in the prone or the lateral decubitus position. The examination begins from the upper popliteal fossa and continues inferiorly till the bifurcation. Posterior tibial vein evaluation usually starts posterior to the medial malleolus of tibia, where it is visualised as paired structure along side the artery of the same name. The examination is then continued upward till the tibio-peroneal trunk. Peroneal veins can be visualised lateral to the posterior tibial vessels; they most often lie in relation to the posterior surface of the fibula. Anterior tibial veins are scanned in the supine position of the leg between the anterior surface of the tibia and fibula. They are difficult to evaluate in the superior part as they may be obscured by bony outlines of the tibia and fibula.

Saphenofemoral junction It is identified just below the groin. Examination in oblique plane may be required for proper visualisation. A valve may be identified at this level. The great saphenous vein is followed into the upper thigh. *Small saphenous vein* may be seen in the popliteal fossa. It is followed upwards till its entry in the Popliteal vein. Gastrocnemius vein may cause confusion, but the small saphenous vein can be followed from the popliteal vein into the subcutaneous plane, while the gastrocnemius vein is limited to the muscle plane. *The perforating veins* are not seen in the normal patients.

Gray scale examination should include assessment of compressibility, presence of thrombus and presence of valves. Evaluation of flow dynamics like phasicity, augmentation, competence of valves can be done by colour Doppler. Spectral analysis is performed to confirm and document the findings visualized on CDFI.

Upper Limb

Upper limb veins are examined in the supine position with head tilted away from the side being examined. The subclavian vein is seen above the sternoclavicular joint at the root of neck, its junction with the internal jugular vein may be seen in some patients. CDFI and Duplex evaluation is done in this medial portion, as the vein is not amenable to compression by the transducer. A phasic flow should be seen in the normal vein. Middle portion is not directly accessible due to overlying clavicle; patency of this segment can be ascertained by presence of normal flow in the proximal and distal segments. Lateral portion of the subclavian vein continues as the axillary vein. Junction of the cephalic and axillary vein is seen at the outer end of the first rib. Axillary vein is examined by raising the arm and resting it on the examination table with palm facing upwards. Distally the examination continues till the brachial venous bifurcation. Examination of the

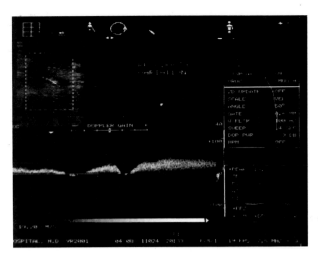

Figure 18.1

Normal venous waveform; Pulse Doppler image of common femoral vein shows low velocity monophasic flow with respiratory variation (phasicity)

Radial and Ulnar veins should be started at the wrist and the veins should be followed proximally along their accompanying arteries.

Examination of the neck veins is also performed along with proximal veins of the upper limbs, as the pathology may involve both of them simultaneously. Internal jugular vein is traced from the root of neck to the angle of mandible. The vein is located anterolateral to the common carotid artery. Doppler evaluation shows prominent bi-directional flow due to transmitted cardiac pulsation. External jugular vein is smaller in size than the internal jugular vein. It lies lateral to the internal jugular vein along the posterior border of the sternocleidomastoid muscle.

Characteristics of A Normal Vein

On gray scale imaging a normal vein has echo free lumen. Walls are thin and may be slightly echogenic. Venous valvular leaflets may be seen as thin echogenic structures in the lumen. On pulsed Doppler, monophasic, low velocity blood flow is seen. Mild fluctuation in velocity is seen with phase of respiratory cycle, slow flow is seen during inspiration and faster flow during expiration*(phasicity)*(Fig. 18.1). In normal upper limb veins, spontaneous phasic flow is seen with bi-directional pattern. The retrograde component is due to contraction of the heart. Various manoeuvres are employed to demonstrates patency and normal haemodynamics:

Compression (Figs 18.2a and b) Gentle pressure over the vein by the transducer causes apposition of the

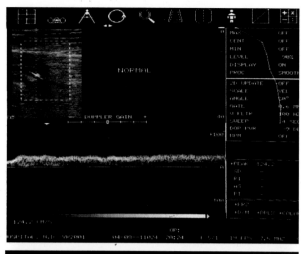

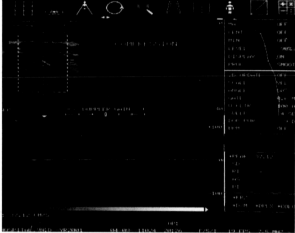

Figures 18.2a and b
(a) Transverse section through upper thigh shows common femoral vein (arrowhead), and (b) on applying gentle transducer pressure, venous lumen is obliterated

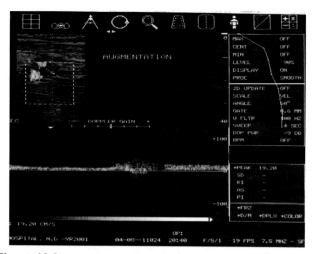

Figure 18.3
Longitudinal pulse Doppler image femoral vein showing augmentation of blood flow (arrow) on compression of distal lower limb

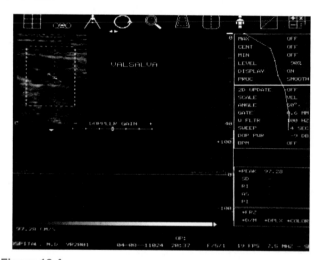

Figure 18.4
Longitudinal pulse Doppler image of superficial femoral vein showing progressive decrease in venous flow on performing Valsalva manoeuvre

wall and obliteration of the lumen in a normal vein. This finding can be easily appreciated on gray scale imaging in transverse plane. Complete obliteration of lumen on mild compression effectively rules out acute thrombosis.

Augmentation (Fig. 18.3) This refers to increase in the blood flow in the vein when distal limb is compressed by hand. This feature can be seen on both on CDFI and pulsed Doppler and is suggestive of patency of venous segment between site of compression and examination. Weak augmentation may be seen in partial thrombosis, or development of venous collateral in the settings of acute thrombosis.

Valsalva manoeuvre (Fig. 18.4) The patient is asked to take a deep breath and bear down. This causes increase in the intra-abdominal pressure and retards the venous return towards the heart. Pooling of blood occurs in the abdominopelvic and proximal lower extremity veins, causing their dilatation. This feature can be appreciated on gray scale imaging. On CDFI, decrease in colour is seen followed by complete cessation. On pulsed Doppler complete cessation of the flow can be documented. A positive test in the femoral veins is indicative of patency of proximal venous system. This manoeuvre is also used to establish the competence of the saphenofemoral junction.

Lower Extremity Deep Venous Thrombosis

Detection of deep vein thrombosis accounts for majority of venous system examinations. Detection of this entity is important because it can cause pulmonary embolism.

Clinical considerations Acute deep venous thrombosis is the most common indoor vascular disorder. In the initial stages the thrombus develops in the calf veins. Approximately 40 per cent of these thrombi resolve spontaneously, 40 per cent organize focally. Proximal progression in the popliteal and femoral veins occurs in only 20 per cent of the cases. Acute thrombus is loosely attached and has tendency to embolize. Conditions and factors, which predispose to thrombosis include:

- Prolonged bed-rest
- Malignancy, particularly in pancreas, lung or gastro-intestinal tract
- Administration of oestrogens including oral contraceptives
- Disseminated intravascular coagulation
- Post-partum period, and
- Paralysis.

Symptoms and signs of the deep venous thrombosis consist of pain, swelling and erythema. These features are however non-specific and may be seen in a large number of local and systemic conditions. Most of the patients are asymptomatic and development of pulmonary embolization may be the first clue to the presence of thrombosis. Lack of specificity of clinical evaluation along with risk of severe life-threatening complication associated with the deep venous thrombosis has prompted search for a non-invasive technique which provides accurate diagnosis in this condition. Impedance plethysmography measures venous capacitance and the rate of venous outflow from the lower extremities. In expert hands it has sensitivity ranging from 87 to 100 per cent and specificity ranging from 92 to 100 per cent for detection of DVT above the knee. Its sensitivity for detection of isolated calf vein thrombosis is 17-33 per cent. Multiple radionuclide techniques have been developed but have not been sufficiently accurate to mandate a role in the diagnostic evaluation. A large number of studies have proven the sonography as the ideal and in most cases the only technique required for the diagnosis. Gray scale US supplanted with Doppler flow assessment has proved to be extremely accurate (sensitivity, 88-100%; specificity, 92-100%) for detection of femoro-popliteal DVT and occlusive thrombosis of the external and common iliac veins. One significant limitation of standard duplex sonography has been the difficulty in identifying and assessing the deep veins of the calf. A second limitation has been the inability to directly image the common and external iliac veins because of their depth from the skin and presence of overlying bowel gas. CDFI vividly displays venous blood flow, thus allowing direct imaging of the entire venous system. Unlike other non-invasive methods, CDFI allows calf veins to be readily examined in most patients. Also evaluation of the abdominal veins is better as compared to other modalities. MRI may detect DVT with equal ease, it also has the additional advantage of assessing deep abdominal and pelvic veins, but its relatively steep cost and limited availability is a major limiting factor.

Sonographic and Doppler Findings

Lack of venous compression is the most sensitive and specific finding with a sensitivity of 93 per cent and specificity of 97 per cent. It is not necessary to compress every continuous millimeter of the venous lumen searching for the clot. In the symptomatic patient, clot usually involves whole or multiple venous segments. Direct visualization of thrombus is a highly specific finding but it is not seen in all cases, as an acute thrombus may be completely anechoic. Increase in the diameter of the thrombosed vein is also seen. Change in venous calibre with respiration and increase in size in response to the valsalva manoeuvre are lost. Several pitfalls may occur during venous evaluation include:

- Improper technique
- In patients with large extremities evaluation may be difficult
- Recanalization of the vessel causing residual wall thickening
- Subacute clot may not distend the vein
- Normal Valsalva manoeuvre is seen in partially occluding thrombus; also this manoeuvre has limited value below the knee.

Gray scale imaging may be unable to visualize some parts of the deep venous system; the problem areas include calf veins, adductor canal where compression is difficult and pelvic veins, which may be obscured by the overlying bowel gas. Pulsed and colour Doppler imaging play a significant role in evaluating these areas. Pulsed Doppler should be performed along with gray scale imaging. Absence of flow is seen in cases of thrombosis. Loss of phasicity

KEY POINTS

Deep venous thrombosis: sonographic and doppler findings

- Lack of venous compression, direct visualization of the thrombus. In a thrombus completely filling the lumen, No colour is seen on CDFI, No signals are seen on pulsed doppler interrogation.
- CDFI is better for evaluation of the pelvic veins, adductor canal region and the calf veins.
- Loss of phasicity and absence of normal response on the Valsalva's maneuver suggests obstruction in the proximal venous system.
- Lack of augmentation is seen in obstruction of the distal venous system.
- Partially occluding thrombus is best evaluated with the CDFI.

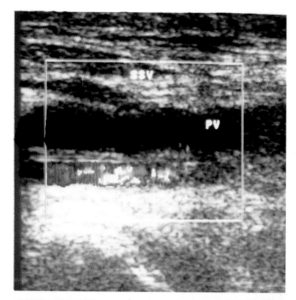

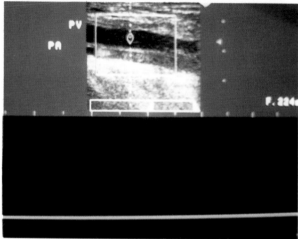

Figures 18.5a and b
Colour doppler in a patient with limb swelling shows enlarged popliteal vein with absent colour, and (b) spectral tracing from the vein revealed absence of flow

in a patent segment is suggestive of proximal thrombosis. Lack of augmentation on distal compression point toward obstruction in the distal venous system. On colour Doppler, venous thrombosis is seen as an area of colour void (Figs 18.5a and b). Partial nonoccluding thrombus, which may not be detected on gray scale and Duplex sonography is well demonstrated on CDFI. Gray scale imaging along with Duplex and colour Doppler also help by providing alternative diagnosis in patient with limb swelling, these conditions include Baker's cyst, aneurysm and lymphadenopathy, etc.

When lower extremity venous thrombosis is noted, the upper extent of the clot should be determined. Clot extending above the inguinal ligament necessitates assessment of the pelvic veins and, if necessary, the inferior vena cava to see the upper margin. This information is necessary to determine the site for filter placement and will also provide the documentation of the present extent of the clot. Resolution of thrombus can be seen on sequential studies (Fig. 18.6).

Chronic Deep Venous Thrombosis (DVT)

The distinction between acute and chronic thrombus is important because of increased tendency of the acute clot to embolize. Acute clot is more likely to progress proximally. Acute thrombus is usually anechoic or hypoechoic with smooth borders. The vein is enlarged in size. With time the thrombus becomes organized. Chronic occlusion causes wall thickening of the involved segments. These changes lead to poor visualization of the clot and incomplete venous compression. CDFI plays a significant role in differentiation of acute and chronic venous thrombi. The features, which may be observed in chronic DVT, include:
- Irregular, echogenic thickening of vein walls
- Reduced calibre
- Atretic venous segments
- Presence of venous collaterals.

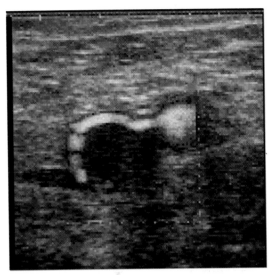

Figure 18.6
Follow-up power doppler in a case of deep vein thrombosis shows partial canalization of lumen

Upper Extremity Thrombosis

Thrombosis of the deep veins is the most common abnormality of the upper extremity venous system. Causes of upper extremity DVT include:

- Acute or repetitive trauma
- Vigorous exercise
- Anatomic abnormalities like cervical rib
- Extrinsic compression by malignancy
- Focal infection
- Intravenous drug abuse
- Indwelling central venous catheters.

Only 10 to 12 per cent of patients with arm DVT develop pulmonary emboli and majority of these are insignificant. Clinical features of DVT in upper limbs are less severe because of development of extensive collateral pathways and lack of hydrostatic pressure. Basic principles for evaluation of the upper extremity are the same as those for the lower limbs. As subclavian and brachiocephalic veins are not easily compressible, Evaluation with CDFI assumes more importance. Venous flow is assessed for phasicity, augmentation and waveform. Features, which may be seen in a case of thrombosis, include:

- Incomplete compression
- Persistent visualisation of filling defect on CDFI
- Absence or reduction of transmitted cardiac pulsations
- Abnormal response to the valsalva manoeuvre
- Detection of large collateral veins

KEY POINTS

Venous insufficiency

- The patient should be examined in erect position with weight transferred to the opposite limb.
- Proximal veins are evaluated with the Valsalva's maneuver while techniques are better for the distal veins.
- A very short period of flow reversal is normal and should not be construed as an evidence of abnormality.

Sensitivity of CDFI for detection of venous thrombosis in upper extremity ranges from 78 to 100 per cent and specificity from 92 to 100 per cent. Lower accuracy is a result of technically difficult examination of the upper limbs.

Venous insufficiency In competence of venous valves may be primary (not preceded by DVT) or it may follow venous valvular damage following DVT (post-phlebitic syndrome). The valvular damage in venous insufficiency leads to valvular in competence. Incompetence may be observed in:

1. Deep venous system
2. Saphenofemoral and/or saphenopopliteal junction and
3. Perforating veins.

Venous incompetence is assessed by examining the patient in erect position, facing the examiner, holding onto a support, to provide stability and eliminate unwanted contraction of the leg muscles. The weight of patient is placed mainly on the opposite limb.

Deep venous system The number of valves in the deep veins increases distally. Hence proximal valvular damage produces more haemodynamic abnormality. For complete assessment the following veins must be examined:

a. Common femoral vein
b. Proximal superficial femoral vein
c. Distal superficial femoral vein
d. The popliteal vein
e. Proximal and distal posterior tibial vein.

Saphenofemoral junction It is visualised in the groin, for Duplex evaluation the sample volume should be placed in the proximal great saphenous vein. Sample volume should include entire lumen, by putting the cursors on the inner walls. For examining *Sapheno Popliteal Junction*, the patient faces away from the examiner and the leg is slightly flexed at the knee. The probe is placed on the skin and its position is adjusted so that three structures can be identified in a sagittal plane: The popliteal artery lying deepest, the popliteal veins lying more superficial to it, and the short saphenous vein most superficial. Because of variation in the anatomy of the sapheno- popliteal junction, careful scanning above and below the popliteal fossa is necessary before individual veins can be identified. Other veins that should be identified and scanned for incompetence, are the gastroenemius veins. They drain into popliteal and/or short saphenous veins. They may be confused with short saphenous vein but can be differentiated from it, as they do not reach the subcutaneous tissue plane, as is the case with short saphenous vein.

Perforating veins It can be identified wih realtime imaging by scanning transversely along the long and short saphenous veins or the posterior arch of the long saphenous vein. For this examination, the patient stands as described previously or sits on a couch with leg positioned vertically over the edge and the foot resting on a stool on which examiner is sitting facing the patient. Perforating veins can be seen dipping from the superficial veins towards the deep system. The probe is rotated in a manner that the superficial and deep veins are visualized in a longitudinal plane with the perforating vein joining the two. All visualized perforators are not in competent. The incompetent perforators usually have a large lumen.

Proximal venous structures like common femoral vein, proximal superficial femoral vein and great saphenous veins are best evaluated using Valsalva's manoeuvre. On performing this manoeuvre, a normal vein shall show progressive reduction followed by cessation of colour on CDFI. In presence of incompetent valves, venous reflux will be seen as change in colour, lasting for variable duration, depending upon the degree of Valvular incompetence.

Distal augmentation manoeuvre is more useful for evaluation of distal femoral vein popliteal vein, posterior tibial vein and sapheno-popliteal junction. Brisk distal compression causes increased antegrade flow in the venous system. The compression is then released. A very short period of flow reversal may be seen in normal veins due to effect of gravity, but this reversal ceases, as the returning blood encounters the first competent venous valve. Incompetent veins have

a greater degree of flow reversal, lasting for a longer period of time. On CDFI, this is seen as change in colour. On pulse Doppler tracing change in flow direction is seen.

In perforating veins normal direction of flow is from the superficial to the deep venous system. Retrograde flow is prevented by the presence of venous valves. In presence of incompetent perforators, flow augmentation causes reflux of blood from deep to superficial venous system. On CDFI, this is seen as flow towards the transducer placed on the skin (normally coded red). Site of incompetent perforators can be marked on skin to enable surgeon to accurately ligate these veins.

Spectral display may be helpful to quantitate the degree of reflux. It may be graded as follows:

Grade I   :   reflux lasting for 1-2 sec.
Grade II   :   reflux lasting for 2-3 sec.
Grade III   :   reflux lasting for 4-6 sec.
Grade IV   :   reflux lasting more than 6 sec.

Preoperative saphenous vein mapping Infra-inguinal bypass procedures, that use an autogenous saphenous vein can be aided by a detailed pre-operative assessment. Better information about the venous anatomy and any anatomic variations results in improved use of veins and precise planning of the specific surgical procedure for the bypass procedure. Duplex scanning along with CDFI has proved to extremely valuable for saphenous vein mapping.

Technique Patient's limb is placed in a dependent position by asking him to stand or sit upright with legs unsupported. The examination starts at the knee. A transverse section is used to localize the great saphenous vein and patency is confirmed by compressing it. Probe is then rotated to get a longitudinal image and its position is marked with a small line by using a water-proof marker. The vein is then traced along its entire course. Coupling gel is used sparingly, so that the skin surface can be marked easily.

Tributaries are more easily seen on transverse images, anterior and posterior tributaries are marked 'A' and 'P'. Veins crossing the main system are marked with 'X' at the crossover point. Site of perforators is also marked. If a double system is found their arrangement is recorded.

When the examination is complete, gel is wiped from the skin, the preliminary map made with water-proof marker is traced using permanent marking ink. This imprint lasts for 3-4 days.

19

Intravascular Ultrasound— Newer Advances, Current Applications and Future Directions

Sanjiv Sharma
Gurpreet Gulati

INTRODUCTION

Catheter-based angiography is still the most valuable modality to make the diagnoses and guide interventional procedures in coronary and peripheral vascular disease. However, it has many limitations, pathologic studies have revealed that angiographic interpretation frequently leads to an under- or overestimation of disease severity.[1-3] Angiography depicts the arteries as a two-dimensional view of the contrast-filled lumen, hence any arbitrary projection can misrepresent the true extent of stenosis, particularly for eccentric lesions.[4] The estimation of degree of stenosis by angiography relies upon comparison with an uninvolved normal segment. Autopsy studies demonstrate that there is no truly normal segment, the disease usually being diffuse in nature. Also, angiography is limited in its ability to assess the disease mechanism and composition of the obstructive lesion.

Over the last few years, intravascular ultrasound (IVUS) has emerged as new technique to assess vascular pathology. It refers to the acquisition of cross-sectional images of the target vessel by an ultrasound probe placed on the tip of an endoluminally positioned catheter.

Rationale for Intravascular Ultrasound Imaging

The application of IVUS to vascular imaging has evolved based upon several characteristics inherent to ultrasound technology. Due to the tomographic orientation of ultrasound, the full circumference of the vessel wall can be visualised and not just a two-dimensional view. This enables comprehensive assessment of angiographically difficult areas such as diffusely diseased arteries, eccentric lesions, ostial stenoses and angiographically foreshortened segments. Also, measurements are performed using an electronically generated scale, thus offering an advantage over angiographic stenosis estimation which needs to be corrected for radiographic magnification.[4,5]

A unique feature of IVUS is its ability to provide qualitative information about plaque composition and its response to interventional strategies. The consistency of plaque (soft, fibrous, calcific or mixed) and its differentiation from thrombus is well demonstrated by IVUS. Various studies have demonstrated a good correlation between the histopathology of the atheromatous plaque and its echogenicity on IVUS.[6,7]

IVUS imaging has been used mainly for coronary interventions. The following description focuses on the present day role of IVUS in imaging and intervention in peripheral vascular disease and its applications in the future.

KEY POINTS

IVUS: General principles
- Very high frequency transducers ranging from 12.5 to 40 MHz are required.
- Phased array and mechanical type of transducers can be used.
- Large elastic arteries have two layered appearance; muscular arteries appear three layered.

Table 19.1	Comparison between phased-array and mechanical IVUS transducers	
	Phased-array transducers	*Mechanical transducers*
	1. Can be coupled with smaller catheters	1. Require relatively larger catheters
	2. Flexible and hence can be guided into smaller and tortuous vessels with ease	2. Stiffer, hence traversing the aortic bifurcation or reaching the visceral vessels is difficult without the use of guiding catheters
	3. Non-uniform rotation in tortuous vessels is not a problem	3. Non-uniform rotation may be a problem due to the presence of a drive cable and moving parts
	4. Can be easily incorporated into interventional devices	4. May be difficult to couple with interventional catheters
	5. Complex in design	5. Designing is comparatively simple
	6. Relatively expensive	6. Less costly

Technical Aspects

The equipment required to perform intravascular ultrasound consists of two major components: a catheter with a miniaturised transducer at its tip and a console containing the electronics necessary to reconstruct the image. Frequency of the ultrasound used is typically centered at 12.5-40 MHz. For peripheral vascular imaging, 20 MHz is the most used frequency. Larger vessels such as the aorta require frequency in the range of 12.5 to 20 MHz. There are two types of catheter systems: those with an end-hole which are delivered over the guidewire, and those which do not have an end-hole and are introduced directly through the sheath. Larger catheters are introduced through larger guiding catheters and sheaths.

Although the reduction in transducer size results in a decrease in resolution, this is partially compensated for the use of higher frequencies. Typically, the wavelength at 30 MHz is 50 μm, yielding a practical axial resolution of 150 μm.[8] Determinants of lateral resolution are more complicated and depend on imaging depth.

Two basic approaches to transducer design have been evaluated: phased-array and mechanical type. In the phased-array systems, multiple transducer elements (32-64) in an annular array are activated sequentially to generate the image. Mechanical probes use a drive cable to rotate a piezoelectric transducer at 1800 rpm, yielding 30 images per second. The advantages and limitations of the two designs are compared in Table 19.1.

Image Interpretation

A well-defined imaging protocol is vital for proper interpretation of IVUS images in the peripheral vascular tree. A slow pullback of the transducer from the distal to the proximal vessels segments is the optimal way to acquire reproducible information about vessel architecture and catheter orientation. Most centres use a motorised pullback system to withdraw the catheter at a predetermined constant rate. Standard perivascular landmarks and side branches as seen on angiography and ultrasound are used to ensure that repeated measurements (e.g. pre- and post-intervention) are assessed at the same position within the artery.

Normal Arterial Anatomy

The generation of ultrasound images is based on the difference in the acoustic impedance of the layers of the vessel wall. Due to this difference, these layers reflect US differently.

Blood

On IVUS images, blood has a characteristic speckled pattern that is constantly changing in echogenecity with the cardiac cycle-being slightly more echogenic during systole.[9] In realtime imaging, sometimes the lumen/intima interface may be difficult to distinguish when the blood flow is slow and stagnant, such as proximal to a severe stenosis. In such situations, the increased backscatter from blood may give the false impression of thrombus or plaque. One more reason for increased backscatter from blood may be the incorrect adjustment of the control for near field gain (time gain compensation or TGC). When the TGC is set too high, blood speckle becomes accentuated, masking the lumen/intima border.[10]

Arterial Wall

The wall of the artery is composed of the intima, internal elastic lamina, media, external elastic lamina, and adventitia (Fig. 19.1). The intima consists of a monolayer of endothelial cells which in itself is beyond the resolution of current ultrasound catheters. However, if there is intimal hyperplasia, it may be detected as a thin echogenic layer (Fig. 19.2).[11] The internal elastic lamina is seen as the innermost thin echogenic layer.[7] Because of its high echogenicity, the actual thickness of the layer may be overestimated (a phenomenon referred to as blooming), which may sometimes make it difficult to distinguish from mild intimal proliferation.[11] The outermost layer, i.e. the adventitia is collagen-rich and is thus bright in appearance.

The echogenicity of the media, depends upon the relative content of smooth muscle on one hand and collagen and elastin on the other. The latter are strongly echoreflective, and in objective terms, the reflectance of collagen is about 1000 times more than that of muscle.[10]. The relative composition of the media is different for the elastic and muscular arteries. The

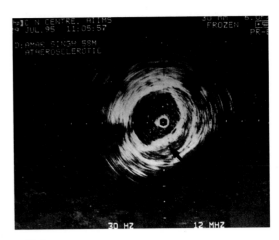

Figure 19.2
IVUS image showing eccentric increase in thickness of inner layer (arrow)-intimal hyperplasia

aorta, pulmonary artery, and the proximal segments of the brachiocephalic, carotid, subclavian and common iliac arteries belong to the elastic type. All other arteries such as the coronary, renal and femoral are the muscular type. The media of the muscular arteries is composed largely of smooth muscle cells, and thus it is poorly echoreflective, forming a large acoustic mismatch between the surrounding layers, resulting in a three-layered appearance on the US image.[12] Large elastic arteries have a media that contains a higher relative amount of collagen and elastin which make this layer strongly echoreflective. Hence, the distinction between the three layers is less marked, resulting in a two-layered appearance.[13]

Appearance on IVUS in Various Disease States

Atherosclerosis Studies have compared the ultrasound appearance of plaques to histology in freshly explanted human arteries.[13,14] Currently IVUS is the most reliable imaging modality that identifies the composition of arterial plaques.

Gussenhoven *et al*[15] proposed that there are essentially four basic relationships between plaque composition and its echogenicity on IVUS: hypoechoic, representing a high lipid content of plaque; soft echoes, representing fibromuscular tissue; hyperechoic, representing collagen-rich (fibrous) plaque; and hyperechoic with lack of through transmission, representing calcium (Fig. 19.3). Hodgson *et al*[16] studied IVUS morphology in human coronary arteries and correlated the image obtained with angiography. They classified IVUS images into 5 morphological subtypes: (a) soft, (b) fibrous, (c) calcific, (d) mixed (Fig. 19.4),

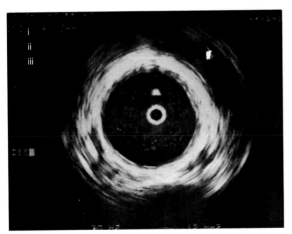

Figure 19.1
IVUS image in a normal subject: 3-layered appearance
  (i) thin inner echogenic layer (internal elastic lamina),
  (ii) middle hypoechoic layer (media),
  (iii) outermost echogenic layer (adventitia). Blood around catheter seen as speckled pattern

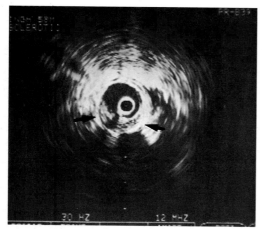

Figure 19.3
Same patient at another level: fibrous plaque (arrow) with outer echogenic line with distal acoustic shadowing (calcium)

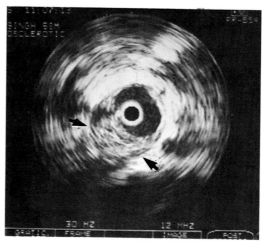

Figure 19.4
IVUS image of aorta in a 58 years old male: arrows point to mixed echogenicity plaque

(e) concentric subintimal thickening. They found that compared with stable angina, patients with unstable angina had more soft lesions (greater lipid content) (74% vs 41%), fewer calcified and mixed plaques (25% vs 59%) and intralesional calcium deposits (16% vs 45%). IVUS demonstrated a greater sensitivity than angiography for identifying unstable lesions (74% vs 40%). These observations have important implications for peripheral vascular disease as well. It is the plaque composition, rather than the stenotic severity, that predicts the vulnerability of a lesion to rupture and produce acute symptoms. This information is most reliably provided by IVUS and no other imaging modality.

Plaque measurements Atheroma area is determined by planimetry of the intimal leading edge and external elastic lamina (EEM), thus including the media in measurements. The media is included due to two reasons: the spread of ultrasound signal of the intimal plaque into the media, obscuring the trailing edge of the intima (known as 'blooming'), and the media not being consistently seen as a truly sonolucent layer. Measurements performed in this manner have shown a close correlation with histological assessment.[14,15]

Plaque burden or "per cent area stenosis" refers to the percentage of the EEM area occupied by the atheroma. This quantitative ultrasound measurements is usually substantially greater than that made on angiography due to two major reasons: the diffuse nature of the disease affecting even the angiographically "normal reference sites", and the expansion of the EEM which occurs as a response to atherosclerosis (known as *positive* remodelling)[17,18] and maintains a constant luminal area during the early stages (Glagov effect).

The majority of plaques are seen to be eccentric in location on IVUS studies. This observation has important implications for guiding interventional procedures, particularly for directional atherectomy and other selective plaque removal techniques.

In some vessel segments, instead of vessel expansion, vessel shrinkage may occur, which has been referred to as de-remodelling or *negative* remodeling. This may actually contribute to luminal stenosis. Recently, this phenomenon has been implicated in restenosis after interventional procedures.[19]

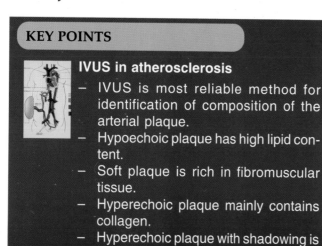

KEY POINTS

IVUS in atherosclerosis

- IVUS is most reliable method for identification of composition of the arterial plaque.
- Hypoechoic plaque has high lipid content.
- Soft plaque is rich in fibromuscular tissue.
- Hyperechoic plaque mainly contains collagen.
- Hyperechoic plaque with shadowing is mainly composed of calcium.
- Unstable plaques are more reliably identified with IVUS as compared to angiography.

Other Disease States

Thrombus Thrombus is echogenic, and may be difficult to distinguish from a noncalcified fibrous plaque or even stagnant blood. It however has a typically scintillating or sparkling pattern on realtime US examination. The presence of microchannels, and an echodensity of less than 50 per cent of the adventitia are important clues to its correct identification.[20,21]

False lumen A false lumen may occur spontaneously or commonly following endovascular interventions. Mistaking a false lumen for true lumen can have serious consequences if the former is selected for stent or stent-graft placement (as in aortic dissections). IVUS may help in such situations by: recognition of the characteristic three-layered appearance of true lumen; identification of side branches taking off from the true lumen; and by the slow flowing, more echogenic blood within the false lumen. In addition, flush injections of contrast may at times reveal the echogenic patterns of the contrast to "hang-up" and take longer to evacuate from the false lumen compared to the true lumen.

Aneurysm A true aneurysm is differentiated histologically from a false aneurysm by the presence of media in the former. IVUS can detect the presence of hypoechoic media to distinguish the two entities, although at times the media may be very thinned out.

Nonspecific aortoarteritis Sharma *et al*[22] reported the IVUS imaging findings in aorta in Takayasu's arteritis.

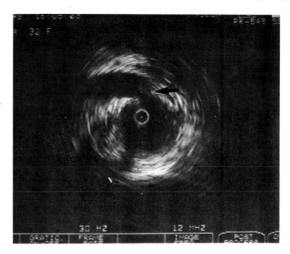

Figure 19.6
Same patient as above: Renal artery take-off (arrow) seen in upper part of image with stenosis at its ostium. Aortic wall shows thick echogenic media

They observed that intima is unaffected and remains thin. There is increase in the echogenicity and thickness of the media. The adventitia is also similarly affected with diffuse periarterial fibrosis (Figs 19.5 and 19.6). Due to these changes, the characteristic three-layered appearance may not be seen at places. There may be calcification. The compliance of the aortic wall may be seen to be lost on realtime imaging. Importantly, these changes were observed even in the angiographically "normal" segments of the vessel, emphasizing the diffuse nature of involvement by the disease.

Clinical Applications

Quantitative ultrasound Angiography permits only monoplanar assessment of the lumen diameter, while IVUS allows planimetric measurement of the artery lumen as well as the vessel wall area. This leads to underestimation of the disease, as has been consistently demonstrated by various studies.

Balloon angioplasty A major mechanism of percutaneous transluminal angioplasty (PTA) is the creation of cracks and dissections of atherosclerotic plaques with localized medial dissection. This has been clearly demonstrated by IVUS studies.[23] Concentric lesions that dissected during PTA achieved a greated lumen gain compared to those that did not dissect or were eccentric in location.[24] The detection a large intimal flap created during PTA mandates a repeat prolonged

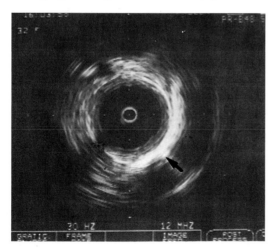

Figure 19.5
Young hypertensive female: thick echogenic media and adventitia (arrow) with thin innermost layer, suggesting aortoarteritis

inflation or stent placement. Hence, the use of IVUS can help determine the end-point of angioplasty.

Accurate determination of balloon size is enhanced by using IVUS to measure vessel diameters. In addition, IVUS can help in selecting an appropriate recanalisation technique by virtue of its ability to differentiate a stenosis produced by thrombus, plaque or mural abnormality.

The amount and distribution of calcium may have a significant impact on the outcome of angioplasty procedures.[25] This can be reliably detected by IVUS. Compliant lesions without a definite fibrocalcific structure are more likely to have elastic recoil following PTA, whereas large calcific deposits may predispose to more severe tearing of the vessel wall.

IVUS is helpful after PTA when pressure gradients still exist despite a satisfactory angiogram as it provides a direct anatomical assessment of the residual stenosis. Angiography consistently underestimates the degree of residual narrowing even when performed in multiple projections.[26]

Stenting Endovascular stenting is performed for complex lesions, total occlusions, or in cases with suboptimal response or obstructive dissection following PTA. Due to the brightly echogenic appearance of the meatal struts, stents are easily recognized on IVUS. IVUS is extremely valuable in assessing the degree of apposition of the stent to the vessel wall, an information not obtained on angiography.[27] In cases with incomplete apposition, balloon dilatation within the stent should be performed. This is important since any space left between the stent and the endothelium will be occupied by thrombus, delaying the ingrowth of the endothelium to cover the inner surface of the stent.

Atherectomy For atherectomy, it is important to know the location and depth of the plaque as well as the presence of significant calcification. Ultrasound imaging can identify superficial calcium, which is associated with poor tissue retrieval. The sizing of the atherectomy device is crucial, since a device which is undersized will leave a significant residual plaque burden, whereas one that is oversized may share or cut into the media and adventitia, potentially leading to vessel rupture or formation of a pseudoaneurysm. Deep intimal tearing also predisposes to accentuated intimal hyperplasia and significant restenosis following the procedure.[25,28] In this respect, the planimetric information obtained from IVUS is helpful to select the ideal size of the atherectomy device.

The most striking finding from IVUS studies in the context of directional atherectomy is the substantial residual plaque burden following the procedure, consistently demonstrated with IVUS in cases where the angiographic result seems to be optimal.[29] This has called attention to the issue of more aggressive plaque removal on the basis of ultrasound imaging, allowing the safe use of larger burrs with a greater subsequent lumen gain.

Stent graft placement For endovascular treatment of aneurysms, it is imperative to know the diameter of proximal and distal neck is order to select the correct size of the stent graft. If the device is too small, endoleaks may occur post-procedure from the proximal or the distal end. This sizing is accurately done with the cross-sectional measurement performed with IVUS. Also, during the procedure the complete apposition of the stent struts or hooks to the vessel wall can be confirmed with IVUS imaging. This cannot be accurately assessed with angiography.

For stent graft placed for aortic dissection, the sealing of the site of entry tear is most reliably confirmed only with ultrasound imaging.

Vena cava filter Whenever technical problems (filter tilting or filter migration) or complications (caval thrombosis or recurrent pulmonary embolism) of filter placement are suspected, IVUS may be used to complement or obviate cavography. It is also possible to perform the entire procedure under ultrasound guidance, since the identification of renal veins is easy with IVUS.

Mechanisms of restenosis-insights with IVUS imaging In the early years of interventional cardiology, it was believed that the predominant mechanisms of restenosis was intimal hyperplasia. Following angioplasty, this would occur with a deep extension of the dissection, exposing the media to blood and initiating an aggressive platelet response which results in intimal proliferation.[25] With atherectomy, IVUS may sometimes demonstrate a scalloped outline of the lumen, predisposing to increased local turbulence which causes greater platelet aggregation and restenosis.[30] However, Pasterkamp *et al*[31] studied peripheral vessels with IVUS and observed that shrinkage of the vessel or *negative* remodeling was another major mechanism contributing to late lumen loss. In another study on coronary interventions,[32] decrease in the EEM area contributed to 70 per cent of the lumen loss, whereas intimal proliferation was responsible for only 23 per cent of the loss.

The restenotic response occurring following stent placement is different in that it is primarily due to neointimal hyperplasia. This is probably because stents can resist the remodelling process.[33] This, combined with the fact that stents result in greater initial luminal expansion, contributes to a lower late restenosis rate with stenting compared to balloon angioplasty or atherectomy.

Miscellaneous Applications

a. In case of aortic dissection, IVUS has been to be superior to angiography and transoesophageal echocardiography in identifying the points of entry and re-entry.[34]

b. Percutaneous fenestration of aortic dissection has been accomplished successfully using IVUS as the guiding imaging modality. Identification of the highly echogenic needle as it passes from one lumen into the other is easily monitored with ultrasound.

c. IVUS can be employed for assessing progression of plaque, where it is superior to angiography.[35]

d. Tissue characterization is possible with ultrasound imaging based on the differential acoustic impedance properties of the various layers of the vessel wall. This may have a role in patients with Marfan's syndrome (abnormalities in the elastin content) where IVUS may be used for diagnosis and follow-up.[36]

e. IVUS has the capability to study the cardiac chambers, wall motion abnormalities and valve movements.[37]

f. Endoluminal sonography has been used for evaluation of gastrointestinal and genitourinary tracts as well as tracheobronchial tree to image a variety of abnormalities.[38-40]

i. Uses in the gastrointestinal tract include distinguishing between various submucosal lesions, assessing the severity of oesophageal varices and evaluating fibrosis in scleroderma.

ii. In the genitourinary tract, endoluminal US has been applied to diagnose upper urinary tract calculi, tumors and mural abnormalities as well as an adjunct to endourological procedures. It has been experimentally employed in the imaging of tubal abnormalities.

iii. In the tracheobronchial tree, it has been applied as a guide to biopsy of lymph nodes and tumors not visualized on routine bronchoscopy.

Limitations of Intravascular Ultrasound

1. With the current resolution and processing available with IVUS devices, it may be difficult to differentiate a thrombus superimposed upon plaque from a soft, lipid laden plaque.

2. In tortuous vessel anatomy, there may under or overestimation of disease due to inability to maintain a constant catheter-vessel coaxial alignment.

3. Calcific/fibrous lesions may cause echo dropouts, hindering the visualizing of underlying plaque.

4. The high cost of equipment may be inhibitory to a majority of interventionists, who are still not comfortable with its use.

Future Directions

New and creative areas of IVUS applications are being explored. Doppler capabilities are being incorporated within IVUS catheters to allow for simultaneous haemodynamic assessment of stenosis. Realtime three-dimensional reconstruction of IVUS data, by providing information about spatial relationships of anatomical structures may enhance the capabilities of IVUS.

Continued improvements in transducer design and technology will allow for better resolution and penetration of US waves. Improvements in catheter trackability and steerability should allow for easier catheterization of tortuous vessels and side branches that are presently difficult to select.

One of the key issues, for the future of intravascular US to be incorporated as an integral part of the interventional radiologist's armamentarium is the demonstration of a clear clinical benefit.[41] Two kinds of studies are currently being initiated, those that analyze the effect that IVUS imaging has on decision making of the operator during the therapeutic procedure, and those that evaluate the impact of this modality on the long-term outcome of endovascular interventions. There are also studies engaged in developing and testing prototypes of combined imaging/stent delivery and imaging/atherectomy devices. These would significantly reduce the procedure time and give an "online" assessment of plaque orientation and changes occurring with the device. Ultrasound may have the potential to be used for pulverizing plaque or thrombus, creating a channel whereby a subsequent angioplasty can be performed. It may even be used as a sole therapeutic modality using higher energies, thus bringing down the cost and time of lysis procedures.

Endoluminal sonography, particularly three-dimensional reconstruction algorithms may open new vistas in gastroenterology imaging such as in treatment of inflammatory bowel disease, staging of rectosigmoid neoplasia and pancreatobiliary disease processes. It may be an adjunct to imaging and intervention in endometrial, cervical and prostatic tumors.

REFERENCES

1. Vlodaver Z, Frech R, Van Tassel RA *et al*: Correlations of the antemortem arteriogram and the postmortem specimen. *Circulation* **47**: 162-69, 1973.
2. Isner JM, Kishel J, Kent KM *et al*: Accuracy of angiographic determination of left main coronary arterial narrowing: Angiographic-histologic correlative analysis in 28 patients. *Circulation* **63**: 1056-64, 1981.
3. White CW, Wright CB, Doty DB *et al*: Does visual interpretation of the coronary arteriogram predict the physiologic importance of a coronary stenosis? *N Engl J Med* **310**: 819-24, 1984.
4. Nishimora RA, Welch TJ, Stanson AW *et al*: Intravascular US of the distal aorta and iliac vessels: Initial feasibility studies. *Radiology* **176**: 523-25, 1990.
5. Davidson CJ, Sheikh KH, Harrison JK *et al*: Intravascular ultrasonography versus digital subtraction angiography: A human *in vivo* comparison of vessel size and morphology. *J Am Coll Cardiol* **16**: 633-36, 1990.
6. Yock PG, Linker DT, White NW *et al*: Clinical applications of intravascular ultrasound imaging in atherectomy. *Int J Cardiac Imag* **4**: 117-25, 1989.
7. Tobis JM, Mallery J, Mahon D *et al*: Intravascular ultrasound imaging of human coronary arteries *in vivo*. Analysis of tissue characterizations with comparison to *in vitro* histological specimens. *Circulation* **43**: 913-26, 1991.
8. Nissen SE, Yock P: Intravascular ultrasound: Novel pathophysiological insights and current clinical applications. *Circulation* **103**: 604-16, 2001.
9. Yamada EG, Fitzgerald PJ, Sudhir K *et al*: Intravascular ultrasound imaging of blood. The effect of hematocrit and flow on backscatter. *J Am Soc Echo* **5**: 385, 1992.
10. Metz JA, Yock PG, Fitzgerald PJ: Intravascular ultrasound: Basic interpretation. *Card Clin* **15(1)**: 1-15, 1997.
11. Tobis JM, Mahon D, Goldberg SL *et al*: Lessons from intravascular ultrasonography: Observations during interventional angioplasty procedures. *J Clin Ultrasound* **21**: 589-607, 1993.
12. Fitzgerald PJ, St. Goar FG, Connolly AJ *et al*: Intravascular ultrasound imaging of coronary arteries. Is three layers norm? *Circulation* **86**: 154-58, 1992.
13. Nishimura RA, Edwards WD, Warnes CA *et al*: Intravascular ultrasound imaging: *In vitro* validation and pathologic correlation. *J Am Coll Cardiol* **16**: 145-54, 1990.
14. Gussenhoven EJ, Essed CE, Lancee CT *et al*: Arterial wall characteristics determined by intravascular ultrasound imaging: as *in vitro* study. *J Am Coll Cardiol* **14**: 947-52, 1989.
15. Gussenhoven WJ, Essed CE, Frietman P *et al*: Intravascular echographic assessment of vessel wall characteristics: A correlation with histology. *Int J Cardiac Imag* **4**: 105-16, 1989.
16. Hodgson J MCB, Reddy KG, Suneja R *et al*: Intracoronay ultrasound imaging. Correlation of plaque morphology with angiography, clinical syndrome and procedural results in patients undergoing coronary angioplasty. *J Am Coll Cardiol* **21**: 35-44, 1993.
17. Glagov S, Weinsenberg E, Zarins CK *et al*: Compensatory enlargement of human atherosclerotic arteries. *N Engl J Med* **316**: 1371, 1987.
18. Kakuta T, Curries JW, Haudenschild CC *et al*: Differences in compensatory vessel enlargement, not intimal formation, account for restenosis after angioplasty in the hypercholesterolemic rabbit model. *Circulation* **89**: 2809, 1994.
19. Kimura T, Kaburagi S, Tamura T *et al*: Remodeling of human coronary angioplasty or atherectomy. *Circulation* **96**: 475-483, 1997.
20. Chemarin-Alibelli MJ, Pieraggi MT *et al*: Identification of coronary thrombus after myocardial infarction by intracoronary ultrasound compared with histology of tissues sampled by atherectomy. *Am J Cardiol* **77**: 344, 1996.
21. Lee DY, Eigler N, Fishbein MC *et al*: Identification of intracoronary thrombus and demonstration of thrombectomy by intravascular ultrasound imaging. *Am J Cardiol* **73**: 522, 1994.
22. Sharma S, Sharma S, Taneja K *et al*: Morphological mural changes in the aorta in non-specific aortoarteritis (Takayasu's arteritis): Assessment by intravascular ultrasound imaging. *Clin Radiol* **53**: 37-43, 1998.
23. Isner JM, Rosenfield K, Losordo DW *et al*: Percutaneous intravascular US as adjunct to catheter-based interventions: Preliminary experience in patients with peripheral vascular disease. *Radiology* **175**: 61-70, 1990.
24. Fitzgerald PJ, Yock PG, Guide Trial Investigators: Discrepancies between angiographic and intravascular ultrasound appearance of coronary lesions undergoing intervention. A report of Phase 1 of the Guide trial. *J Am Coll Cardiol* **134A**: 738-44, 1993.
25. Steele PM *et al*: Balloon angioplasty: natural history of the pathophysiological response to injury in a pig model. *Circ Res* **57**: 105-12, 1985.
26. Ehlrich S, Honye J, Mahon D *et al*: Unrecognized stenosis by angiography documented by intravascular ultrasound. *Cathet Cardiovasc Diagn* **3**: 198-201, 1991.
27. Yock PG, Fitzgerald PJ, Linker DT *et al*: Intravascular ultrasound guidance for catheter-based coronary interventions. *J Am Coll Cardiol* **17**: 39B-49B, 1991.

28. Backa D, Polnitz AV, Nerlich A *et al*: Histologic comparison of atherectomy biopsies from coronary and peripheral arteries, abstracted. *Circulation* **82(Suppl III)**: III-324, 1995.

29. Matar FA, Mintz GS, Pinnow E *et al*: Multivariate predictors of intravascular ultrasound end points after directional coronary atherectomy. *J Am Coll Cardiol* **25**: 318-24, 1995.

30. Tobis JM *et al*: Intravascular ultrasound cross-section imaging before and after balloon angioplasty *in vitro*. *Circulation* **80**: 873-82, 1990.

31. Pasterkamp G, Wensing PJ, Post MJ *et al*: Paradoxical arterial wall shrinkage may contribute to luminal narrowing to human atherosclerotic femoral arteries. *Circulation* **91**: 1444-49, 1995.

32. Mintz GS, Kent KM, Pichard AD *et al*: Contribution of inadequate arterial remodeling to the development of focal coronary artery stenosis: an intravascular ultrasound study. *Circulation* **95**: 1791-98, 1997.

33. Painter JA, Mintz GS, Wong SC *et al*: Serial intravascular ultrasound studies fail to show evidence of chronic Palmaz-Schatz stent recoil. *Am J Cardiol* **75**: 398-400, 1995.

34. Ayala D, Chandrasekaran K, Ross J Jr, *et al*: MHz intravascular ultrasonography in the diagnosis of aortic dissection: Comparison to transesophageal echocardiography and aortography (abstract). *Circulation* **88**: 0522, 1993.

35. Hausmann D *et al*: Accuracy of intravascular ultrasound to assess progression of experimental aortic atherosclerosis (abstract). *Circulation* **88**: 2699, 1993.

36. Recchia D *et al*: Quantification of abnormal aortic elastin content and organization in Marfan syndrome with ultrasonic tissue characterization (abstract). *Circulation* **88**: 3119, 1993.

37. Pandian NG *et al*: Intracardiac echocardiography: current developments. *Int J Card Imag* **6**: 207-19, 1991.

38. Liu JB, Goldberg BB: Endoluminal vascular and nonvascular sonography: past, present and future. *Am J Roentgenol* **165(4)**: 765-74, 1995.

39. Liu JB, Goldberg BB: 2-D and 3-D endoluminal ultrasound: vascular and nonvascular applications. *Ultrasound Med Biol* **25(2)**: 159-73, 1999.

40. Goldberg BB, Liu JB, Merton DA *et al*: Endoluminal US: experiments with nonvascular uses in animals. *Radiology* **175(1)**: 39-43, 1990.

41. Fitzgerald PJ, Yock PG: Mechanism and outcomes of angioplasty and atherectomy assessed by intravascular ultrasound imaging. *J Clin Ultrasound* **21**: 579-88, 1993.

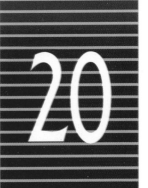

20

Role of Colour Flow and Doppler in Obstetrics, Gynaecology and Infertility

Narendra Malhotra
Jaideep Malhotra
Vanaj Mathur
Sakshi Mittal

INTRODUCTION

Doppler Ultrasound offers a very efficient non-invasive technology to study the circulatory system. This method allows an insight into uterine, ovarian, tubal, and other important pelvic vessels. The excellent reproducibility of the technique and the ability to visualize smallest of the vessels in the ovary, uterus, endometrium and conditions such as ectopic pregnancy makes it an excellent diagnostic tool with high degree of accuracy. The sensitivity and specificity of the diagnosis is increased and great help is obtained in the evaluation of gynaecological malignancy.

The technology of colour flow imaging deals with two points:
a. Imaging problems
b. Clinical uses.

Imaging Problems

When the first colour flow imaging was used, the images were too fascinating and different from the gray scale and duplex images that many thought that it was not ultrasound. Yet like duplex and B mode imaging, colour flow has its own problems despite the bright and dynamic images. These are as follows:

1. *Tissue attenuation* Muscle, fat, plaque, and connective tissue rapidly attenuate signals. Though, these signals are very small, the echo signals from blood vessels are smaller.

2. *Accurate blood flow sampling* It will depend upon pulsed Doppler sample volume geometry. The same flow will have a different frequency mix as the sample volume shape changes.

3. *Colour flow imaging system* It detects moving blood in colour. This is easy to do when blood is the only echo source within the scanning field, which obviously is not leading to a complex mixing of signals at blood vessel interface. Strong tissue signals mix with peak blood signals. The walls are not always still either. The technology must be able to adequately separate moving blood from sometimes moving soft tissues. It must also separate different patterns in blood movements.

Colour flow scanning takes us away from conventional imaging approaches to vessels and organs in the sense that B-mode imaging traditionally seeks out the specular reflections of a structure. The ultrasound beam is perpendicular to the flow pattern in the vessel; on the other hand Doppler needs an angle away from 90°, preferably less than 60° for greatest accuracy (Fig. 20.1a).

Clinical Uses

Colour flow imaging specifically visualises the vascular system. The word "vascular" not only includes the heart, carotids or aorta but a huge system spread all over the body with systemic, neural and hormonal controls. The vascular system of the body responds to stress, trauma, drugs and hosts a very complex biochemistry for clot and thrombus formation. A successful vascular image system must be able to portray changes due to normal regulation, drugs and diseases. It must also do more than just put colour on the display. Hence, if a colour flow imaging has to function as an effective clinical tool it must be able to detect disease and evaluate the extent of the disease.

Hence, in the arterial and venous system, colour flow imaging should be able to tell us the condition of the wall, the lumen (stenosis), the intima, should be able to detect a plaque, predict the blood flows and over, and above it should be able to identify and neovascularisation.

The Doppler Signal

When an ultrasound beam is transmitted towards the blood flow in a vessel, it is scattered in all directions and back scattered to the transducer. The moving RBC cause Doppler shift of the scattered ultrasound. This velocity of blood flow can be determined using certain equations, if the values of the angle and of the Doppler signal are known. The processing of the Doppler signal unroles sequential steps of amplification, demodulation, spectral processing and display (Fig. 20.1a).

The spectral analysis of Doppler signal involves processing, quantification of the frequency and power content of the signal. The vertical axis of the sonogram shows the magnitude of the frequency shift and horizontal axis represents the temporal change. Brightness of the spectrum is an indication of power of the spectrum.

In order to quantify the volatile resistance, various indices have been proposed (Fig. 20.1b).

1. **PI (Pulsatility Index)** $= \dfrac{\text{Peak Systolic Velocity} - \text{End Diastolic Velocity}}{\text{Mean Velocity}}$

(Gosling and King 1975)

2. **RI (Resistance Index)** $= \dfrac{\text{Peak Systolic Velocity} - \text{End Diastolic Velocity}}{\text{End Diastolic Velocity}}$

(Bourcelot 1974)

3. **Systolic/Diastolic Ratio** $= \dfrac{\text{Peak Systolic Velocity}}{\text{End Diastolic Velocity}}$

(Stuart et al 1980)

The higher the value of these indices more the impedance to blood flow and perfusion of the particular area. In order to understand the pathological features of different gynaecological conditions one has to know about the indices of various vessels.

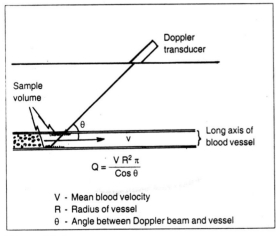

Figure 20.1a
Doppler measurement of blood flow

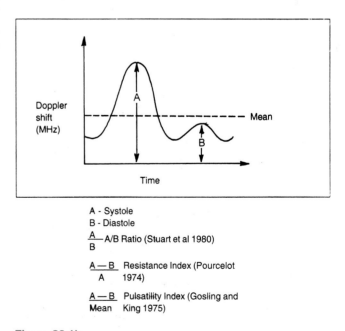

Figure 20.1b
Flow velocity wave form

How the Colour Image is Formed?

Colour images are of two type: (i) Asynchronous and (ii) Synchronous imaging. In asynchronous imaging, the gray scale and Doppler information are gathered at different times. In contrast, synchronous imaging information is gathered simultaneously.

Asynchronous Colour Flow Imaging

Two images are produced during scanning and are later super imposed. The gray scale comes from a real time image. The Doppler image comes from steering another ultrasound beam at an angle to the array (0-45°). The image is composed in a digital scan converter. Two different frequencies can be used for the two image components; a system could have gray scale at 5 MHz and colour at 3 MHz.

Synchronous Colour Flow Imaging

Simultaneous processing for amplitude, phase and frequency is achieved by the same echo signal. This technology is so different that it is known as angiodynagraphy. The linear array sends a dynamically focused beam, which is perpendicular to the vessels. This is good for imaging but not for Doppler. To provide the Doppler angle needed to visualise blood flow, a wedge stand off site between the array surface and the skin surface. The image is divided into a set of sample bits, which are same in the field of view. Within this site the system looks at the echo signal amplitude in one path, at the phase and frequency in the other.

The machine now builds the image on a pixel basis, testing exit for evidence of motion and its direction. If motion exits at a pixel, it is coloured, otherwise it takes on a gray scale proportionate to the echo signal strength. Having set out the image formation the next step is colour coding of the pixels, in which motion was detected.

Colour Coding the Information

'Gray's Anatomy' colour code is used by all of the colour flow imaging systems. Flow in one direction is red, and in the opposite direction, it is blue. Now, because all of us are tuned to the fact that all red vessels are arteries and blue vessels are veins, it is all too easy to read the image the wrong way. Even the most skilled readers fall prey to this reading error from time to time. It is to be noted and clarified that colour indicates and represents existence of motion and direction

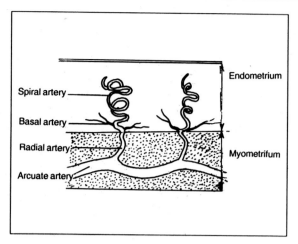

Figure 20.2
Vasculature of uterine wall

of flow, not the vessel type. Colour shows where flow exists in the image and its direction with respect to the transducer.

COLOUR DOPPLER IN GYNAECOLOGY

Main Uterine Vessels

The colour doppler signal from the main uterine vessels may be seen in all patients lateral to the cervix. The small branches of uterine artery can be followed by searching the corpus ascending along the lateral wall (Fig. 20.2). Waveform analysis shows high velocity and high resistance flow. The RI depends on the age, phase of menstrual cycle and any special condition such as pregnancy or tumour.

RI of uterine artery are as follows:
a. In early proliferative phase 0.88 ± 0.04 (Fig. 20.3a)
b. Ssecretory phase 0.84 ± 0.04 (Fig. 20.3b)
c. Radial vessels 0.78 ± 0.10 (Fig. 20.3c)
d. Spiral vessels 0.54 ± 0.03

Ovarian Vessels

It is difficult to visualise the ovarian vessels but an experienced operator, using modern colour doppler unit can detect them in most patients in the lateral upper pole of the ovary (Figs 20.4a to c).

Colour flow is usually not prominent, velocity is low and resistance varies according to the menstrual cycle. A low velocity, high impedance pattern is seen during the follicular phase. At ovulation, there is maximum increase in the velocity and RI decrease, reaching a dip of 0.44 ± 0.09 four to five days later and slowly increases by 0.04-0.05 before menstruation.

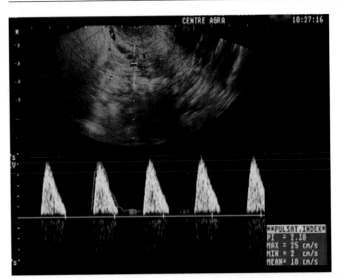

Figure 20.3a
Uterine artery waveform during the early proliferative phase

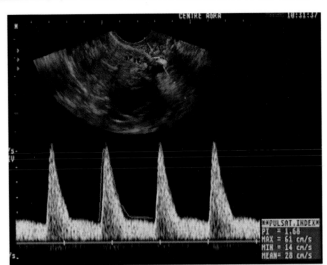

Figure 20.3b
At day ten of menstrual cycle

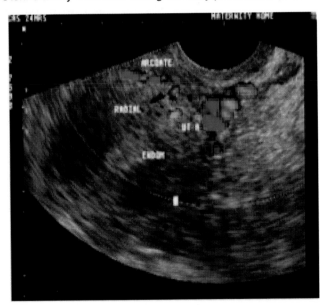

Figure 20.3c
Color Doppler showing uterine, arcuate and radial artery

Active Ovary	:	RI	0.44 ± 0.09
		PSV	$(27 \pm 10 \text{ cm/sec})$
Inactive Ovary	:	RI	0.76 ± 0.22
		PSV	$(8.9 \pm 3.8 \text{ cm/sec})$

Iliac Flow

The common and external iliac arteries show plug flow, a window under the waveform and a reversed component during diastole. The internal iliac vessel in contrast has a parabolic flow with an even distribution of velocities within the waveform.

Ovarian Masses

Neovascularisation

The importance of neovascularisation remains in the hypothesis that increased cell population must be preceeded by the production of new vessels. Such abnormal vascular morphology can be used as a valuable marker for the presence of a malignant tumor. New vessels are continually produced at the periphery of the tumour and act as marker for continued growth and proliferation. The amount and vascularity of the stroma vary greatly in different tumours. In general, rapidly growing tumors particularly sarcomas have a highly vascular stroma with little connective tissue. More slowly growing tumors are less well vascularised.

Intratumoral blood flows displayed on Colour Doppler image indicate that there is flow rapid enough to be detected. The presence of AV communications should be an important factor that produces sufficient velocity above the minimal threshold on Colour Doppler Imaging. The technique may be helpful in demonstrating pelvic tumours with rapid blood flow and in providing haemodynamic information. Colour Doppler can also depict the haemodynamic characteristic of the tumour, allowing echo sources of the hypo-echoic zones to be separated into compartment, vessels and the blood pooling or haemorrhage surrounding them.

The goal of Transvaginal Colour Doppler sonography should be to identify ovarian tumors which are not significantly enlarged. TV-CD is a non-invasive

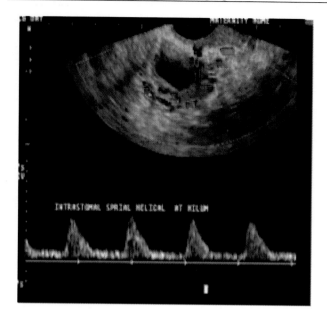

Figure 20.4a
Ovarian arterial flow pattern. Intrastromal color flow is also noted.

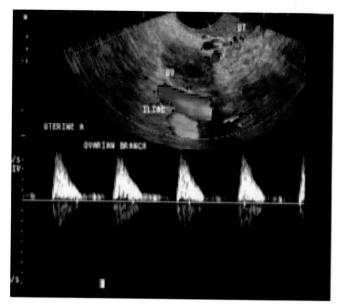

Figure 20.4b
Ovarian branch of uterine artery

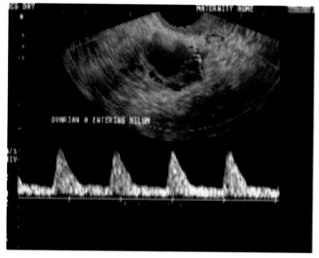

Figure 20.4c
Spectral waveform of the ovarian artery

method and its diagnostic sensitivity, specificity and accuracy seem to be clinically good enough for its to be a potential technique for use in a screening programme.

Several authors have attempted to improve their diagnosis of ovarian cancer by considering the flow characteristics using the RI or PI. Kurjak and Zalud used an RI of 0.4 as a cutoff and found that all 624 benign masses had an RI of > 0.4 and that 54 of 56 cancers had an RI of less than 0.4. However, there is a considerable overlap between benign and malignant

impedance and it is now generally becoming recognized that we must consider the morphology in addition to the impedance estimate.

The other lesions which demonstrate low impedance high diastolic flow are tuboovarian abscesses, actively haemorrhagic corpus luteum (Fig. 20.5a), and some dermoids (Fig. 20.5b). If the waveform has a diastolic notch, the possibility of it being benign are more. Malignant tumors tend to demonstrate colour flow in the central portion, increased flow is seen in the papillary excrescences or in irregular areas of the wall in a malignant mass.

In endometriosis low impedance flow is seen when there is haemorrhage in the menstrual phase of cycle.

Fibroids

Colour flow doppler and spectral doppler findings are variable in uterine fibroids reflecting their natural history with growth followed by episodes of degeneration. The vascularity in fibroids is typically peripheral with very high velocities and low resistance (Figs 20.6a and b). In contrast the centre of fibroids is often avascular and necrotic. A pedunculated fibroid can simulate an ovarian cancer. On endovaginal colour flow copious vascularity may be seen with perfusion characteristics identical to those in ovarian cancer. The pitfall can be avoided by demonstrating the connecting pedicle.

There is an increase in blood flow and a decrease in impedance in both uterine arteries in patients with

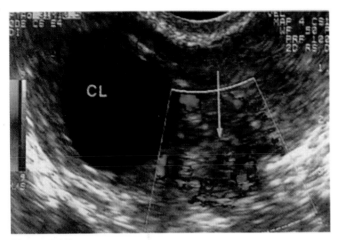

Figure 20.5a
Color flow pattern of the corpus luteum

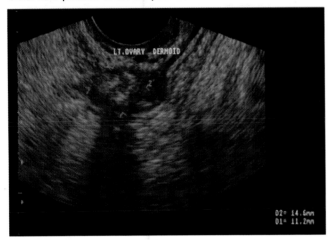

Figure 20.5b
Grey scale image showing an ovarian dermoid

fibroids. The degree of vascularity of a fibroid can determine how the patient should be managed, i.e. when myomectomy should be offered and by which route, whether GnRH agonists should be given or when hysterectomy should be performed. As a general rule of thumb vascularity of fibroids is greater.

Premenopausally and on HRT

Adenexal Ovarian Torsion

One of the major applications of colour doppler is in the diagnosis of ovarian torsion. Although ovary has a dual blood supply, torsion typically affects flow from both ovarian artery and from abdominal branch of uterine artery. The typical appearance is enlarged ovary, which may demonstrate irregular solid areas related to haemorrhage which may precipitate torsion initially. There is no visible arterial flow within the

KEY POINTS

- Normal uterine arteries-low velocity and high resistance flow. Resistance varies with period of menstruation.
- In-active ovarian flow is low velocity with high resistance, active ovarian flow is high velocity with low resistance.
- Malignant lesions more commonly show central vascularity with low impedance, high diastolic flow.
- Fibroids show peripheral vascularity with low impedance, high diastolic flow.
- Fibroids show peripheral vascularity with high resistance flow.
- In ovarian torsion, no visible arterial flow. Endometriosis show scattered flow patterns. High resistance flow is seen within the hilar vessels.
- High velocity, low impedance flow is seen in molar pregnancy due to extensive arterio venous communications.

ovary and high resistance flow in hilar vessels. This early diagnosis can save the organ and allow laparoscopic untwisting which is a relatively simple procedure.

Endometrioses

Colour Doppler may demonstrate flow within these apparent solid structures thereby confirming the diagnosis. The vessels at the periphery of the endometriotic cyst show relativity high vascular impedance. If inflammatory changes occur there may be altered flow showing reduction in impedance to flow (D/D malignancy).

Gestational Trophoblastic Disease

These include molar pregnancy (both partial and complete), invasive mole and choriocarcinoma. Patients with moles usually present in early pregnancy as a threatened abortion and serum HCG levels are found to be greater than 100,000 U/Lt. Examination of the uterus by Endovaginal Ultrasound discloses echogenic contents, and the application of colour flow shows these contents to be highly vascular with placenta like flow. If a normal gestation is seen within uterus, the

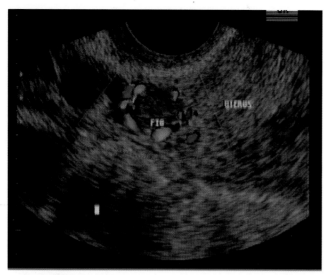

Figure 20.6a
Color doppler demonstrates peripheral vascularity in a fibroid

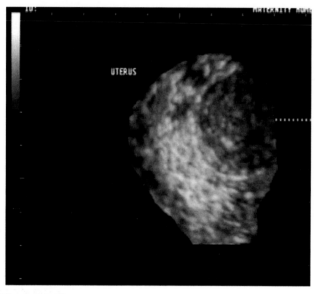

Figure 20.6b
3D image of a uterine fibroid

serum HCG should be repeated because errors in dilutions are not uncommon and may lead to erroneously high serum level.

Colour is extremely helpful in possible recurrence. Myometrial invasion or invasion of adnexa may be seen by the application of colour flow. Moles have extensive arteriovenous communications, which account for high velocity, low impedance flow. Choriocarcinoma displays a typical colour coded 'hot' area representing pre existing and newly formed blood vessels. All these vessels show high velocity low impedance blood flow signals.

Gestational Trophoblastic Tumors

There is reduction in the resistance indices of uterine artery doppler spectra—This pattern correlates well with aggressive trophoblastic tumors and with prognosis. Those tumors exhibiting high resistance index value require massive chemotherapy and fewer treatment cycles.

Ectopic Pregnancy

The advent of colour doppler to TV probe has improved the diagnostic accuracy to almost 98%. Colour flow imaging shows classical "fire ring" with trophoblastic flow pattern (Figs 20.7a to c). Also colour flow help in monitoring medical treatment with methotrexate and in planning medical treatment.

Pelvic Congestion Syndrome

The association between chronic pelvic pain, dyspareunia and pelvic varices has been termed pelvic congestion syndrome. There is dilatation of pelvic veins with congestion of the ovaries with resultant ovarian swelling and cyst formation, occasionally there may be vulvar and leg varices. Dilated pelvic veins can be seen in the absence of symptoms and not all patients with characteristic congestion exhibit the typical ultrasound appearance. Large Serpiginous pelvic veins of a diam > 4 mm with flow velocities < 5 cm/sec in association with cystic ovaries is characteristic. Similarly reversed flow during valsalva which is usually transient, is maintained in this condition with reverse flow of 2 cm/sec or greater.

Colour Doppler sonography is excellent for the diagnosis of uterine and ovarian plexus varicosities. It differentiates arteries from veins.

Malignant Uterine Tumours

Uterine sarcomas appear as in homogeneous mass with increased tumour vascularity showing low impedance flow. In addition, peak systolic velocity also show a decline from normal. Abnormal blood vessels are seen in all cases with sarcoma, whereas only 30 per cent of fibroids show abnormal vessels. Richly vascularised necrotic and large uterine myoma has to be properly evaluated for its blood flow in order to differentiate from sarcomas.

Endometritis and Endometrial Carcinoma

Endometritis results from infection, trauma such as D and C, prolonged labour, premature rupture of

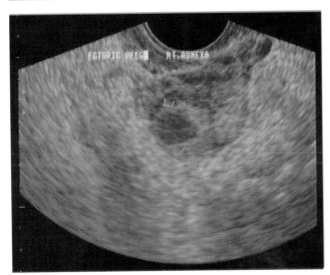

Figure 20.7a
Ectopic pregnancy—Grey scale image showing a complex right adenexal mass

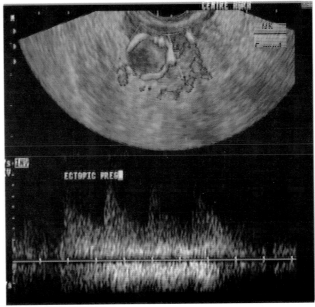

Figure 20.7c
Ectopic pregnancy—Duplex Doppler demonstrates trophoblastic flow pattern

ratio is not clear. In practice any postmenopausal woman presenting with endometrial thickness of > 6 mm needs to undergo biopsy (Fig. 20.8).

It has recently become apparent that tamoxifen may also be associated with some significant endometrial abnormalities. From the NCI report, it appears that the risk of endometrial cancer in patients receiving tamoxifen is apx. three times that of normal population.

Intrauterine Polyp

The diagnosis of intrauterine polyps can be difficult without invasive procedures. Even with endovaginal ultrasound, polyps can be easily missed unless fluid is instilled into the uterine cavity to outline them. Endovaginal colour flow can be helpful where the vascular pedicle can be demonstrated (Fig. 20.9).

Carcinoma of the Cervix

Doppler appears to have little applications in the diagnosis of carcinoma of the cervix. However, cervical carcinoma can be seen on endovaginal ultrasound and neovascularity can be demonstrated.

Sonosalpingography

Tubal patency study by fluid injection through the cervical cannula and observation of fluid dynamics through the fallopian tube and fluid collection in the

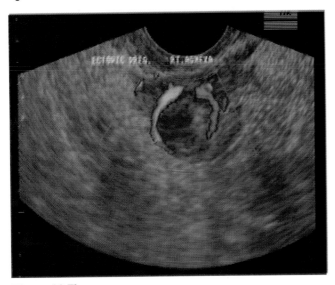

Figure 20.7b
Ectopic pregnancy—On color Doppler "ring of fire" appearance is seen

membranes or retained products of conception. Endometritis may be associated with considerable hyperaemia, this may be of the low impedance pattern described in endometrial carcinoma (Taylor *et al*). In patients with postmenopausal bleeding due to endometrial carcinoma, the mean PI was 0.91 with a range of 0.31-1.49 (Bovine *et al*). Women with other causes for postmenopausal bleeding had a mean PI of 3.83 with a range of 1.95-6.40. Unfortunately due to the confusion with similar flow found in both hyperplasia of endometrium and in endometritis the value of this

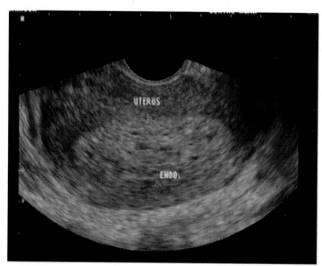

Figure 20.8
Increased endometrial thickness in a case of endometrial hyperplasia

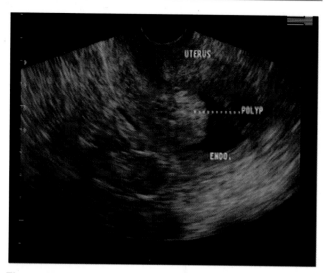

Figure 20.9
Endometrial polyp seen as a localised echogenic lesion in the endometrium

pelvis is a common, noninvasive and useful test. Colour Doppler helps easy identification of flow of fluid through the tubes and also facilitates location of free spill of fluid into the peritoneal cavity (Waterfall Sign).

During the same procedure if 200-250 cc of fluid is injected via the Foley's, then the adnexa and POD can be evaluated for adhesions.

ROLE OF COLOUR DOPPLER IN INFERTILITY

Introduction

The advent of transvaginal Colour Doppler Sonography has added a new dimension to the diagnosis and treatment of infertile female. Colour Doppler innovation is a unique non-invasive technology to investigate the circulation of organs like uterus and ovaries. Dynamic changes occur almost every day of the menstrual cycle in a reproductively active female. These events are picked up very well by transvaginal Colour Doppler and definite conclusions can be drawn regarding the diagnosis, prognosis and treatment of infertile patients. As the vaginal probe lies close to the organs of interest various vessels supplying these structure can be studied in detail like the uterine artery, ovarian artery and their branches.

Study of Menstrual Cycle by Colour Doppler

It is very important to study the whole of the menstrual cycle by transvaginal colour doppler during the evaluation of infertility. It provides vital information about follicular dynamics like blood flow to the grow-

ing follicle, the vascular supply of the endometrium and corpus luteum vascularization which are very important for a successful outcome in terms of pregnancy.

Changes in the Ovary

The ovaries are situated on either side of the uterus and measure about 2.2 to 5.5 cms in length, 1.5 to 2.0 cms in width and 1.5 to 3.0 cms in depth and are recognized by the presence of follicle of different sizes. The blood supply is by ovarian artery via the infundibulo-pelvic ligament and ovarian branch of the uterine artery. There is anastamosis between the two sources of blood supply. The primary and secondary branches of the ovarian artery grow along with the development of the follicle. Dominant follicle within the ovary can be recognized by transvaginal colour doppler by day 8th or 10th of the cycle by a ring of angiogenesis around it, when compared to the subordinate follicles which do not demonstrate this (Fig. 20.10). These vessels become more abundant and prominent as the follicle grows to about 20-24 mm in size.

The Phases are described as early follicular (Day 5-7), late follicular (Day 11-13), early luteal (Day 15-17) and late luteal (Day 26-28). In general the index values are high in the early part of menstrual cycle and fall as ovulation approaches. According to Kurjak *et al* the RI in the early proliferative phase is 0.54 +/- 0.04 and declines the day before ovulation (LH Peak) when it is about 0.44 +/- 0.04.

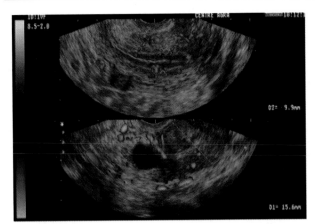

Figure 20.10
Color Doppler showing ring of angiogenesis around the dominant follicle of the ovary. Vascularity is also seen in the endometrium

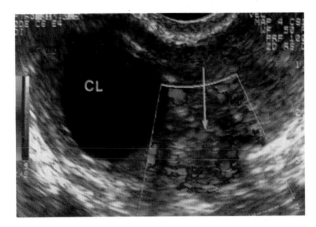

Figure 20.11
Color Doppler image of corpus luteum

This is the best time for administration of surrogate HCG. The increase in peak systolic velocity with a relatively constant is a particularly interesting finding that might herald impending ovulation. It is hoped that information on ovarian perfusion may be used to predict ovulation and to investigate ovulatory dysfunction. The lowest RI values were obtained during the mid luteal phase (RI 0.42 $\pm$ 0.06) with a return to higher vascular resitance (0.50 $\pm$ 0.04) during the late luteal phase.

The dominant ovary corpus luteum show a low impedance waveform with a RI of 0.39 – 0.49, characteristic of blood flow in early pregnancy (Fig. 20.11). The contralateral ovary show a high impedance flow with a RI of 0.69–1.00 characteristic of non dominant ovary (Kurjak *et al*). If the ovary having corpus luteum shows high RI (> 0.50) it is associated with nonviable outcome.

Luteal Phase Changes in Ovarian Vascularity

The functional capacity of the corpus luteum is assessed by the low impedance flow and the abundance of vessels arounds it Mature corpus luteum is a highly vascularized structure with a low RI of 0.44 +/– 0.04. In patients with corpus luteum deficiency the vascularity is not optimal and the RI is raised to around 0.59, with decreased diastolic flow. If pregnancy occurs then low RI of 0.50 continues.

Secretory Changes in the Endometium

Michael Applebaum in his study with transvaginal colour doppler divided the endometrium and peri-endometrial areas into 4 zones. In the study conducted

by him no pregnancy was reported in IVF patients unless vascularity was demonstrated in Zone III or IV prior to transfer.

Doppler Assessment of Uterine and Ovarian Flow in Infertility and IVF

Goswamy *et al* found absent diastolic flow in infertility patients and with severe problems and even reversal of diastolic flow.

Role of Ultrasound and Colour Doppler in Endometrial Evaluation

Ultrasound (TVS) offers a simple, reliable, reproducible, quick and non invasive method for assessing the female pelvis.

Uterine Perfusion

The uterine Artery give rise to the radial arteries which are oriented circumferentially in the outer third of the myometrium. These vessels give rise to the radial arteries, which after crossing the myometrium-endometrium border, further branch and give rise to the basal arteries and the spiral arteries.

The RI in the uterine artery hovers around 0.88 $\pm$ 0.04 until day 13 of the 28 day menstrual cycle (Figs 20.12 and 13). Increased uterine Artery impedance is seen 3 days after the LH peak (day 16). This is explained by increased contractility and compression of vessels traversing the uterine wall which decrease their diameter and consequently cause higher resistance to flow. Lowest blood flow impedance occurs during peak luteal (RI = 0.84 $\pm$ 0.04) during which implantation is likely to occur. RI of radial vessels is 0.78 $\pm$ 0.10.

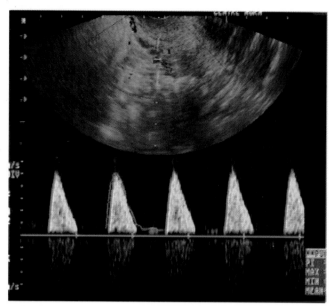

Figure 20.12

Uterine artery flow at second day of menstrual cycle

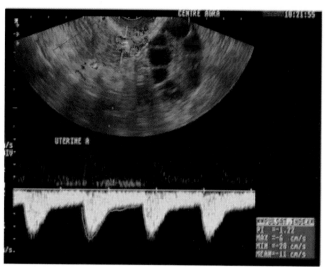

Figure 20.13

Uterine artery flow at day ten showing low impedance flow

Blood flow velocity waveform changes in the spiral arteries during normal ovulatory cycles are characteristics of by lower velocity and lower impedance to blood flow than are those observed in the uterine arteries with larger diameter. It seems that features of endometrial blood flow may be used to predict the implantation success rate and to reveal unexplained infertility problems more precisely than evaluationof the main uterine artery alone.

Changes in the Endometrium

Michael Applebaum in his study with transvaginal colour doppler divided the endometrium and periendometrial areas into 4 zones. In the study conducted by him no pregnancy was reported in IVF patients unless vascularity was demonstrated in Zone III or with in Zone III or IV prior to transfer.

Zone 1 : 2 mm thick area surrounding the hyperechoic outer layer of the endometrium.

Zone 2 : The hyperechoic outer layer of the endometrium.

Zone 3 : The hypoechoic inner layer of the endometrium.

Zone 4 : The endometrial cavity.

Ultrasound Technique for Uterine Biophysical Profile

To perform the UBP special care should be taken. The following guidelines are recommended: (Applebaum 1996).

1. To determine the presence of a 5-line appearance, information from both the transabdominal and transvaginal studies may be useful. For example, although a 5-line appearance may be noted transabdominally, it may not always be possible to see it endovaginally due to uterine position (and vice versa). In this case, a 5-line appearance is considered to be present and endometrial vascular penetration may be estimated when performing the endovaginal study.

2. Perform the Doppler study slowly. The flow of blood in the endometrium is of low velocity, it may take time for the ultrasound machine to register the presence of blood flow and create the image. If one sweeps through the endometrium too quickly, flow may not be seen. Additionally endometrial blood flow has a mercurial personality-it may appear as if it comes and goes. It may also appear in some areas and not others. Do not observe hastily.

3. Endeavor to make the endometrium as specular a reflector as possible. Use the techniques of manual manipulation of the anatomy and probe pressure to achieve this.

4. Scan endovaginally both coronally and sagittally. There may be a difference in how well the blood flow is imaged.

5. When measuring the endometrium in the A-P dimension, try to obtain the value when no contraction affecting it is present. Contractions may affect this value. Also when possible, obtain the measurement in a standard plan such as when both the endometrial and cervical canals continuous.

The Uterine Biophysical Profile

In our experience, certain sonographic qualities of the uterus are noted during the normal mid-cycle. These include:

1. Endometrial thickness in greatest AP diamension of 7 mm or greater (full-thickness measurement).
2. A layered ("5 line") appearance to the endometrium.
3. Blood flow within zone 3 using colour Doppler technique.
4. Myometrial contractions causing a wave like motion of the endometrium.
5. Uterine artery blood flow, as measured by PI, less than 3.0.
6. Homogeneous myometrial echogenicity.
7. Myometrial blood flow seen on gray-scal examination (internal to the arcuate vessels).

The uterine scoring system for reproduction ("USSR") comprises evaluation of the following parameters:

1. Endometrial thickness (full-thickness measured from the myometrial-endometrial junction to the endometrial-myometrial junction).
2. Endometrial layering (i.e., a 5-line appearance).
3. Myometrial contractions seen as endometrial motion.
4. Myometrial echogenicity.
5. Uterine artery Doppler flow evaluation.
6. Endometrial blood flow.
7. Gray-scale myometrial blood flow.

Each parameter is scored as follows:

1. Endometrial thickness
   a. < 7 mm = 0
   b. 7-9 mm = 2
   c. 10-14 mm = 3
   d. >14 mm = 1
2. Endometrial layering
   a. no layering = 0
   b. hazy 5-line appearance = 1
   c. distinct 5-line appearance = 3
3. Myometrial contractions (seen as wave-like endometrial motion high-speed playback from videotape)
   a. < 3 contractions in 2 minutes (real-time) = 0
   b. > = 3 contractions in 2 minutes (real-time) = 3
4. Myometrial echogenicity
   a. coarse/inhomogeneous echogenicity = 1
   b. relatively homogeneous echogenicity = 2
5. Uterine artery Doppler flow
   a. PI-2.99-3.0 = 0
   b. PI-2.49 = 0
   c. PI <2 = 2
6. Endometrial blood flow within Zone 3
   a. absent = 0
   b. present, but sparse = 2
   c. present multifocally = 5
7. Myometrial blood flow internal to the arcuate vessels seen on gray-scale examination
   a. absent = 0
   b. present = 2

The values assume a technically adequate ultrasound examination with no abnormalities of uterine shape or development, no other gross uterine abnormalities (e.g. significant masses) and a normal ovairan cycle (e.g. without evidence of ovarian-ultrine dyscoordination). A male factor component to the infertility is not present.

In our limited experience (Applebaum)[1] with this system thus far, a USSR "perfect score" of 20 has been associated with conception 100% of the time. [The number of patients in which we predicted successful conception cycles based upon the UBP and USSR perfect score was 5. The group included 2 spontaneous cycles (non-IVF, non-IUI), 2 IUI and 1 IVF]. Scores of 17-19 (10 patients) have been associated with conception 80% of the time. Scores of 14-16 (10 patients) have a 60% chance, while scores of 13 or less (25 patients) have resulted in no pregnancies.

Absent endometrial flow, espite highest values for the other parameters, has always been associated with no conception.

ROLE OF TRANSVAGINAL COLOUR DOPPLER IN OTHER CONDITIONS ASSOCIATED WITH INFERTILITY

Luteinized Unruptured Follicle

This condition is recognized by serial ultrasonography to monitor the growth of follicle, with failure to see expected changes at the time of ovulation.

The typical blood flow pattern seen in the corpus luteum is absent.

In LUF syndrome, no difference in terms of intraovarian RI was obtained after the LH peak. Similar RI values were obtained during the follicular and luteal phases (0.55 ± 0.04 Vs 0.54 ± 0.06). There was no difference between the sides in terms of intraovarian vascular resistance.

Luteal Phase Defect

This is due to decreased vascularisation of corpus luteum. The three to seven fold increase in blood supply is necessary to deliver the steroid precusors to ovary and removal of progestrone as shown in experimental animals.

In the LPD group no difference was obtained in terms of intraovarian RI during the follicular pahse. The mean RI throughout the luteal phase (0.56 ± 0.04) was significantly higher compared to that in the normal women. Fushemole did not show any difference between the easly, middle and late luteal pahse. In the LPD group on difference occured in terms of intraovarian RI between the sides.

Fibroid

To define the borders of fibroid colour doppler is of real help as the vascular supply at the periphery of the leiomyoma can be delineated very well. Good vascularity denotes a favourable response to GnRH if used before laparoscopic surgery.

Endometriosis

On gray scale scan endometrioma is seen as a homogeneously echogenic intraovarian mass. Colour doppler may demonstrate the flow around and not within the endometriotic cyst.

Tubal Causes

During active phase of PID low impedance blood flow signals are usually detected and after effective antibiotic therapy flow tends to return to normal. Int he absence of this change surgery is indicated.

Polycystic Ovarian Disease (PCOD) (Fig. 20.14)

Contrary to the normal ovarian blood flow which is seen around the growing follicle PCOD subjects show abundantly vascularised stroma. Waveforms obtained from the ovarian tissue showed a mean resistance index of 0.54 without cyclical change between repeated examinations.

Patients of PCOD with RI less than 0.54, if gonadotrophins are administred will land into ovarian hyperstimulation syndrome.

Uterine Factor

The possibility of decreased uterine blood flow may be associated with infertility as already discussed in proceeding paragraphs Gowswamy *et al* depicted in their study that uterine artery indices which were high in failed IVF cases improved after the patients were put on oral oestrogen therapy and pregnancy rate

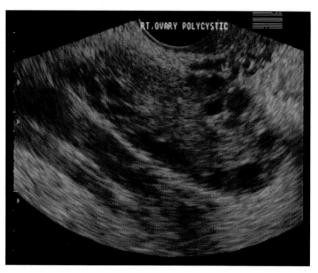

Figure 20.14
PCOD: grey scale image showing an enlarged right ovary (volume: 28.78ml) with small peripheral follicles and increased stromal echogenecity

improved when compared to those who did not get this treatment.

Colour Doppler in In vitro Fertilization

Colour Doppler could prove valuable in the prediction of the response of patients to ovarian stimulation in assisted conception, assessment of oocyte quality based on peri follicular flow and parameters influencing implantation following embryo transfer.

a. *Prediction of patient response to ovulation stimulation:* It is seen that women with greater ovarian stomal peak systolic blood flow velocity have increased intraovarian perfusion (Fig. 20.15). Thus, in response to the same dose of gonadotrophin administration, a larger amount is delivered to the target cells. In women with PCOD ovaries a higher stromal blood flow velocity is seen not only at the baseline scan but also during the entire menstrual cycle Colour Doppler therefore offers valuable information regarding the dose of gonadotrophin required for successful ovarian stimulation in assisted conception.

In a stimulated cycle resistance of the intraovarian vessels measured by transvaginal colour doppler correlates well with number of follicles, that is those with more than 15 mm size. This correlation exists even during the early follicular phase, when follicular recruitment and development have just started. This suggest that vascularization of the

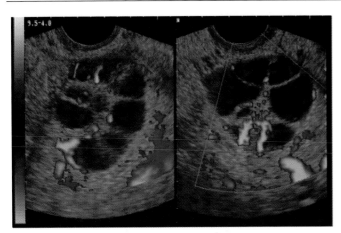

Figure 20.15
Intraovarian perfusion seen in a case of ovarian stimulation

follicles may play a role in their maturation from early follicular phase onwards. This study in the early follicular phase can prevent ovarian hyper stimulation syndrome (OHSS).

b. *Colour Doppler and its contribution towards in vitro fertilization* During stimulation protocols colour doppler ultrasound has its greatest contribution in monitoring follicular development and guiding oocyte harvesting procedures. The use of colour doppler ultrasound can occasionally be of help as it avoids accidental puncture of iliac vessels and also vessels on the surface of ovary.

c. *Follicular characteristics assessment in predicting oocyte quality:* A rapid rise in blood flow velocity in the perifollicular and ovarian stromal vessels is seen at the time of LH surge. These charges are as a result of neoangiogenesis occuring during late follicular development. A marked increase in peak systolic velocity around the follicle, in the presence of a relatively constant pulsatility index could be a sign of folicle maturity and herald impending ovulation. Administration of HCG resulted in a rapid increase in peak velocities. Nargund et al showed that oocytes obtained from highly vascularised follicle were of higher quality and were more likely to fertilize and result in pregnancy. From the available data, it appears that assessment of perfollicular vascular perfusion could lead to a better selection of oocytes and ultimately a higher pregnancy rate.

d. *Implantation:* Steer and Colleagues noted that the lowest uterine artery PI was found 9 days after the LH peak, which is consistent with maximum

uterine perfusion at the time of peak luteal function and expected implantation.

They also showed that uterine artery impendance was different in the mid luteal phase in women with subinfertility compared with those with normal fertility. They grouped the patients according to whether the PI was low (1-1.99), medium (2-2.99) or high (>3.0). There were no pregnancies in high PI group and the PI was significantly lower in women who become pregnant as compared with those who did not.

In a recent work by Campbell it is possible to calculate the probability of pregnancy by using PI values of uterine artery on the day Embryo Transfer. Highest probability of pregnancy was predicted for patients who had medium values for PI. Those with high PI had failure rate upto 35 percent.

The ability to predict implantation before the administration of hCG allows the clinician the option to delay giving hCG until the uterine artery PI improves. An alternative approach would be to try to improve uterine perfusion by the administration of glyceryl trinitrate (GTN). It has been suggested that administration of GTN may increase pregnancy rates in women with poor uterine perfusion.

Conclusion

The role of this new modality in the evaluation of an infertile female is becoming more important as various centres are coming out with a multitude of studies indicating its superior accuracy and excellent reproducibility.

TUBAL EVALUATION

Introduction

Endosonography as a tool for checking the patency of fallopian tubes was an expected development with great strides taken within the field of Gynaecology. Sonosalpingography also known as 'Sion Test' used transvaginal sonography to confirm the tubal patency by visualizing the spill of fluid from the fimbrial end of fallopian tubes (Figs 20.16 and 17). Fallopian tubes are isoechoic and cannot be normally seen on Ultrasound unless pathological or fluid surrounds the tubes. We propose to perform this test not as a substitute for hysterosalpingagraphy or laparoscopy but as a noninvasive, cheap outdoor screening procedure in patients of infertility.

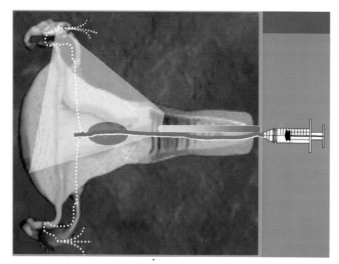

Figure 20.16
Sonosalpingography technique

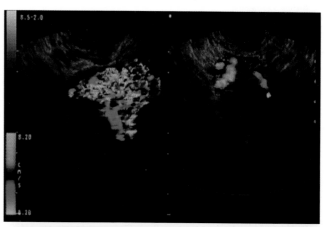

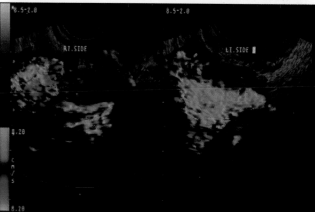

Figures 20.18a and b
Spill from the fimbrial end on both sides confirming the tubal patency

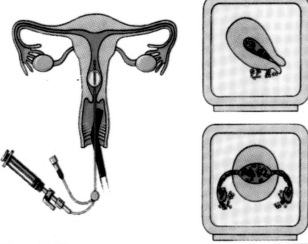

Figure 20.17
Sonosalpingography with echovist

Sonosalpingography

We used this test as a basic screening test for evaluating tubal patency in all.

Number 8 Fr. foleys cath, is put inside the uterine cavity the bulb is inflated with 2 ml of distilled water. Prior to procedure the patient is asked to evacuate the bladder and baseline vaginal scan is performed. 20-60 ml of solution containing ciplox, hylase and dexamethasone is taken in 50 ml catheter tip syringe and pushed via foleys catheter and spill is studied from the fimbrial end (Figs 20.18a and b) .

We have done the 'Sion Procedure' in the patients of suspected pelvic factors. In this we have flooded the pelvis using the same fluid about 200-300 ml, pushed via foley's catheter and visualized the fallopian tubes (Fig. 20.19).

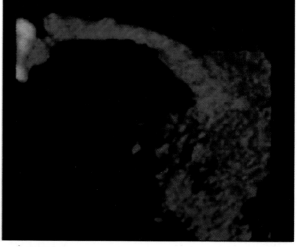

Figure 20.19
3D color tubes

KEY POINTS

I. COLOR DOPPLER IN INFERTILITY

- Doppler indices of ovarian and uterine perfusion change with the phases of menstrual cycle.

OVARIAN ARTERY

- Follicular phase — Low velocity, high impedance pattern, RI (early proliferative phase) = 0.54+/-0.04

  Day 8-10, dominant follicle shows a ring of angiogenesis around it
- At ovulation — High velocity , low impedance flow

  RI (a day before ovulation) = 0.44+/-0.04

  PSV =27+/-10 cm/sec
- Luteal phase dominant ovary with corpus luteum shows RI =0.39-0.49

  RI > 0.5 has a nonviable outcome.

UTERINE ARTERY

- High velocity, high resistance flow
- RI depends on age and phase of menstrual cycle
- RI (proliferative phase 1-13 days) = 0.88+/-0.04
- RI (day 16 that ie 3 days after LH surge) increases
- RI (peak luteal phase) = 0.84+/-0.04 (leads to successful implantation)

UTERINE BIOPHYSICAL PROFILE (UBP)

- Done during mid cycle phase
- USSR scores the following parameters to determine the success of natural or artificial conception:
  - Endometrial thickness
  - Endometrial layering
  - Myometrial contraction
  - Uterine artery doppler flow
  - Endometrial blood flow within zone 3
  - Myometrial blood flow to arcuate vessels on gray scale
- Score of 20-100% conception
- Score of 13 or less-No conception occurs

II. TVCD IN OTHER CONDITIONS ASSOCIATED WITH INFERTILITY

- Intraovarian RI remaining same before and after LH peak signifying luteinized unruptured follicle
- RI (luteal phase) of 0.56+/- 0.04 (more than in normal women) suggests a luteal phase defect
- Good peripheral vascularity in fibroid denotes a favourable response to GnRH
- In PCOD, there is vascular stroma which shows mean RI of 0.54 with no cyclical changes
- Role of doppler in Invitro fertilization: the dose of gonadotropin directly corresponds to the ovarian stromal PSV, the marked increase in PSV around follicle and a constant pulsatility index signifies follicle maturity and impending ovulation, 9 days after LH peak showed lowest uterine PI (i.e. maximum uterine perfusion) and good chances of implantation.

SSG/ Sion Test

- non invasive modality to assess the tubal patency
- 20-60 ml of solution (ciplox, hylase and dexamethasone)is instilled via a foleys catheter placed in the uterine cavity
- visualisation of spill from the fimbrial end establishes tubal patency
- flooding the pelvis with 200-300 ml of fluid helps in detecting adhesions.

Aims and Objectives

The present study was conducted with the aim to study the tubal patency using sonosalpingography as a first screening method. The patients were further followed up by Hysterosalpingography and Laparoscopy. 'Sion Procedure' was done in only suspected cases of having adhesions and tubal pathology.

Observations (Tables 20.1 to 20.5)

Case Distriubtion							
Table 20.1	Total cases	Infertility		Posi- tive	Sion test	Nega- tive	Sion test
		Primary	Secondary				
	200	160	40	135	10	25	30

Negative Sion Test (n = 55)		
Table 20.2	Total cases	Hysterosalpingography
		Tubal block	Patent tube
	55	51	4

Laparoscopy		
Table 20.3	Total cases	Diagnostic laparoscopy
		Tubal patency	Tubal block
	20 selected randomly	17	3

Sion procedure suspected pelvic factor			
Table 20.4	Cases	Adhesions	Fimbrial path	Normal
	25 random	5	2	18

Suspected pelvic factors (n = 25) laparoscopy			
Table 20.5	Cases	Adhesions	Fimbrial path	Normal
	24	6	2	16

Results and Discussions

As it is very evident from the above tables that sonosalpingography is a good noninvasive screening test for judging the tubal patency. The findings of sonosalpingography were further confirmed by hysterosalpingography. In patients where a tubal pathology was suspected, sion procedure was done and we found that out 25 patients of suspected pelvic factor problem 5 had adhesions, 2 had fimbrial pathology. The same group of patients were further followed up by diagnostic laparoscopy and we could additionally pick one more case of adhesions. Since last 6 years we are evaluating all cases of infertility by colour doppler (Medison 7700 and Voluson 530 D).

Optimal Conditions for Embryo Transfer

The lower the PI value in uterine artery more the chance of pregnancy. Steer et al. have shown that if PI is > 3 before ET no pregnancy results.

CONCLUSION

The role of this new modality in the evaluation of an infertile female is becoming more important as various centres are coming out with a multitude of studies indicating its superior accuracy and excellent reproducibility.

COLOUR IN RELATION TO OBSTETRICS

The minimum frequency of transducer should be 7.5 MHz in early prgnancy (upto 8 weeks) and 5 MHz in 9-13 weeks pregnancy. The vaginal probe should have dynamic focusing and produce minimal artifacts. The transducer should have colour sensitivity to demonstrate small vessels with low velocity blood flow, which characterize the trophoblast. An update duplex Doppler or a triplex Doppler capability is essential for displaying Doppler waveforms and for calculating the Resistance Index (RI) and Pulsatility index (PI) and also the A/B ratio (peak systolic/End Diastolic Ratio).

The same is achieved after 14 weeks by TAS. Although no significant difference has been obtained in the value of these indices in clinical practice, but most workers prefer Pourcelot Index (PI) over RI. Decreased values of RI reflect less peripheral vascular resistance.

Changes in Pregnancy

1. Gravid uterus shows a generalized increase in vascularity in the myometrium.
2. The decidua (Endometrium) shows no evidence of flow before implantation.
3. An area of vascularity is demonstrated in the hyper echoic decidua on days 26-28 post LMP (implantation site signal).
4. Chorionic sac stage (29-34 days) is characterised by multiple areas of vascularity in the decidua trophoblast layers and adjacent myometrium.
5. CDS picks up diastolic flow of small vessels with low impedance characteristic of Trophoblastic invasion even before embryo is sighted (Fig. 20.20).

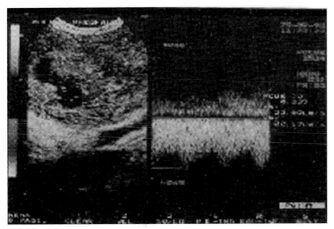

Figure 20.20
Trophoblastic flow detected in early pregnancy reveals low impedance pattern

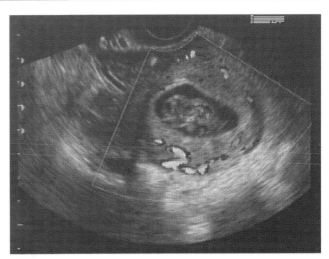

Figure 20.21a
Color Doppler at nine weeks of gestation

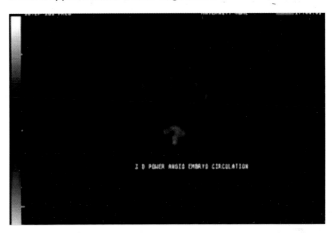

Figure 20.21b
3D power angio of the uterus showing early embryonic circulation

6. Once embryo is seen (34-39 days) a distinct colour signal is seen in its cardiovascular system and is referred to as the embryonic heart beat.
7. As the embryo grows, cardiovascular system will be seen on CDS-the aorta, vena cava, intracranial and hepatic circulation. The umbilical cord, placenta vitelline (yolk sac) circulation becomes visible at 8-9 weeks gestation (Figs 20.21a and b).
8. Triplex TV-Doppler (colour flow plus duplex) can determine various indices in the pelvic vessels during the first trimester.

Problems in Acquiring and Interpreting the Waveforms

Artifactual Loss of End Diastolic Frequencies

This may be due to:

a. A high angle between the ultrasound beam and the vessel that results in very low frequencies disappearing below the height of the vessel wall filter. If end-diastolic frequencies appear absent one should reduce the vessel wall filter to its lowest setting (usually 50 Hz) or remove it if possible. Then one should alter the angle of the probe relative to maternal abdomen and if end diastolic frequencies are still absent one should then attempt to obtain the signal from a different site within the uterus as this is likely to result in a different angle of insonation. One should also ensure that foetus is not breathing by demonstrating a smooth waveform of the umbilical vein in the opposite channel. We do not report absence of end diastolic frequencies until this has been demonstrated on two successive days.

The alternative is to submit the woman to a duplex, pulsed Doppler examination.

b. *Foetal breathing movements* These cause wild fluctuations in the signal from umbilical artery and are readily recognisable by being unable to demonstrate a steady state in the umbilical vein that is recorded in the other channel. After a little practice, they can also be recognized from the arterial signal. The only course to take if the foetus is breathing is to wait until this stops.

Failure to Obtain a Signal

This may be due to:

a. *Incorrect machine settings* This is usually recognised by having a signal that is not displayed on the screen. First one must check that the frequency range is not too high or low-4 MHz is a good starting point. If the screen is still blank then turn up the gain slowly. If the screen is saturated with white noise then turn the gain down slowly until the waveform appears. If the there is still no visual signal then ensure that balance setting is not turned to one extreme such that one channel of the spectrum analyser is obliterated.

b. Foetal death
c. Maternal obesity
d. Oligohydramnios.

   In the latter three situations, use a real time transducer to check that the foetus is still alive and then to locate a loop of cord. Mark the spot on the maternal abdomen with a finger and then replace the real time transducer with the Doppler probe. One cannot undertake real time imaging and acquire Doppler signals simultaneously, as the signals interfere with each other. In pulsed Doppler machines the real time imaging is usually frozen when the Doppler signal is being acquired.

Duplex Evaluation in Normal and High Risk Pregnancy

Fetal growth depends on a study supply of nutrients and oxygen from the mother; a normal uteroplacental and fetoplacental circulation is necessary for this to occur. In recent years, however Doppler ultrasound has given us a non-invasive method of evaluating blood flow in the fetoplacental and uteroplacental circulation in normal and complicated pregnancies.

Utero-placental Circulation

During pregnancy there is hyperplasia and hypertrophy of the uterine wall and the arterioles elongate and coil (Fig. 20.22). At the base of placenta there is thinning of endometrium with invasion of trophoblast. The trophoblastic invasion leads to stripping off the muscular elastic coat of spiral arteries by the 20th postmenstrual week. This decreases the resistance to blood flow progressing from the radials artery into the intervillous spaces. The pressure falls about 70-80 mm in the former to 10 mm Hg in the later.

Feto-placental Circulation (Fig. 20.23)

The branches of the umbilical artery and umbilical vein radiate out from the site of insertion of the cord along the fetal surface of placenta beneath the amnion.

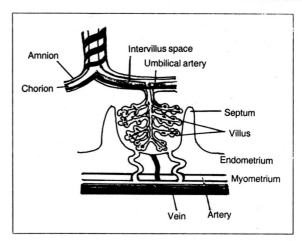

Figure 20.22
Line diagram showing normal utero-placental vasculature

Branches of the artery along with an accompanying vein penetrate the chorionic plate and enter the main stem chorionic villi. Ther they divided to supply individual chorionic villi. It is at this level that the exchange of nutrients and waste products takes place between the fetal and maternal circulations. The unit composed of the main stem chorionic villus and its branches is called the "Fetal Cotyledon". It is this capillary bed that produces the most resistance to pulsatile blood flow. As pregnancy advances, the size of the chorionic villi increase, whereas their number decreases. This is accompained by a reduction inthe thickness of the tissue layer between the fetal capillaries and the maternal intervillous spaces. These changes allow for more efficient exchange between the two circulations. The fetal circulation is characterized by a high blood flow and a low vascular resis-

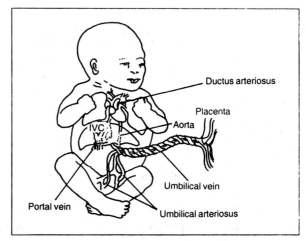

Figure 20.23
Line diagram showing normal fetal circulation

tance. Umbilical blood flow increases with gestational age and pressure gradient driving the blood from the descending aorta through the placenta and back to inferior vena cava.

Umbilical flow velocity waveforms before 14 weeks of gestation are typically characterised by the absence of end diastolic velocities. Diastolic flow is incomplete until 14 weeks of gestation. After this, pan diastolic frequencies are consistently present. Intraplacental waveforms with foetal characteristics can be identified and clearly differentiated from the beginning of the 2nd trimester.

The appearance of end diastolic frequencies in the umbilical circulation coincide with an abrupt and significant increase in uterine artery peak systolic velocity together with presence of continuous intervillous flow within the placenta. The establishment of the intervillous circulation may be associated with change in the pressure gradient due to the expansion of the intervillous space and/or with modification in blood gases and metabolite concentrations which in turn may explain the rapid appearance of end diastolic frequencies in the umbilical circulation.

Abnormal 1st Trimester

Colour flow can be used very effectively in:

1. *Complete versus incomplete abortion* Dillon *et al* reported that 24 hours after an abortion persistent placental flow was seen in half the patients, which resolved spontaneously over the next few days. Although, there are several possible ways to interpret these findings, the most likely explanation is that many therapeutic abortions are incomplete and spontaneously proceed to completion without further intervention. Thus, the decision about further intervention following therapeutic abortion should be made on the basis of patients symptoms and signs and not on the ground of demonstration of intrauterine placental alone flow. However, there should be no placental flow 1 week after an abortion and demonstration of low impedance flow indicates the need for D and C. The intrauterine appearances are unimpressive for, retained products. However, the presence of low impedance flow correctly predicted retained product of conception and indicated the need for repeat D and C. It should be stressed that clinical correlation is important for correct diagnosis because endometritis can give rise to similar low impedance endometrial flow as described earlier.

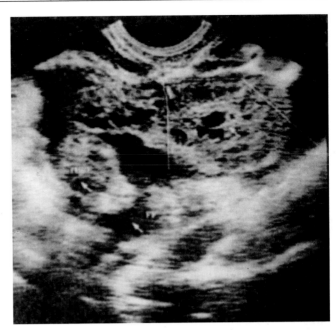

Figure 20.24
Grey scale image showing small ectopic gestation

2. *Ectopic pregnancy* The process of ectopic placentation is morphologically similar whether it occurs in the uterus or in the fallopian tube (Fig. 20.24). The chorion villi with the intervening intervillous space are well seen within the fallopian tube. High velocity, low-impedance flow is seen in the tubal mass. On colour flow a solid adnexal mass shows pronounced vascularity, which identifies it as an ectopic gestation (Figs 20.25a and b).

Care must be exercised in the differentiation between placental flow in the tube and luteal flow in the ovary. In 85 per cent of ectopic gestations, the pregnancy is on the same side as the corpus which can be used to guide the initial examination. Women are also accurate at realizing their ectopic by the side of their pelvic pain. In practice, it is necessary to identify the ovary by its specific morphology and to look for a vascular area, usually medial to the side of luteal flow, which can therefore be identified as the ectopic gestation.

Taylor *et al* showed in his series of ectopic pregnancy, no placental flow was detected in about 18 per cent cases. These avascular ectopics probably represent nonviable gestations. It is notable that they display low S. HCG values indicating the limited activity of the trophoblast failing to thrive in the hostile environment of the tube. Such gestations may be especially suitable for medical therapy.

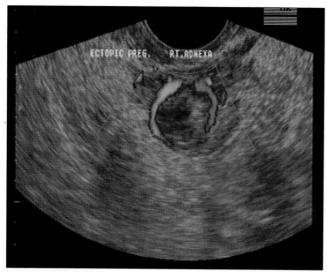

Figure 20.25a
On color Doppler "ring of fire" appearance is seen in ectopic gestation

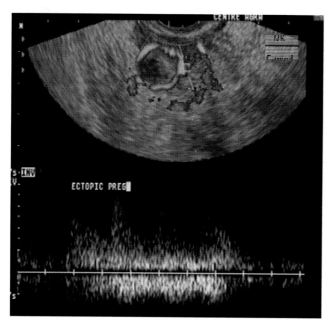

Figure 20.25b
Duplex Doppler demonstrates trophoblastic flow pattern

3. *Recognition of pseudosacs* (Fig. 20.26) A pseudosac displays the normal high impedance flow from the endometrium, whereas the abnormal gestational sac shows the high velocity, low impedance flow of the placental interface. It should be noted that the absence of an embryo does not affect the presence of placental flow because placental low results from pressure gradient between the maternal tubal arteries and the low

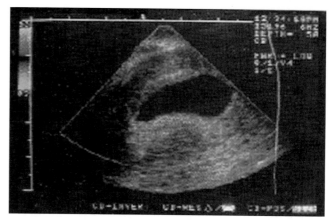

Figure 20.26
Grey scale image showing an empty gestational sac

resistance of the intervillous space. This depends on trophoblastic activity and not on the presence of foetus.

4. *Molar pregnancy (Discussed earlier)* ·

Second and Third Trimester

In second and third trimester of pregnancy colour flow offers a very exciting avenue to study umbilical and placental haemodynamics. Along with foetal circulation this has proved to be very useful in assessing IUGR foetus and foetal anomalies.

Indications for umbilical artery waveform:

- Assessment and continued monitoring of the foetus that has been demonstrated to be small for gestational age on realtime ultrasound.
- Assessment of the foetus of a mother with systemic lupus erythematosus (SLE) and PET.
- In conjunction with utero placental waveforms in the assessment of oligohydramnios.
- Assessment of differing of sizes or growth patterns in twins.

The following are specially examined:

1. *Uterine artery* (Figs 20.27 and 28) Diastolic Notch of uterine artery disappears by 24 weeks (Figs 20.29a and b) and RI drops from 0.84 to 0.56 RI of radial branch is 0.33 and that of spiral branch is 0.32. The placentation process continues until 24-26th week of pregnancy, after which there is only a small decrease in values in the main uterine branch reflecting the sum of the radial and spiral vessels. If the notch has not been lost by 24-26 weeks most women will develop a hypertensive complication of pregnancy. After delivery, the uterine artery does not return to its pre-pregnant level for 4-6 weeks.

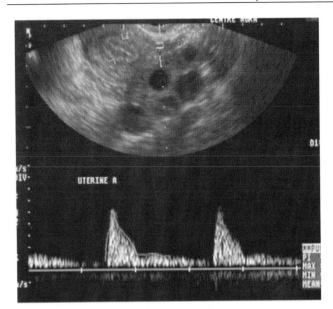

Figure 20.27
Flow pattern of uterine artery in nonpregnant state

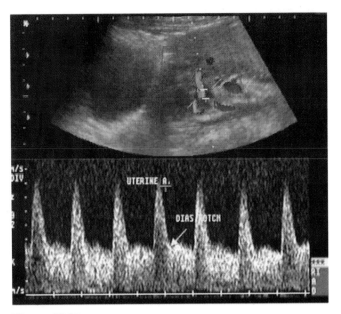

Figure 20.29a
Uterine artery flow pattern before 24weeks of gestation shows a diastolic notch

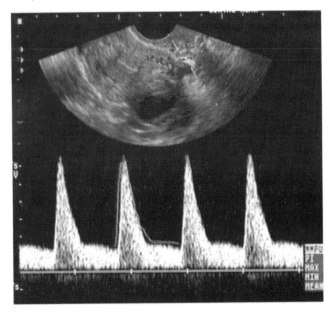

Figure 20.28
Flow pattern of uterine artery in pregnancy

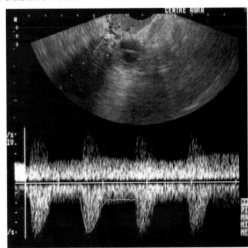

Figure 20.29b
The notch normally disappears by 24-26 weeks of gestation

Impaired uterine artery flow velocity is identified by (a) Persistent abnormal index (b)A persistent notch (c) A significant difference between the Indices in two vessels. The upper limit of S/D ratio is approximately 2.6 and the difference between two vessels should not exceed 1.

Adverse outcomes associated with abnormal uterine artery flow velocity include (a) preecclampsia (b) Fetal growth retardation and its sequeale.

2. *Umbilical A* With the aid of colour flow, the umbilical arteries can be detected as early as 6-8 weeks (Fig. 20.30). Doppler flow velocity profile shows only the systolic or ventricular component. By 20 weeks, all fetuses should have end-diastolic flow (Fig. 20.31). As pregnancy advances there is increasing end diastolic flow velocity with lesser changes in systolic peak velocity. A mature umbilical artery flow velocity waveform is usually achieved by 28-30 weeks but some fetuses may

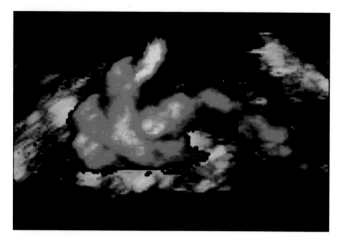

Figure 20.30
Power Doppler at 7weeks showing two arteries and one vein in the umbilical cord

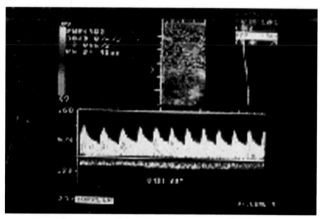

Figure 20.31
Normal umbilical artery flow pattern reveals a low resistance flow

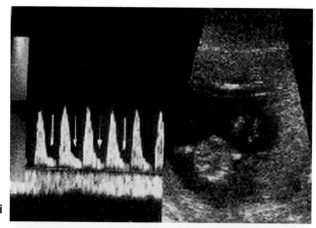

i

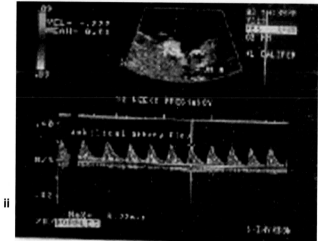

ii

Figure 20.32a(i, ii)
Doppler at 30weeks of gestation shows reduced diastolic flow in the umbilical artery signifying placental insufficiency

show a delayed maturation such as in twins. The indices are highest at the fetal abdomen and are lowest at the cord insertion into the placenta. Those at the mid cord or placental insertion are clinically reliable. Normal resistance index is between 0.5 to 0.7 and S/D ratio is < = 3.

Absent end diastolic velocity is clearly abnormal and a S/D ratio > 4.0 is probably going to stay in the elevated range. Decreased diastolic flow (RI > 0.7) in adicates early placental insufficiency (Figs 20.32a to c). When there is a reversal of flow, it may be a clinical emergency because most of these fetuses die within 2 weeks (Fig. 20.32d).

3. *Foetal descending thoracic aorta* (Fig. 20.33)
Normal flow wave pattern shows an RI = 0.82 ± 0.1 and a PI = 1.83 ± 0.3 (Fig. 20.34).

Significance of aortic flow is that there is increase in RI and PI of growth retarded fetuses. High PI in suggestive of foetal acidaemia.

Absent end-diastolic flow is suggestive of perinatal complication such as respiratory distress syndrome, necrotizing enterocolitis, renal failure.

4. *Foetal middle cerebral artery* (Figs 20.35 and 36)
Normal resistance index of MCA is > 0.7 and pulsatility index is > 1.3. Foetus with mild hypoxia (reduced umbilical artery flow velocity) will dilate its cerebral vessels as compensatory response (brain sparing effect-RI < 0.7) seen in asymmetrical growth retardation. When hypoxia worsens the cerebral vessels lose their autonomic reactivity and return to previous state. This is an alarming sign. The preterminal flow pattern shows absent diastolic flow in the umbilical artery, aorta, vena cava and umbilical vein pulsations.

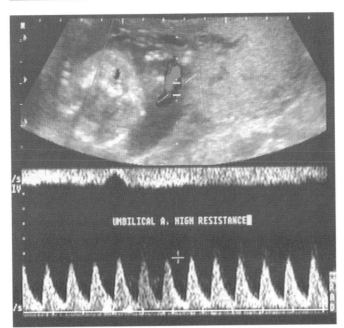

Figure 20.32b
RI in umbilical artery is more than 0.7 indicating decreased diastolic flow

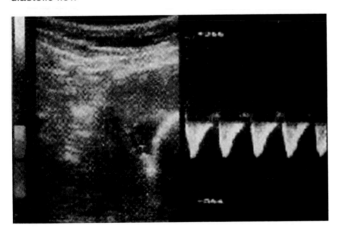

Figure 20.32c
Umbilical artery waveform in a case of IUGR

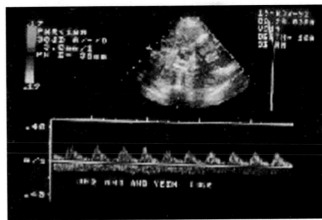

Figure 20.32d
Reversal of diastolic flow in umbilical artery signifying impending fetal death

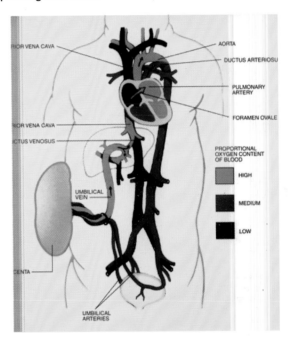

Figure 20.33
Line diagram showing normal fetal vasculature

In the growth retarted fetus that appears normal, the first question to ask is, what is the state of umbilical and uterine circulation? The next question is, is the foetus hypoxpemic? This is determined by middle cerebral doppler. The foetus with signigicant reduction of umbilical flow should have dilated cerebrals. If it does not, it is critically ill or not hypoxic. If it is not hypoxic, it may have congenital heart disease and the reduced peripheral flow is caused by reduced forward flow, not increased resistance. Careful evaluation of the heart then becomes imperative.

5. *Fetal venous circulation* Doppler evaluation of foetal venous circulation specially of the ductus venosus, hepatic veins and umblical veins gives an idea of fetal hypoxic and acidotic state (Figs 20.37a). Absent diastolic velocities and reversal of blood flow in ductus venous is an absolute indication of delivery (Fig. 20.37b).

6. *Fetal echocardiography:* A detailed foetal echo study will reflect earliest changes in the fetal circulation (Figs 20.38a and b).

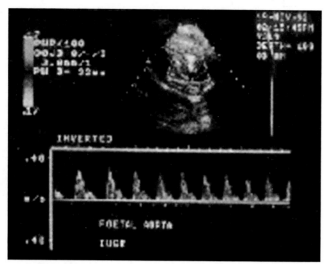

Figure 20.34
Flow pattern of aorta in IUGR showing loss of end diastolic flow

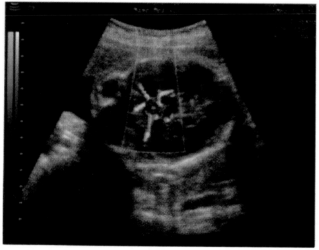

Figure 20.35
Doppler showing fetal circle of Willis

Limitation of Umbilical Artery Waveform

Umbilical artery waveforms are of little or no value as a screening test for the small for gestational foetus and do not appear to predict unexplained antepartum stillbirths. They are also not predictive of placental abruption.

The role of umbilical artery waveform is not established in foetuses of insulin dependent diabetes and foetal death has been reported within 24 hours of obtaining normal umbilical artery waveforms from the foetus of such women. The place of umbilical artery waveforms in antepartum haemorrhage and preterm labour or rupture of the membranes is unknown.

KEY POINTS

- 7.5 MHz is used in early pregnancy (upto 8 weeks) and 5 MHz in 9-13 weeks of pregnancy. TVS is used after 14 weeks.
- Gravid uterus shows generalized increased in vascularity of myometrium, an areas of vascularity is demonstrated in the hyperechoic decidua on days 26-28 post LMP (Implantation site signs).
- Placental flow even after 1 week of therapeutic abortion is an indication for dilatation and curettage.
- A solid adenexal mass with pronounced vascularity showing high velocity, low impedance flow suggests and ectopic gestation.
- Pseudosacs display high impedance flow.
- Uterine diastolic notch is seen normally upto 20-22 weeks after which it disappears. Persistence beyond 4 weeks of gestation with high RI suggests pre ecclampsia, IUGR and placental abruption.
- Umbilical artery flow pattern > 26 weeks of gestation show RI < 0.70 and PI < 1.5. Reduced/absent/Reversal of diastolic flow indicate IUGR.
- Normal flow pattern show RI = 0.82 ± 0.1 and PI = 1.83 ± 0.3 in Descending thoracic aorta. Increased Resistance suggests IUGR.
- Middle cerebral artery show brain sparing effect (increased diastolic flow in IUGR

Interpretations of Waveforms

1. In the absence of acute incident such as a placental abruption, a small for gestational age foetus with normal umbilical artery waveforms will not develop loss of end diastolic frequencies within a 7 days period so that monitoring may be performed weekly.
2. Only 10 per cent of foetuses that are demonstrated to be asymmetrically small for gestational age on real time ultrasound will demonstrate loss of end diastolic frequencies at any time during their pregnancy.

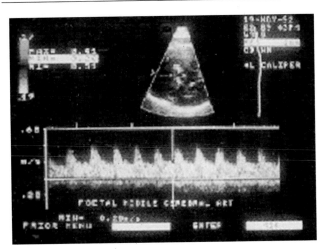

Figure 20.36
Duplex Doppler showing fetal middle cerebral artery

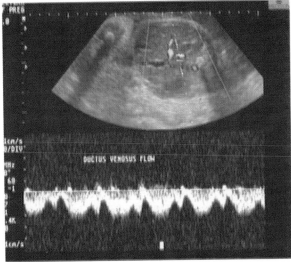

Figure 20.37a
Duplex Doppler showing normal pulsatile flow in ductus venosus

3. Loss of end diastolic frequencies is associated with an 85 per cent chance that the foetus will be acidotic.

4. The finding of a symmetrically small for date foetus with absent and diastolic frequencies in the umbilical artery but with normal uteroplacental waveforms suggest the possibility of a primary foetal cause for the growth retardation such as a chromosomal abnormality or a TORCH virus infection.

5. Foetuses demonstrating absence of end diastolic frequencies but which are managed along standard clinical lines have a 40 per cent chance of dying and at least a 25 per cent morbidity rate from necrotising enterocolitis, haemorrhage or coagulation failure after birth. The time between loss of end diastolic frequencies and fetal death appears to differ for each foetus. Following loss of end-diastolic frequencies there are no other reliable changes in the waveform that help in deciding when to deliver the baby.

6. Reversed frequencies in end diastole are only observed in a few fetuses prior to death. This finding should be considered as a preterminal condition. Few foetuses if any will survive without some form of therapeutic intervention.

7. Loss of end diastolic frequencies precedes changes in the cardio to cography by some 7-42 days in foetuses that have been shown to be small for gestational age on real time ultrasound. In the absence of maternal hypertension many centres would toco monitor small for gestational age fetuses solely with Doppler ultrasound. The ocurrence of CTG deceleration not related to contractions, together with absent end diastolic frequencies carries an extremely poor prognosis.

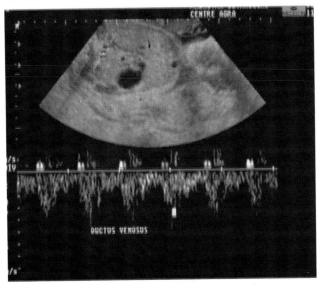

Figure 20.37b
Increased reversed flow in ductus venosus in fetal distress

Current Recommendations

It is probably reasonable for the clinicians to deliver all small for gestational age foetuses that present with absent (Reversed) end diastolic frequencies after 28 weeks. In units with neonatal intensive care facilities the perinatal mortality for infants that are more than 28 weeks gestations is less than 10 per cent with about a 6 per cent chance of handicap in survivors. If these foetuses are managed along standard clinical lines a mortality rate of about 40 per cent with a 25 per cent chance of severe handicap can be expected.

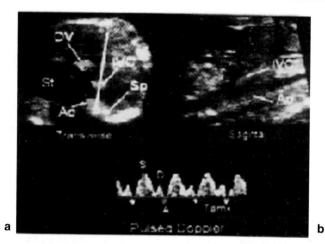
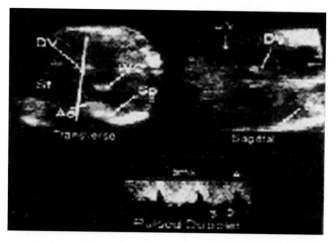

Figures 20.38a and b
Fetal echocardiography

At less than 28 weeks gestation these foetuses should probably be referred to a regional centre for detailed studies of the foetal circulation and possibly cordocentesis with an aim to therapy that may improve foetal oxygenation and growth.

CONCLUSIONS

Today the advent of colour flow imaging, doppler and power anio have opened up a new diagnostic horizon for understanding physiology and vascular pathology of gynaecology, infertility and uteroplacatal and fetal circulation.

The diagnostic ability with use of doppler in routine practise has increased(Tables 20.6 to 8).

"See better with sound
Use colour to improve your image
Explore the 3rd and 4th Dimension
Practise better medicine with better images"

Data analysis 5 years MNMH—Agra		
Table 20.6	• Total deliveries	6500
	• Total Deliveries	6500
	• Ultrasound Scans	4320
	• Diabetes	87
	• PIH	213
	• High risk Pts	456
	• Abnormal Doppler	123
	• IUFD and Perinatal Deaths	65
	• NICU Addmissions	125

Doppler in IUGR and perinatal salvage				
Table 20.7	• Parameter		Normal	Abnorm
	• All IUGR	R	91.67%	69.4%
		M	87%	60%
	• > 1300 gms	R	100%	93.7%
		M	95%	90%
	• < 1300 gms	R	50%	20%
		M	40%	18%

Doppler indices and perinatal mortality	
Table 20.8	• Normal Uterine and Umblical	Nil
	• High Umbilical Resistance	10%
	• Absent Diastolic Umbilical flow	40%
	• Abnormal Uterine and Umbilical	65%
	• Abnormal Ductus	90%

BIBLIOGRAPHY

1. Stuart Campbell: Ultrasound in obstetrics and gynae-cology: Recent advances. *Clinics in Obstetrics and Gynaecology.* WB Saunders Company Ltd, **10**: 1983.
2. Peter W Callen: *Ultrasonography in obstetrics and gynae-cology,* WB Saunders Company Ltd.
3. Asim Kurjak, Ivica Zalud: Doppler and Colour Flow Imaging. *Transvaginal Ultrasound.* Mosby Year Book (Ch-15), 285-94,1992.
4. Bourne TH: Transvaginal Colour Doppler in Gynaecology. *Ultrasound Obstet Gynecol* **1**: 359-73, 1991.
5. Kujak A *et al*: Transvaginal Colour Doppler in Pelvic Tumor Vaecularity: Lesions teamed and future challanges. *Ultrasound Obstet Gynecol* **6**: 145-49, 1995.
6. Steer CB *et al*: Transvaginal Colour Doppler Imaging of the Uterine Arteries during Ovarian and Menstrual Cycles. *Human Repord* **5**: 391-95, 1990.
7. Kenneth JW Taylor, Peter N Burns, Peters NT: *Wells Clinical Applications of Doppler Ultrasound* (2nd edn). Raven.

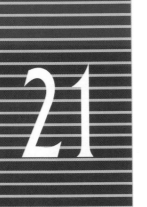

21

Gray Scale Ultrasonography and Colour Doppler Study in Fracture Healing

OP Sharma

Fracture healing starts from haematoma formation around fracture site to its organization followed by early callus, bone callus and finally its remodelling. Derangement in this chain can occur at early stage to result into abnormal union or mal-union. The basic method to monitor the fracture healing is by conventional radiograph but recently developed non-invasive, non-radiation technique i.e. ultrasound provides reliable information regarding healing process like—

1. They may quantitated the state of fracture healing.
2. Early diagnosis of disturbed union.
3. Time of exact surgical intervention.
4. Treatment/diagnostic procedure is performed without adding further trauma to fracture site.

After the recent advancement in ultrasonographic technique, Goldberg *et al.* (1975)[1] have advocated its extensive use. Realtime ultrasonography using high frequency linear array transducer is the best imaging procedure for evaluation of osseous and soft tissue pathology of extremity.

Experimental Study

Rabbit have been used for the purpose and fracture has been created in bilateral ulna and followed them for 6-8 weeks. In union group the abnormal mobility persisted for about 3rd to 4th week though around 2nd week there was mild resistance to mobility which progressively increased and after 4th week fracture was no longer mobile. The bony swelling that appeared around 3rd week due to callus formation, increased in size and then slightly decreased in size which was because of remodelling defect. The fracture union and remodelling was complete in rabbit by 8 weeks (Table 21.1).

Clinical Study

Thirty eight patients of present study, including delayed union (5), non-union (8) and fresh fractures (25) were studied. In normal union group patients for about 10 days following fracture treatment neither the radiographic nor the USG showed any evidence of callus formation. But between 2nd and 3rd week USG revealed hyperechoic area in the fracture gap, at this stage there was no evidence of new bone formation in the radiograph. At 5-6 weeks time increase in number and intensity of hyperechoic spots were noted which was more in the centre than at periphery. Radiography at this stage revealed fuzzy fracture margin indicative of fracture healing. Scan at the time of 8-12 weeks showed increase in intensity and number of hyperechoic spot or zones bridging the fracture gap (Figs 21.1a and b). Radiograph at this stage showed well-formed bridging callus, which appeared increasing until the fracture line was obscured and remodelling has started. The fracture, which was treated with intra-medullary

Table shows comparison of US and Radiographic findings with duration				
Table 21.1	*Days after surgery*	*Healing phase evaluated*	*Radiographic findings*	*Ultrasonography findings*
	5-7 days	Stage of organised haematoma	Clear-cut fracture line, no callus	Hypoechoic gap
	10-14 days	Stage of early callus	Fracture line visible No e/o callus	Hyperechoic shadow in fracture gap and around it indicating early callus
	17-20 days	Stage of bridging callus	Haziness of fracture indicating early callus	↑ in amount and intensity of shadow, hyper-reflecting line indicating bridging callus
	24-28 days	Stage of union	Callus seen bridging the fracture ends	↑ in intensity of hyper-reflecting line
	5-8 weeks	Stage of remodelling	Initial increase in amount of callus and later reorganization	Not much ↑ in hyperecho-, genecity minimal remodelling could be assessed

nail, revealed delayed union on radiograph but USG was able to predict the callus formation. Intra medullary nail was discernible in the earlier stage of fracture healing which was obscured in later stage through all the three portals, due to callus obstructing the entry of ultrasound waves. Five cases had evidence of delayed union with feature of nonvisulisation of callus formation either on radiography or on USG even at 8-12 weeks. The site studied were femur (1), tibia (2), humours (1) and radius (1). At 12 weeks there was steady increase in hyperechoic foci at fracture site and no callus on radiograph (Figs 21.2a and b).

The cases of non-union did show some callus at early stage but the progress was arrested. And USG also showed some hyperechoic shadows at early stage but progress in term of amount and intensity was absent. The cases of non-union to start with USG

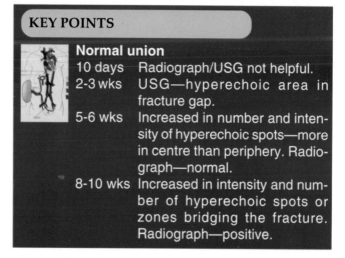

KEY POINTS

Normal union
10 days — Radiograph/USG not helpful.
2-3 wks — USG—hyperechoic area in fracture gap.
5-6 wks — Increased in number and intensity of hyperechoic spots—more in centre than periphery. Radiograph—normal.
8-10 wks — Increased in intensity and number of hyperechoic spots or zones bridging the fracture. Radiograph—positive.

revealed a gap between fracture ends with hypoechoic zone in between (Figs 21.3a and b).

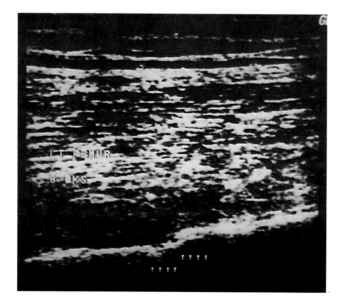

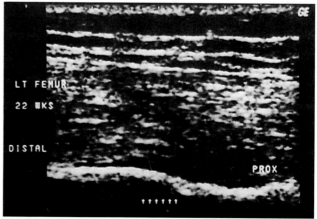

Figures 21.1a and b
USG scan at 8-12 weeks interval shows increased intensity and number of hyperechoic spots (zone) bridging the fracture gap. Radiograph also revealed bridging callus

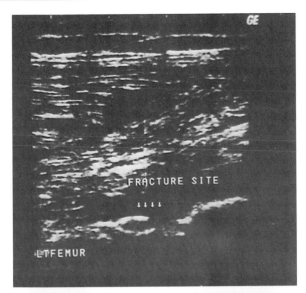

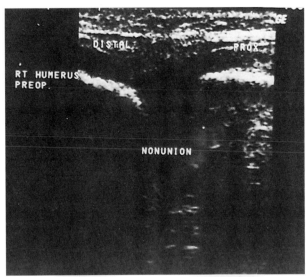

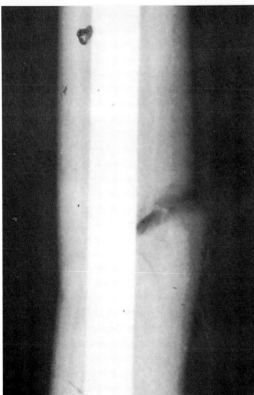

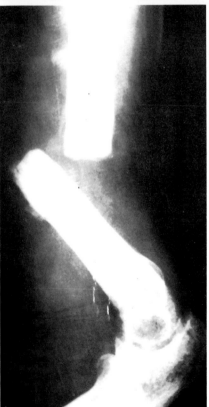

Figures 21.2a and b
USG shows hyperechoic zone but radiograph did not reveal any evidence of callus formation in a cases of delayed union

Figures 21.3a and b
In a case of non-union USG as well as radiograph revealed no evidence of callus formation

Routine radiography does not permit the minor changes in fracture healing during early stage while the ultrasonography through its potential of early assessment of the presence or absence of callus at the fracture site can be used to predict the need for secondary surgical procedure.

Colour Doppler was employed to optimize detection of weak and slow flow signals expected from small vessels. Sagittal and axial scan were employed with caution not to have more pressure by transducer to the tissue to avoid obliteration of small superficial vessels. Colour Doppler was only able to image anterolateral and antero-medial side of fracture while gray scale sonography could utilize all the three portal, i.e. anterior portal also.

In control subject the bone surface appeared smooth specular reflector with acoustic shadowing. No Doppler signal were observed on periosteal surface or within surrounding tissue.

At first examination (10 days after trauma) gray scale sonography demonstrated a small hypoechoic haematoma surrounding the fracture site. The flow signals were not detected by colour Doppler imaging at this stage except a few scattered colour dots within periosseous soft tissue 1-2 cm from fracture. Special analysis from periosseous soft tissue varied with RI ranging from 0.51 to 0.81 visible at the level of periosteum. Within the fracture site small colour dots could be appreciated with RI in same range.

Second examination (6 weeks) revealed absence of haematoma, there was increase a flow signals within the periosseous soft tissue with small linear vessel (approx. 1 mm in diameter) 0.40 to 0.65.

Third examination (10 weeks) had flow signals in small tortuous vessel at the fracture site. The signals had RI ranging from 0.32 to 0.51.

Fourth examination (15 weeks) showed small hyperechoic streaks at fracture site. Persistence of vascular flow with RI of 0.40 to 0.63, was also observed.

Fifth examination (18-19 weeks) showed a well-developed callus with good flow on earlier examination and flow signal around it had almost completely disappeared.

Sixth examination (24 weeks) showed no flow either within or around the healed lesion except for small colour dots in periosseous soft tissue RI from colour dots 0.50-0.77. Fracture cases of delayed union had no flow in fracture site or in periosteum at earlier examination but of small vessels in periosseous tissues successive exam revealed few colour dots within fracture site with gradual increase of RI 0.70-0.80. Gray scale sonography and radiography did not show sign of callus and labelled as delayed union.

However, venous signals could rarely be seen only in those case who had well developed callus.

Earliest changes during new bone formation are development of small blood vessels. The capillary surrounding the fracture site show signs of neo-angiogenesis, which is accompanied by osteoblast proliferation, in first week after bone fracture. This process may be identified on gray scale sonography about 3 weeks after fracture while conventional radio-

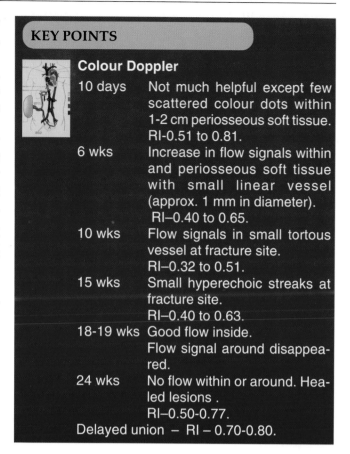

KEY POINTS

Colour Doppler

10 days	Not much helpful except few scattered colour dots within 1-2 cm periosseous soft tissue. RI-0.51 to 0.81.
6 wks	Increase in flow signals within and periosseous soft tissue with small linear vessel (approx. 1 mm in diameter). RI-0.40 to 0.65.
10 wks	Flow signals in small tortous vessel at fracture site. RI-0.32 to 0.51.
15 wks	Small hyperechoic streaks at fracture site. RI-0.40 to 0.63.
18-19 wks	Good flow inside. Flow signal around disappeared.
24 wks	No flow within or around. Healed lesions. RI-0.50-0.77.
Delayed union – RI – 0.70-0.80.	

graphy cannot visualize the repair process until 30-40 days after trauma.

Two main vascular phenomenon occur after a bone fracture. First, at the time of trauma, the normal blood supply to fracture site is disrupted with formation of haematoma. Then blood vessel rapidly reach this tissue coming both from peripheral soft tissue to periosteal portion of callus and from medullary circulation endosteal callus. Histologically newly formed capillaries care be recognized as early as 7 days after fracture and many vessels are seen at 9 days. Presence of many vessels progressively increase of RI, and development of telesystolic notch within spectral waveform indicates normal callus formation. Identification of only 1 or 2 vascular signals at 4th weeks and lack of development of telesystolic notch were considered sign of delayed fracture healing (Callioada *et al* 1993).[2]

Initial decrease in RI in-patient with normal callus development is due to impressive neoangiogenesis during the early weeks afte fracture, the neoangio-genesis lowers the resistance through the overall increase in vascular calibres. Gradual increase in resistance is likely related to degree of vascularity decreasing. Patient with delayed healing probably have less angiogenesis and thus higher resistance. In addition, the scarce vascularity in the non-union group makes Doppler evaluation technically difficult. Early demonstration of delayed healing can help guide treatment changes (Caruso *et al* 2000).[3] Additional studies are needed to show whether the colour Doppler imaging can demonstrate the return of vascularization after change in therapy and whether the patient outcome is affected by the use of this technique. At present, conventional radiography remains the primary technique for evaluating callus formation.

REFERENCES

1. Goldberg: *Textbook of Diagnosis Uses of Ultrasound* 1975.
2. Callioada F, Bottinelli O, Sala G: Color doppler differential diagnosis between normally and delayed healing bone fracture. *Radiology* **189**: 209, 1993.
3. Caruso G, Lagalla R, Derchi L *et al:* Monitoring of fracture calluses with color doppler sonography. *J of Clinical Ultrasound* **28**: 20, 2000.

Index